Sports Cardiology

Massimo Fioranelli • Gaetano Frajese
Editors

Sports Cardiology

From Diagnosis to Clinical Management

Forewords by Jacob Shani and Moussa Mansour

Springer

Editors
Massimo Fioranelli
Head of Heart Center
Casa di Cura Mater Dei
Rome, Italy

Scientific Director of the
Centro Studi in Scienze della Vita
"Guglielmo Marconi" University
Rome, Italy

Gaetano Frajese
Professor of Endocrinology
Director, Postgraduate School in Sports Medicine
"Tor Vergata" University
Rome, Italy

The contents of this book are based on:
Cardiologia dello sport. M. Fioranelli, G. Frajese (a cura di)
© Springer-Verlag Italia 2011

ISBN 978-88-470-3910-0
DOI 10.1007/978-88-470-2775-6
ISBN 978-88-470-2775-6 (eBook)

Springer Milan Dordrecht Heidelberg London New York

7 6 5 4 3 2 1 2012 2013 2014

Cover design: Ikona S.r.l., Milano

Typesetting: Ikona S.r.l., Milano

Springer-Verlag Italia S.r.l. – Via Decembrio 28 – I-20137 Milan
Springer is a part of Springer Science+Business Media (www.springer.com)

I dedicate this book to all my colleagues, who are excellent cardiologists; their professional and personal commitment has enabled the development of the Mater Dei Heart Center:

Maria Bianchi, Caterina Bisceglia, Valentina Boccadamo, Fiorella Caranci, Giovanna Giubilato, Carlo Gonnella, Roberto Leo, Antonio Lucifero, Enrica Mariano, Augusto Mazzetti, Francesco Perna, Emiliano Pica, Maddalena Piro and Vittoria Rizzello

Massimo Fioranelli

Foreword

The field of sports cardiology gained notoriety over the last few years when several well-known athletes have succumbed to sudden cardiac death. The media attention to these events has inflamed the controversy of whether better screening would have prevented any of the deaths or whether the time has come for nations and health organization to agree on an universal approach.

Unfortunately there is no universal approach to screen athletes or the general population. There is no accepted method of screening people of different ages that want to participate in athletic activity. The challenges to the physicians who have to decide whether to approve or deny the participation and the right to compete are great.

The International Olympic Committee (IOC) has recommended, but not mandated, that all countries screen their athletes to minimize the risk of sudden death. According to the IOC, if the twelve lead ECG raises the suspicion of an underlining serious problem in an athlete, further testing should be performed. In many screening programs, the work up also includes an echocardiogram. By contrast, the American Heart Association, (AHA) and the American College of Cardiology (ACC) do not recommend the use of ECG for cardiovascular screening of athletes at any level. The Canadian Heart and Stroke Foundation also has no screening recommendations for athletes nor does the Canadian Academy of Sports and Exercise Medicine.

At the far end of the spectrum is the Italian model, in which individuals are not allowed to participate in minor sports unless they have had a family history taken, physical examination and twelve lead ECG. In the United States and Canada the sports medicine community had not embraced mandatory ECG screening because of concerns about cost, access, and risk of false positives, that leave some healthy kids on the side lines. Instead North American doctors typically rely on information from family history and physical exam to guide decisions.

In this volume the Editors managed to put together a textbook and a reference for physicians and people who have interest in sports medicine. To my knowledge there is no other textbooks such as this. All the issues that involve cardiac activity and sports from arrhythmia and sudden death to mechanical and hemodynamic issues are addressed.

This book is unique, because it is concise, accurate and extremely helpful in making decisions. Both the general practitioner as well as the cardiologist will find this textbook a useful resource and reference when they deal with patients with or without cardiac issues, who want to participate in athletic activity. Through the collective efforts of all the Authors and the Editors, they were able to catalog the knowledge of this very important branch of medicine that impacts enormously the quality of life of the general populations, and athletes in particular.

Jacob Shani, MD, FACP, FACC, FSCAI
Chairman Cardiac Institute
Director, Division of Cardiology
Program Director, Cardiovascular Disease
and Interventional Cardiology
Professor of Medicine, Maimonides Medical Center
New York, USA

Foreword

Earlier this year and within the span of few weeks, two European football players, Fabrice Muamba and Piermario Morosini sustained sudden cardiac arrests, sending shock waves across the athletic and medical communities. These and other similar events over recent years have fueled an increased interest in sports cardiology. This field has been overlooked for years, which resulted in a poor understanding of the prevention and management of cardiac conditions among athletes.

This book, edited by Massimo Fioranelli and Gaetano Frajese, is a comprehensive practical guideline to sports cardiology. The areas covered include all aspects of this field, from history and physical examination to advanced imaging. The chapters are concise and clear, making this book an important tool for practicing cardiologists who will find themselves increasingly faced with situations requiring proficiency in the prevention, diagnosis and treatment of cardiac diseases in athletes.

Moussa Mansour, MD, FHRS, FACC
Director, Cardiac Electrophysiology Laboratory
Director, Atrial Fibrillation Program
Massachusetts General Hospital
Cardiac Arrhythmia Service
Boston, USA

Preface

Physical activity and health are now inseparable terms; regular exercise, like a pharmacological intervention, is a powerful tool of prevention and treatment for many cardiovascular diseases. In addition, the psychophysical well-being that comes from sport drives many individuals, including the elderly, to initiate and continue the practice of many sports.

The athlete's cardiovascular adaptation is sometimes a thin line between physiology and pathology, and often makes it difficult to assess the individual risk.

Whenever an athlete dies on the playing fields, cardiologists are called upon to answer the usual questions: what was the cause of death, and why was not possible to prevent it?

This whole issue revolves around the professional competence of the modern cardiologist and the limitations of current screening procedures.

If this is an objective difficulty, amplified by the media's widespread reporting of just a few fatal accidents, there are also clinical settings with less media attention but which are not free from reflection or from medical and legal implications.

The constant evolution of knowledge in the field of cardiovascular pathophysiology and the stressful pace of the work force the clinical cardiologist and the sports physician to rapidly and continuously update their knowledge.

As with other specializations, and maybe more so, the modern cardiologist has a variety of skills that make it even more important to integrate news with everyday clinical practice; we therefore require tools that can assist doctors in making clinical decisions.

This book is developed for these requirements and is characterized on the one hand by a systematic review of indications for modern non-invasive and invasive diagnosis, and on the other hand on the clinical approach to most cardiovascular problems that affect athletes.

Particular care has been take to cover modern interventional therapies ranging from coronary artery interventions to issues related to closure of the patent foramen ovale, precautions to observe in patients with antiarrhythmic devices, and safety precautions for sporting activity in patients with congenital heart disease.

I hope that this book can help the modern sports physicians in the daily task of solving clinical problems.

Massimo Fioranelli

Contents

Contributors

Gennaro Alfano Electrophysiology Department, Policlinico Casilino, Rome, Italy

Paolo Angelini Medical Director, Center for Coronary Artery Anomalies, Texas Heart Institute at St. Luke's Episcopal Hospital, Houston, USA

Pier Paolo Bassareo Department of Cardiovascular and Neurological Sciences, University of Cagliari, Cagliari, Italy

Maria Bianchi Heart Center, Casa di Cura Mater Dei, Rome, Italy

Caterina Bisceglia Electrophysiology Department, "San Raffaele" University Hospital, Milan, Italy

Valentina Boccadamo Heart Center, Casa di Cura Mater Dei, Rome, Italy

Leonardo Calò Electrophysiology Department, Policlinico Casilino, Rome, Italy

Fiorella Caranci Heart Center, Casa di Cura Mater Dei, Rome, Italy

Maria Antonietta Carbone Cardiology Department, "San Carlo di Nancy" Hospital, Rome, Italy

Ilaria D'Angeli Heart Center, Casa di Cura Mater Dei, Rome, Italy

Ilaria Dato Cardiovascular and Neurological Department, San Donato Hospital, Arezzo, Italy

Lucia de Luca Electrophysiology Department, Policlinico Casilino, Rome, Italy

Fabrizio D'Errico Cardiology Department, "San Carlo di Nancy" Hospital, Rome, Italy

Ermenegildo de Ruvo Electrophysiology Department, Policlinico Casilino, Rome, Italy

Alessandro Fagagnini Electrophysiology Department, Policlinico Casilino, Rome, Italy

Elisa Fedele Medicine and Surgery, Università Cattolica del Sacro Cuore, Rome, Italy

Massimo Fioranelli Head of Heart Center, Casa di Cura Mater Dei, Rome, Italy, Scientific Director of the Centro Studi in Scienze della Vita, "Guglielmo Marconi" University, Rome, Italy

Gaetano Frajese Professor of Endocrinology, Director, Postgraduate School in Sports Medicine, "Tor Vergata" University, Rome, Italy

Leda Galiuto Medicine and Surgery, Università Cattolica del Sacro Cuore, Rome, Italy

Giovanna Giubilato Heart Center, Casa di Cura Mater Dei, Rome, Italy

Carlo Gonnella Cardiology Department, "San Carlo di Nancy" Hospital, Rome, Italy

Paolo Gozzo General Surgery, University of Rome "La Sapienza", Rome, Italy

Fabrizio Guarracini Electrophysiology Department, Policlinico Casilino, Rome, Italy

Emanuele Guerra Internal Medicine Unit, Department of Health Sciences, Università degli Studi di Roma "Foro Italico", Rome, Italy

Eduardo A. Hernandez Baylor College of Medicine, Houston, USA

Luigi Irace Vascular Surgery, University of Rome "La Sapienza", Rome, Italy

Filippo Lamberti Electrophysiology Department, "San Eugenio" Hospital, Rome, Italy

Milena Leo Cardiology Department, Policlinico Gemelli, Rome, Italy

Roberto Leo Internal Medicine, "Tor Vergata" University, Rome, Italy

Chiara Leuzzi Interventional Cardiology, Policlinico Universitario, Modena, Italy

Gabriella Locorotondo Medicine and Surgery, Università Cattolica del Sacro Cuore, Rome, Italy

J. Alberto Lopez Baylor College of Medicine, Houston, USA

Antonio Lucifero Heart Center, Casa di Cura Mater Dei, Rome, Italy

Enrica Mariano Interventional Cardiology Unit, "Tor Vergata" University, Rome, Italy

Ombretta Martinelli Department of General Surgery, University of Rome "La Sapienza", Rome, Italy

Annamaria Martino Electrophysiology Department, Policlinico Casilino, Rome, Italy

Augusto Mazzetti Heart Center, Casa di Cura Mater Dei, Rome, Italy

Warren H. Moore Baylor College of Medicine, Houston, USA

Serafino Orazi Head of Cardiology Department, Ospedale Civile di Rieti, Rieti, Italy

Armando Passeri Heart Center, Casa di Cura Mater Dei, Rome, Italy

Paolo Pavone Radiology Department, Casa di Cura Mater Dei, Rome, Italy

Francesco Perna Heart Center, Casa di Cura Mater Dei, Rome, Italy

Emiliano Pica Heart Center, Casa di Cura Mater Dei, Rome, Italy

Giuseppe Picciolo Cardiac Intensive Care, AOU Policlinico S. Martino, Messina, Italy

Mara Piccoli Cardiology Unit, Policlinico "Luigi di Liegro", Rome, Italy

Fabio Pigozzi Internal Medicine Unit, Department of Health Sciences, Università degli Studi di Roma "Foro Italico", Rome, Italy

Maddalena Piro Heart Center, Casa di Cura Mater Dei, Rome, Italy

Bruno Pironi Interventional cardiology, "M.G.Vannini" Hospital, Rome, Italy

Italo Porto Cardiovascular and Neurological Department, San Donato Hospital, Arezzo, Italy

Marco Rebecchi Electrophysiology Department, Policlinico Casilino, Rome, Italy

Vittoria Rizzello "S.Giovanni-Addolorata" Hospital, Rome, Italy

Fabiana Rollini Interventional Cardiology, Policlinico Universitario, Modena, Italy

Massimo Sangiorgi Interventional Cardiology, Policlinico Universitario, Modena, Italy

Luigi Sciarra Electrophysiology Department, Policlinico Casilino, Rome, Italy

Antonella Sette Electrophysiology Department, Policlinico Casilino, Rome, Italy

Nishant R. Shah Texas Heart Institute, Baylor College of Medicine, Houston, USA

Fabio Sperandii Internal Medicine Unit, Department of Health Sciences, Università degli Studi di Roma "Foro Italico", Rome, Italy

Antonella Tommasino Cardiology Department, Ospedale Civile di Rieti, Rieti, Italy

Stefano Tonioni Cardiology Department, "San Carlo di Nancy" Hospital, Rome, Italy

Claudia Tota Electrophysiology Department, Policlinico Casilino, Rome, Italy

Rocco Vergallo Cardiovascular and Neurological Department, San Donato Hospital, Arezzo, Italy

Part I

Cadiovascular Diagnostics

Medical History and Physical Examination in Sports Medicine

1

Milena Leo, Francesco Perna, Roberto Leo
and Massimo Fioranelli

1.1 Introduction

Medical history and physical examination are recognized worldwide as the milestone of athletes' preparticipation cardiovascular screening. They are defined as the systematic medical practice of evaluating large populations of athletes before sports participation in order to identify (or raise suspicion of) those abnormalities that might undergo disease progression or sudden cardiac death.

Although this screening process traditionally involves the evaluation of several organs, it mainly focuses on cardiovascular diseases and especially on sudden death, a tragic event bearing a considerable impact on the lay and medical communities, as well as on the general population, because athletes are usually young and considered the healthiest part of society [1].

Intense athletic training and competition act as a trigger to increase the risk of sudden cardiac death or disease progression in susceptible athletes with underlying heart disease (although quantification of that risk remains elusive). Most cardiac sudden deaths in young athletes occur during sports training or competition. Therefore, a relationship has been drawn between intense physical activity and arrhythmic sudden death. The risk of sudden death, however, appears to be unrelated to the level of athletic competition (i.e., high school, college, or professional). Indeed, early identification of relevant diseases may well prevent some instances of sudden death after temporary or permanent withdrawal from sports or targeted therapeutic interventions [2,3].

To date, there is universal agreement about the need to screen athletes for suspected heart disease before participation in competitive sport, but recommendations about the methods (European Society of Cardiology (ESC), International Olympic Committee (IOC), American Heart Association (AHA) preparticipation screening scientific statement) and the actual clinical practice vary greatly [4-6]. Noninvasive tests, such as electrocardiogram or echocardiogram, could raise the chances of detecting cardiovascular abnormalities, such as hypertrophic cardiomyopathy (HCM). However, according to some authors, such screening proposals would be hard to achieve and too expensive for most schools. This is further hampered by the fact that sudden cardiac death is an infrequent event in athletes (1:200,000) and that only a small proportion of those participating in team sports are at risk from misdiagnosed cardiovascular disease. The causes of sudden death during sporting activity are strictly related to the participants' age. Atherosclerotic coronary artery disease accounts for the vast majority of fatalities in adults (age > 35 years), while cardiomyopathies, such as HCM or arrhythmogenic right ventricular cardiomyopathy/dysplasia, have been consistently observed as the leading cause of cardiac arrest in younger athletes. Other, less common cardiovascular causes for sport-related sudden death in young athletes include premature atherosclerotic coronary artery disease, congenital coronary anomalies, myocarditis, dilated cardiomyopathy, mitral valve prolapse, conduction system diseases, Wolff-Parkinson-White (WPW) syndrome, ion channel

M. Leo (✉)
Cardiology Department
Policlinico Gemelli, Rome, Italy

M. Fioranelli and G. Frajese (eds.), *Sports Cardiology*,
DOI: 10.1007/978-88-470-2775-6_1,

diseases (long QT syndrome, catecholaminergic polymorphic ventricular tachycardia, Brugada syndrome), spontaneous aortic rupture complicating Marfan's syndrome or bicuspid aortic valve [7].

Therefore, personal and family history and physical examination may be good starting points in athletes' screening for the prevention of sudden cardiac death [8].

1.2 Family History

Most cases of non-traumatic sudden death in athletes are genetically determined diseases with an autosomal dominant pattern of inheritance, and therefore the importance of family history in identifying affected athletes should be emphasized.

According to the AHA statements, ESC recommendations and COCIS (Italian) guidelines for preparticipation screening [4,6,9], the main topics to be investigated are:

- premature, sudden and unexpected death (before the age of 50 due to heart disease, in at least 1 relative);
- disability from heart disease in a close relative (need for pacemaker or cardioverter-defibrillator implantation, cardiac surgery or transplantation, myocardial infarction before 55 years in men or 65 years in women);
- family history of hypertrophic or dilated cardiomyopathy, long-QT syndrome or other ion channel diseases, Marfan's syndrome, or clinically relevant arrhythmias.

1.3 Personal Medical History

Personal medical history is essential to define the athlete's cardiovascular risk and to guide the subsequent physical examination.

For this purpose, the most important topics to be investigated are:

- presence of ischemic risk factors such as diabetes mellitus, hypertension, dyslipidemia, smoking;
- history of cardiovascular diseases, including transient ischemic attacks, stroke, peripheral vascular disease and peripheral edema;
- history of previous accidents, especially with chest contusion;
- medications or drug abuse;
- prior identification of heart murmurs or elevated blood pressure values;
- typical cardiac symptoms, such as chest pain, tightness or discomfort, dyspnea, palpitations and syncope, as described below in detail.

It is important to correlate symptoms to the patient's baseline level of physical activity in order to better assess his/her real condition and to identify the best type of management [4,6,9].

1.3.1 Chest Pain

Chest pain is a very common symptom, but is difficult to evaluate. Many diseases can lead to chest pain:

- cardiac diseases: stable angina, acute coronary syndromes (ACS), coronary vasospasm (Prinzmetal's angina), hypertrophic cardiomyopathy, aortic stenosis, arrhythmias, aortic dissection, mitral valve disease, pericarditis;
- respiratory diseases: pneumothorax, pulmonary embolism, pneumonia, pleurisy, lung cancer;
- musculoskeletal diseases: costochondritis, Tietze's syndrome, trauma, rib pain (including fracture, bone metastases, osteoporosis), radicular pain, nonspecific musculoskeletal pain (e.g. fibromyalgia);
- breast disease;
- gastrointestinal diseases: gastro-oesophageal reflux disease, oesophageal rupture, oesophageal spasm, peptic ulcer disease, cholecystitis, pancreatitis, gastritis;
- skin diseases: herpes zoster infection;
- psychiatric diseases: e.g. anxiety, depression, panic attack;
- others: sickle cell crisis, diabetic mononeuritis, tabes dorsalis.

The nature of pain (weight, burning, stabbing, discomfort), as well as its location (middle of the chest, upper abdomen, neck, jaw, left arm, left shoulder), radiation (neck, jaw, back, left or right arm), frequency, intensity, duration, aggravating and relieving factors, correlation with exercise, associated symptoms (e.g. nausea and/or vomiting, sweating, dizziness, and palpitations) are useful features to observe in order to clarify the underlying cause.

Common causes of chest pain in athletes are:

- panic attacks, especially in women, typically associated with palpitations, tingling limbs, dizziness, shortness of breath, sometimes before or soon after stressful activity. A positive screening for previous panic attacks is highly sensitive to diagnosis of actual panic disorder but should not preclude a complete cardiac examination;
- gastro-oesophageal reflux disease, often due to excessive swallowing of air during exercise, or consumption of fizzy drinks or meals that are rich in fat;
- myopericarditis: to be suspected in the case of recent fever or flu, presence of burning, sometimes oppressive, chest pain, which varies with a change in body position or breathing;
- cocaine abuse;
- pleuropericarditis, typically involving posterior, stabbing chest pain, which varies depending on breathing, and is associated with fever or cough;
- spontaneous pneumothorax, typically occurring during exercise with acute and intense dyspnea, common in tall athletes, with marfanoid habitus;
- ischemic heart disease, typically induced by exercise and attenuated while resting, and often associated with icy sweating and general discomfort. It should be suspected in particular in adult athletes.

Less common, but not less important causes of chest pain in athletes are hypertrophic cardiomyopathy, aortic stenosis, coronary artery abnormalities such as myocardial bridge: all those diseases present with effort-related chest pain, dyspnea, or recurrent syncope. In these cases physical examination and additional tests, such as ECG and echocardiogram, are crucial for correct diagnosis.

1.3.2 Dyspnea

Dyspnea is the subjective discomfort of experiencing one's own breathing. It is a normal symptom on heavy exertion, even in well trained athletes, but it can suggest underlying pathological conditions if it occurs at rest or during ordinary physical activity.

Many diseases can cause it: respiratory diseases such as asthma, pneumothorax, chronic obstructive pulmonary disease, pneumonia, interstitial lung disease, cardiac diseases such as ischemia, congestive heart failure, psychogenic causes, neurological diseases. Treatment typically depends on the underlying cause.

Depending on how it was triggered, it may be classified as acute dyspnea, i.e. severe shortness of breath lasting several minutes or hours, or chronic dyspnea, which lasts for several weeks or months.

It may be further distinguished as inspiratory, expiratory or mixed dyspnea, according to the corresponding phase of the respiratory cycle.

According to the *New York Heart Association* (NYHA), dyspnea may be classified into four categories on the basis of the extent of the subject's functional limitation:

- class I: the subject has no dyspnea;
- class II: dyspnea appears during moderate exertion, with only slight limitation during ordinary activity;
- class III: dyspnea is associated with mild exertion, with marked limitation even during less-than-ordinary activity so that the patient feels comfortable only at rest;
- class IV: dyspnea is also present at rest, with severe limitation of daily activities.

Common causes of dyspnea in athletes are:

- panic attacks: dyspnea typically occurs at rest in this case, but not during exercise;
- exercise asthma, with prevalent expiratory dyspnea due to bronchospasm; it is not related to the level of physical activity; predisposing factors are cold, wet weather, and family or personal history of allergies;
- exercise laryngospasm, which is common in women, and is typically resolved by reassurance and anxiolytics;
- spontaneous pneumothorax, which is more common in tall athletes, with marfanoid habitus, typically occurring together with acute and intense dyspnea during exercise.

Other important causes, even though less frequent, are hypertrophic cardiomyopathy, aortic stenosis, ischemic heart disease (especially in adult athletes), and all other cardiac diseases that lead to congestive heart failure.

1.3.3 Palpitations

Palpitations involve an unpleasant awareness of one's own heartbeat. When describing palpitations, patients use terms such as skipping, racing, fluttering, pounding or stopping of the heart. Palpitations may result from an irregular heartbeat, from rapid acceleration or slowing of the heart, or from increased forcefulness of cardiac contraction. Such perceptions also depend on how patients experience their own body sensations. They are a common symptom, both in people with healthy and diseased hearts.

On the basis of the clinical presentation (means of onset and interruption, duration, frequency of episodes, correlation with physical activity, associated symptoms) it is possible to distinguish between three forms of palpitations: anxiety palpitations, extrasystolic palpitations and palpitations due to prolonged supraventricular or ventricular arrhythmias.

Anxiety palpitations are frequent in athletes, especially in women, before and during competitions: they are typically described as a form of agony, associated with a slightly higher than normal heart rate, with a gradual start and end, and no association with any organic disease.

Extrasystolic palpitations are described as an intermittent perception of a missing heartbeat or heart drop that lasts a few seconds but can recur more or less frequently in a day. Both premature supraventricular and ventricular complexes can cause this symptom. Extrasystolic palpitations are usually a benign condition, but, if frequent, they can be related to cardiac diseases such as ischemic heart disease, hypertrophic cardiomyopathy, arrhythmogenic right ventricular disease, Brugada syndrome, long QT syndrome or mitral valve prolapse. Additional tests may therefore be required.

Tachyarrhythmias other than premature complexes generally cause a prolonged feeling of accelerated, regular or irregular heartbeat that can be well tolerated or rather associated with dyspnea, dizziness, light-headedness and chest pain. The onset and end of tachyarrhythmia can be more or less abrupt. Moreover, tachyarrhythmias can be related to physical activity or they can take place at rest, and they can arise both in normal hearts (typically atrioventricular nodal re-entrant tachycardia, WPW syndrome, some cases of atrial fibrillation, or right ventricular outflow tract tachycardia) and in diseased hearts (ischemic heart disease, hypertrophic cardiomyopathy, other cardiomyopathies, arrhythmogenic right ventricular disease, Brugada syndrome, QT long syndrome or mitral valve prolapse). Furthermore, gastrointestinal diseases such as hiatal hernia, thyroid dysfunction, anemic status, coffee and other stimulant abuse, or smoking may be predisposing factors for arrhythmias. In such cases additional tests are required as well.

1.3.4 Syncope and Presyncope

Syncope is a transient loss of consciousness and postural tone characterized by rapid onset, short duration and spontaneous recovery due to global cerebral hypoperfusion that is most often the result of hypotension. Many forms of syncope are preceded by a prodromal state, known as *presyncope*, characterized by lightheadedness, dizziness, temporary loss of vision or hearing, pain, nausea, abdominal discomfort, weakness, sweating, palpitations and other phenomena.

Syncope is a common condition in both the general population and athletes.

Neurally-mediated syncope is the most common type of syncope observed among athletes. It is characterized by peripheral vasodilation, decreased blood pressure, along with bradycardia, and is caused by an increase in the parasympathetic tone and concomitant inhibition of sympathetic output. It generally occurs in susceptible people under physically stressful conditions (strenuous effort, dehydration, hunger or hypoglycemia).

However, cardiogenic syncope must be investigated. It is due to left ventricular ejection obstruction (such as in aortic stenosis or obstructive hypertrophic cardiomyopathy), arrhythmias, pulmonary embolism or hypertension, aortic dissection, congenital coronary anomalies.

Differential diagnosis is important in order to identify and treat the underlying cause.

Furthermore, regardless of its cause, syncope may result in physical injury such as head trauma: it is therefore important to clarify the circumstances of onset and the association with physical activity in order to avoid accidents during exertion.

1.4 Physical Examination

Important information about athletes' preparticipation cardiovascular evaluation comes from a careful and precise physical examination. It includes a general inspection of the patient, measurement of arterial blood pressure in both arms and one or both lower extremities, examination of the arterial pulse and dynamic cardiac auscultation. Based on the results of this inexpensive evaluation, a definite diagnosis can often be made. Selected non-invasive and invasive tests are therefore performed only when appropriate.

1.4.1 General Inspection

Visual inspection of the athlete may provide important information.

First of all, it gives the physician an idea about the general health status of the athlete, his/her physical development and habitus.

Furthermore, careful observation of the athlete may provide clues for the diagnosis of underlying heart diseases.

Xanthoma, xanthelasma or arcus senilis may be signs of familial hyperlipidemia and therefore of premature coronary artery disease.

Edema, cyanosis and breathlessness, though rare in athletes, may suggest heart failure.

Observation of the skin, thorax and extremities may provide clues for the diagnosis of congenital heart diseases, which are often unknown in young athletes.

Bilateral prominence of the anterior chest with bulging of the upper two-thirds of the sternum is common in children with a large ventricular septal defects; a unilateral bulge at the fourth and fifth intercostal spaces at the lower left sternal border is found in adults with ventricular septal defect.

Furthermore, clubbed fingers or cyanosis of the skin or nails suggest congenital heart disease with right-to-left blood shunt.

Underdeveloped musculature in the lower extremities compared to the upper extremities can occur in patients suffering from coarctation of the aorta.

Among those syndromes associated with congenital heart disease, special attention must be paid to *Marfan's syndrome*. It is an autosomal dominant disorder suggested by skeletal features such as increased height, long fingers (*arachnodactyly*), lax joints, kyphoscoliosis, pectus excavatum or carinatum, an elongated face, high-arched palate and flat feet, bilateral subluxation of the lens, severe myopia and blue sclera. Patients with Marfan's syndrome usually have mitral valve prolapse, mitral regurgitation, calcified mitral annulus, mitral chord rupture, dilated aortic root, prolapse of the aortic cusps or aortic dissection.

Patients with *Ehlers-Danlos syndrome* have hyperextensible joints and hyperelastic and friable skin often associated with arterial dilation and rupture, aortic regurgitation or mitral valve prolapse.

1.4.2 Arterial Blood Pressure Measurement

Arterial blood pressure measurement is fundamental because the prevalence of hypertension is growing among athletes, thus carrying a higher cardiovascular risk.

When measuring blood pressure, care should be taken to:

- allow the athlete to sit quietly for several minutes;
- carry out at least two measurements 1-2 minutes apart;
- perform measurements in both arms to detect possible differences due to supravalvular aortic stenosis or subclavian steal syndrome;
- carry out measurements in both arms and at least one leg to detect possible differences caused by peripheral vascular disease or, especially in

younger athletes, coarctation of the aorta.

For practical reasons, hypertensive patients are categorized according to precise thresholds as indicated by ESC and AHA guidelines. However, the real threshold for defining hypertension must be considered flexibly, based on the overall cardiovascular risk of each individual.

It is important to remember that many factors may contribute to variations in blood pressure during daily activities: body posture, status of cerebral or gastrointestinal activity, emotional or painful stimuli, environmental factors such as temperature and noise levels, smoking, coffee, alcohol and other drugs with direct or neurally mediated vasomotor properties.

Furthermore, isotonic exercise in both the supine and upright positions produces a moderate increase in blood pressure; sustained isometric muscular contractions produce an abrupt increase in systolic, mean and diastolic blood pressure that depends on the strength of the contraction. This may have important implications for physical activity restrictions in hypertensive patients.

1.4.3 Arterial Pulses Palpation

Palpation of peripheral arterial pulses is a basic and important element of an athlete's physical examination for several reasons.

First of all, palpation of the radial pulse allows for quick evaluation of the patient's heart rate and rhythm.

Secondly, simultaneous palpation of both the radial pulse and femoral pulse is useful as screening for coarctation of the aorta. If the femoral pulse is reduced or delayed with respect to the radial pulse, further evaluation is needed.

Moreover, evaluation of arterial pulse characteristics may indicate the presence of important heart diseases. A normal arterial pulse has a smooth rapid upstroke, a smooth peak, and a more gradual downstroke. Hyperkinetic arterial pulses are common in athletes with marked bradycardia and an extremely large stroke volume. In contrast, hypokinetic arterial pulse is less frequent and indicates a condition of diminished stroke volume, for example hypovolemia, left ventricular failure, mitral or aortic valve stenosis. The finding of a *bisferiens* pulse, with a waveform characterized by two positive waves during systole, suggests the diagnosis of hypertrophic cardiomyopathy or, less frequently, aortic regurgitation with or without aortic stenosis. The *parvus et tardus* pulse, a small pulse with a delayed systolic peak, is typical of aortic stenosis. A *pulsus alternans*, characterized by regular alternation of the systolic peak in pressure pulses, indicates severe depression of left ventricular performance. Conditions such as asthma, obstructive airways disease and cardiac tamponade are often associated with a *paradoxical pulse*, defined as a marked decrease in pulse amplitude or a decrease in systolic arterial pressure by more than 10 mmHg during normal quiet inspiration.

1.4.4 Cardiac Auscultation

Cardiac assessment should be performed in a quiet setting to facilitate auscultation. The assessment should include a brief visual inspection of the precordium to search for asymmetry and abnormal impulses. Precordial palpation can detect thrills, abnormal apical impulse location and parasternal heave.

The physician should then carefully auscultate for heart sounds, heart murmurs and extracardiac sounds.

The four *primary areas of cardiac auscultation* are: 1) the primary and secondary aortic areas in the second right interspace and the third left interspace adjacent to the sternum, respectively; 2) the pulmonary area in the second left interspace; 3) the tricuspid area in the fourth and fifth interspaces adjacent to the left sternal border; 4) the mitral area at the cardiac apex. Furthermore, in case of heart murmurs, cardiac auscultation should be enlarged to additional areas (such as the neck, posterior thorax, right sternal border and epigastrium) to which it typically radiates.

It is important to adopt a systematic approach to auscultation: in each area one should first listen to the heart sounds, then heart murmurs during systole and diastole respectively, trying to record the time of appearance, the pitch and other characteristics.

The patient should be auscultated in the left lateral decubitus position and, when possible, also while standing, squatting and during and after the *Valsalva manoeuvre* and the *handgrip manoeuvre*, in order to assess sound and murmur changes according to preloading and afterloading variations.

Moreover, if there are diagnostic clues in the medical history as well as in the examination of arterial, venous and cardiac pulzations, the auscultatory counterparts should be pursued diligently.

1.4.4.1 Heart Sounds

The heart cycle is physiologically marked by two (or three) heart sounds; a fourth heart sound may be present in pathological conditions.

The *first heart sound (S1)* is produced by the closure of the mitral valve (M1) followed after only 20 to 30 ms by the closure of the tricuspid valve (T1), so that at the apex in a normal subject only a single sound is usually heard. Wide splitting of S1 because of a delay in T1 can be a sign of *Ebstein's anomaly* of the tricuspid valve, often misdiagnosed in children, right bundle branch block, or ectopic beats originating from the left ventricle. Similarly, ectopic beats originating from the right ventricle, mitral valve stenosis, or left atrial mixoma causing mitral obstruction, will produce reversed splitting of S1 (T1, M1) due to a delay in mitral valve closure and left ventricular contraction. S1 intensity is higher in the case of tachycardia and lower in the case of bradycardia or I grade atrioventricular block, which is often found in athletes.

The *second heart sound (S2)* involves closure of the aortic valve (A2) followed by closure of the pulmonary valve (P2). Inspiration causes increased blood flow into the pulmonary vascular bed, delaying the closure of the pulmonary valve slightly. This inspiratory widening of S2 (*physiological split*) is generally a reassuring sign during the athlete's cardiac examination. A *fixed split* of S2 (because of a P2 delay over 40 ms during both inspiration and expiration) can be a sign of congenital heart disease with pulmonary hyperflow such as an atrial septal defect: in this case cardiac auscultation in the standing position is useful because it can modify S2 by reducing venous blood return. A *paradoxical split* (i.e. narrowing on inspiration) can be a sign of severe aortic stenosis, hypertrophic cardiomyopathy or left bundle branch block.

S1 is separated from S2 by a small pause corresponding to the systole, while S2 is separated from S1 by a large pause corresponding to the diastole.

The *third heart sound (S3)* is related to the early diastolic filling of the ventricles. It is a common benign event in children, adolescents and young adults, but it is rarely present in adults aged over 40. It is also common in endurance athletes with left ventricular dilation and bradycardia. S3 can be heard at the apex in the left lateral decubitus position soon after S2; it generally disappears during tachycardia and while standing.

The *forth heart sound (S4)* is related to the late diastolic filling of the ventricles due to atrial contraction. It is always an abnormal finding: it may be heard in the presence of reduced ventricular compliance (such as severe ventricular hypertrophy for aortic stenosis, hypertrophic or hypertensive cardiomiopathy, or ischemic heart disease) or excessively rapid late diastolic filling (secondary to hyperkinetic states or acute atrioventricular valve incompetence) or arrhythmias such as heart block. S4 is best heard at the apex impulse with the patient turned in the left lateral position, occurring shortly before S1.

Other pathological heart sounds are non-ejection clicks and opening snaps.

Non-ejection clicks are mid-systolic sounds produced by prolapse of the mitral or tricuspid valve and are often associated with a systolic regurgitant murmur. The sound has a sharp, high-frequency clicking quality and may be confined to the apex or widely transmitted on the precordium. There may be a single mid-systolic click, or multiple clicks, probably as a result of different leaflets prolapsing in different times. The timing of the click varies considerably with postural changes and this may be helpful in differentiating non-ejection clicks from early ejection sounds, a split S2 or a S3. In general, manoeuvres that decrease LV volume such as sitting or standing or the strain of the Valsalva manoeuvre move the click closer to S1, while manoeuvres that increase LV volume move the click towards S2.

Opening snaps are crisp, sharp sounds typically produced by the opening of a thickened and deformed stenotic atrioventricular valve. It can be heard in the mid-precordial location, usually most clearly in the area extending from the left sternal border to the apex. It immediately precedes the diastolic rumble of valvular stenosis.

1.4.4.2 Heart Murmurs and Extra-cardiac Sounds

Cardiac murmurs are prolonged series of auditory vibrations produced by blood turbulence through cardiac structures or great vessels because of a high flow rate, forward flow through a constricted or irregular orifice, backward flow through an incompetent valve, septal defects or patent ductus arteriosus.

Useful features to examine in order to characterize heart murmurs are:

- the *timing* in the cardiac cycle, in order to distinguish between systolic (falling between S1 and S2), diastolic (falling between S2 and S1) or continuous murmurs: there is seldom any difficulty distinguishing between systole and diastole since systole is considerably shorter with normal heart rates; in the case of rapid heart rates, simultaneous palpation of the lower right carotid artery or identification of second heart sound, the louder sounds at the base are useful in properly locating murmurs in the cardiac cycle;
- the intensity (*loudness*), which is related to the velocity of blood flow across the area of murmur production and to the transmission characteristics of the tissue between the source of the murmur and the stethoscope. For systolic murmurs, the loudness is generally graded from 1 to 6 as described by Freeman and Levine (Table 1.1);
- the frequency (*pitch*), which is directly related to the flow velocity and to the pressure head that drives the blood across the murmur-producing area: this is categorized as high, medium or low;
- the configuration (*shape*), which is determined by the intensity over time; it enables crescendo, decrescendo, crescendo-decrescendo (diamond-shaped) or plateau murmurs to be defined;
- the *quality*, which is described as, for example, blowing, harsh, rumbling or musical;
- the *location* and sites of maximum intensity in the primary cardiac areas, radiation due to the direction of blood flow in other thoracic areas (right of the sternum, epigastrium, posterior thorax or neck).

Table 1.1 Classification of the intensity of heart murmurs as described by Freedman and Levine

Intensity	Characteristics
Grade 1	Just audible with a good stethoscope in a quiet room
Grade 2	Quiet but readily audible with a stethoscope
Grade 3	Easily heard with a stethoscope
Grade 4	A loud, obvious murmur with a palpable thrill
Grade 5	Very loud, heard not only over the pericardium but also elsewhere in the body
Grade 6	Heard with the stethoscope off chest

Many cardiac diseases can produce murmurs: detailed analysis of murmur characteristics is a precious tool for differential diagnosis. The most common cardiac conditions associated with heart murmurs in athletes, especially adults, are reported in Table 1.2.

Moreover, murmurs may occur in the absence of physiological and structural abnormalities in the cardiovascular system when, in early systole, peak flow velocity across the left or right ventricle outflow tract exceeds the murmur threshold, the so-called *innocent murmurs*. They are quite common in young athletes. These murmurs are rigorously systolic, of short duration, almost always less than grade 3 in intensity and vary considerably from one examination to another, with the body position and the level of physical activity. They are best heard at the left sternal border on the third or fourth interspace and are not associated with a thrill or with radiation to the carotid arteries or axillae. Hyperkinetic states such as fever or hyperthyroidism, may increase their intensity. For a murmur to be considered innocent, the examination of the cardiovascular system, and if possible an echocardiogram, should reveal no abnormalities.

Among *extracardiac sounds*, pericardial friction sounds may be heard. They are produced by pericardial leaflets rubbing each other due to inflammation of the pericardial sac. These friction sounds are very high pitched, leathery and scratchy in nature. They seem close to the heart and are best heard with the patient leaning forward or in the knee-chest position, holding breath after forced expiration. The pericardial rub may have three

Table 1.2 Characteristics of heart murmurs in various heart diseases

Disease	Timing	Quality	Shape	Location	Radiation	Other findings
Aortic stenosis	Mid-systolic	Harsh	Diamond	1st-2nd right intercostal spaces	Carotid arteries and cardiac apex (Gallivardin phenomenon)	- intensity not correlated to stenosis gravity and increased by increased cardiac output - single S2 or paradoxical splitting of S2 (A2 is absent or late) - S4 (S3) often heard - *parvus et tardus* pulse - systolic ejection click often precedes the murmur
Hypertrophic cardiomyopathy	Mid-systolic	Harsh	Diamond	Lower left sternal edge	Apex, not carotid arteries	- intensity related to intraventricular gradient (increased by decrease in LV preload and afterload or increase in LV contractility): useful stand-squat-stand position and leg raising manoeuvres - normal S2 - S4 always present - bisferiens pulse
Mitral regurgitation	Holosystolic (mid-late-systolic in acute MRs)	Blowing	Plateau	Apex	Axilla	- intensity is not influenced by respiration - short rumble - loud S3 from LV
Tricuspid regurgitation	Holosystolic (mid-late-systolic in acute TRs)	Soft	Plateau	Lower left sternal border	-	- JVP shows a prominent v wave with a rapid y descent - intensity increases during inspiration (Carvallo's sign) - short rumble - loud S3 from RV
Ventricular septal defect	Systolic	Harsh	Plateau	4th, 5th and 6th intercostal spaces along the sternal border	-	- intensity not influenced by respiration - wide physiological splitting of S2 - S4 often present in case of a large shunt

(cont. →)

Table 1.2 Characteristics of heart murmurs in various heart diseases *(continued)*

Disease	Timing	Quality	Shape	Location	Radiation	Other findings
Mitral stenosis	Diastolic	Rumble	Decrescendo-crescendo	Apex	-	- poor correlation between the intensity of the murmur and the severity of the obstruction - loud S1 - mitral opening snap often precedes the murmur
Aortic regurgitation	Diastolic	Blowing	Decrescendo	1st-2nd right interspace (in case of aortic dilatation) 3rd-4th left interspace (in case of valvular disease)	Apex	- intensity increased by handgrip - Austin-Flint murmur (late-diastolic rumble due to partial mitral valve closure induced by increased LVEDP) often heard in severe AR - S3 often present - Corrigan's pulse (rapid rise and quick collapse) - Musset's sign (bobbing of the head with each heartbeat) - Traube's sign (gunshot sound heard over the femoral artery)
Atrial septal defect	Mid-systolic	Scratchy	Diamond	Left upper sternal border	-	- fixed splitting of S2 - low to medium pitched early diastolic murmur over the lower sternal border (because of increased diastolic flow across the tricuspid valve) often present in case of large shunts - cyanosis and clubbing often present in case of right-to-left shunting

components during the intervals of the cardiac cycle when the heart has the greatest excursions within the pericardial sac: at the time of atrial systole, at the time of ventricular contraction and during rapid early diastolic filling. Pericardial friction sounds are common in cases of pericarditis, a common cause of chest pain and dyspnea in young athletes after seasonal influenza [10-12].

References

1. Maron BJ (2003) Sudden death in young athletes. N Engl J Med 349:1064–1075
2. Maron BJ, Shirani J, Poliac LC, Mathenge R, Roberts WC, Mueller FO (1996) Sudden death in young competitive athletes: clinical, demographic, and pathological profiles. JAMA 276:199–204
3. Corrado D, Basso C, Pavei A, Michieli P, Schiavon M, Thiene G (2006) Trends in sudden cardiovascular death in young competitive athletes after implementation of a preparticipation screening program. JAMA 296:1593–1601
4. Corrado D, Pelliccia A, Bjørnstad HH, Vanhees L, Biffi A, Borjesson M et al (2005) Cardiovascular preparticipation screening of young competitive athletes for prevention of sudden death: proposal for a common European protocol: consensus statement of the Study Group of Sport Cardiology of the Working Group of Cardiac Rehabilitation and Exercise Physiology and the Working Group of Myocardial and Pericardial Diseases of the European Society of Cardiology. Eur Heart J 26:516 –524
5. IOC Medical Commission, International Olympic Committee (2006) Sudden Cardiovascular Death in Sport: Lausanne Recommendations: Preparticipation Cardiovascular Screening. European Journal of Cardiovascular Prevention & Rehabilitation 13:859–875
6. Maron B, Thompson P, Ackerman M, Balady G, Berger S, Cohen D et al (2007) Recommendations and Considerations Related to Preparticipation Screening for Cardiovascular Abnormalities in Competitive Athletes: 2007 AHA Scientific Statement Update Circulation 115:1643–1655
7. Maron BJ, Doerer JJ, Haas TS, Tierney DM, Mueller FO (2009) Sudden deaths in young competitive athletes: analysis of 1866 deaths in the United States, 1980–2006. Circulation 119:1085–1092
8. Giese EA, O'Connor FG, Brennan FH, Depenbrock PJ, Oriscello RG (2007) The athletic preparticipation evaluation: cardiovascular assessment. Am Fam Physician 1;75(7):1008–14
9. Santilli G, Casasco M, et al, Comitato Organizzativo Cardiologico per l'Idoneità allo Sport (COCIS) (2010) Protocolli cardiologici per il giudizio di idoneità allo sport agonistico. Medicina dello Sport Vol 63:1–137
10. Fuster V, Wayne Alexander R, O'Rourke R (2010) Hurst's The Heart 13th edition. McGraw-Hill, New York
11. Brukner P, Khan K (2010) Clinical sports medicine. McGraw-Hill, New York
12. Bell C (2008) Cardiovascular Physiology in exercise and sport. Churchill Livingstone, Philadelphia

Electrocardiographic Signal Analysis

2

Francesco Perna

2.1 ECG Analysis

Despite the well-known benefits of regular physical exercise on the cardiovascular system, there is a small population of young athletes (aged under 35 years) who carry an elevated risk of sudden cardiac death (SCD) during exercise. The annual incidence of SCD in young athletes is about 0.5/100,000 per year in the United States and 2.1/100,000 in Italy, and it occurs in more than 90% of cases during or immediately after physical exercise. Sudden deaths are mostly due to cardiac abnormalities that might be identified, provided that appropriate screening of subjects who are candidate to agonistic sports is carried out. Such a psychologically overwhelming problem as the death of a young athlete during a sport competition led to the development of an effective cardiovascular screening program in Italy, which achieved a 89% reduction of the incidence of SCD over 26 years [1]. On the other hand, there are currently no diagnostic tools that can definitely recognize subjects who are potentially at risk of SCD, especially among people with an apparently normal heart. The aim of this chapter is to describe the main instrumental examinations that are used for non-invasive cardiovascular diagnosis in the athletes, and some non-invasive arrhythmic risk markers that are used in cardiology.

F. Perna (✉)
Heart Center
Casa di Cura Mater Dei
Rome, Italy

2.2 Electrocardiogram

Twelve-lead electrocardiogram (ECG) is currently included, along with the medical history and a physical examination, in the preparticipation cardiovascular screening protocol that is used in Italy. It is worth noting that various potentially life-threatening heart diseases can be diagnosed or at least suspected by surface ECG analysis. Therefore, several consensus groups strongly recommend inclusion of ECG in the screening programs.

2.2.1 Cardiomyopathies

ECG is usually abnormal in subjects with cardiomyopathies, in particular those affected by *hypertrophic cardiomyopathy* (particularly with the obstructive form of the disease) (Fig. 2.1). The most common ECG abnormalities for this disease are:

- signs of left ventricular hypertrophy, in particular Sokolow-Lyon index (R in V5 + S in V1) greater than 35 mm;
- ventricular repolarization abnormalities with signs of ventricular overload (ST segment depression, T wave inversion, or giant negative T waves in the apical variant of the disease);
- left axis deviation;
- pathological (narrow but deep) Q waves in the lateral (I, aVL, V5, V6) or sometimes inferior (II, III, aVF) leads.

Arrhythmogenic right ventricular cardiomyopathy (ARVC) is often suspected when the surface ECG shows:

- inverted T waves in V1-V3 or beyond in indi-

M. Fioranelli and G. Frajese (eds.), *Sports Cardiology*,
DOI: 10.1007/978-88-470-2775-6_2, © Springer-Verlag Italia 2012

viduals ≥ 14 years of age in the absence of right bundle branch block;

- epsilon wave (reproducible low-amplitude signals between end of the QRS complex to the onset of the T wave) in the right precordial leads (V1 to V3);
- non-sustained or sustained ventricular tachycardia of left bundle-branch morphology with superior axis.

T wave inversion in the right precordial leads is common in children aged under 14 years, so this feature is not specific enough to diagnose ARVC in this subgroup. Additional minor criteria to be recognized in ECG, SAECG and Holter ECG, along with non-ECG criteria, can be found in the new task force consensus document [2].

ECG is almost always pathological in *dilated cardiomyopathy*, even though such abnormalities are not specific in the majority of cases; the most common ECG features in this disease are left ventricular hypertrophy, low QRS voltages, left bundle branch block, supraventricular or ventricular premature beats, repolarization abnormalities and non-sinus rhythm.

Myocarditis accounts for 5% of cases of SCD in athletes (up to 20% among young military recruits). There are no specific ECG anomalies in acute myocarditis, and it can sometimes mimic acute myocardial ischemia. The most common traits are: ST segment elevation, T wave inversion, widespread ST segment depression and pathological Q waves.

2.2.2 Ion Channel Diseases

Congenital long QT syndrome (LQTS) is a potentially life-threatening pathological condition that could be identified or suspected by ECG. It accounts for about 1-2% of cases of SCD in athletes, and the underlying arrhythmia is often a polymorphous ventricular tachycardia. This pathology is characterized by a prolonged QT interval on surface ECG. The QT interval should be estimated as a mean value derived from 3-5 cardiac cycles, usually in leads II, V5 and V6, and is measured from the beginning of the earliest onset of the QRS complex to the end of the T-wave. Since the QT interval inversely correlates to the heart rate, it is usually corrected for the heart rate itself using the Bazett formula: $QTc + QT/\sqrt{RR}$. This formula is deemed to be acceptable when the heart rate is between 60 and 100 beats per minute (bpm). As a rule, QTc interval is deemed as pathological if it is greater than 450 ms in men and 470 ms in women. T wave morphology may be altered in patients with different genotypes of congenital LQTS: LQTS1 is characterized by broad-based T-waves, LQTS2 by low-amplitude notched T waves, LQTS3 by late-onset peaked or biphasic T-waves.

Short QT syndrome (SQTS) is an extremely rare inherited ion channel disease that has only recently described. It is characterized by a QTc interval constantly equal or less than 320 ms, T wave morphology abnormalities in the precordial

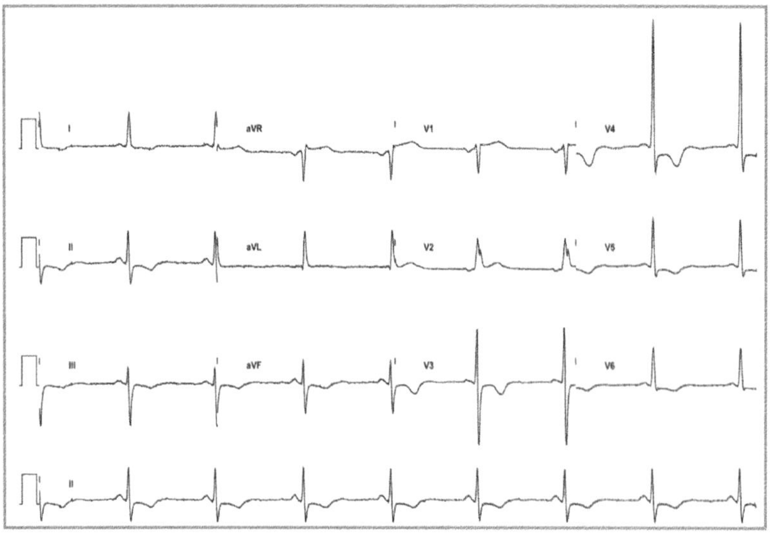

Fig. 2.1 ECG of a patient with hypertrophic cardiomyopathy

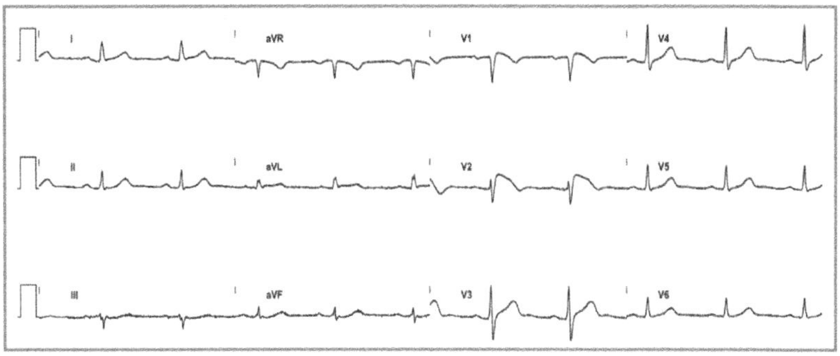

Fig. 2.2 Type 1 Brugada ECG pattern

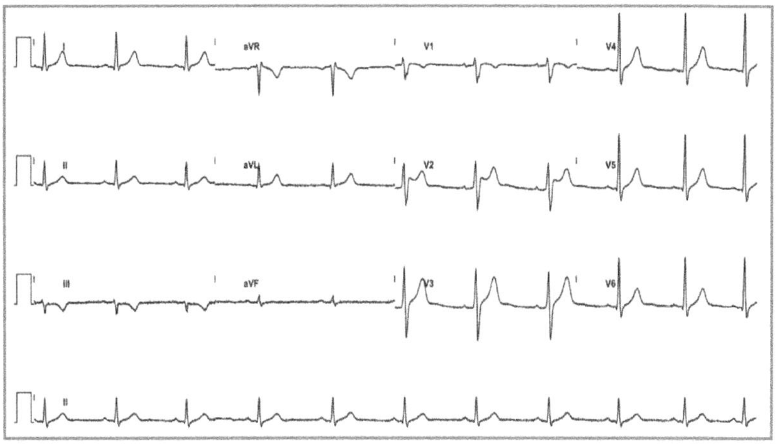

Fig. 2.3 Type 2 Brugada ECG pattern

leads and high incidence of atrial fibrillation, syncope and sudden cardiac death in the absence of structural heart disease. To date, few patients affected by this syndrome have been identified worldwide, including both familiar and sporadic cases [3].

Brugada syndrome is characterized by an ECG pattern of ST segment elevation in V1-V3 associated with documentation of ventricular tachycardia (often polymorphous), ventricular fibrillation, family history of SCD at a young age (< 45 years), otherwise unexplained syncope, nocturnal agonal respiration, in subjects with otherwise normal heart. There are three ST elevation patterns in the right precordial leads (V1-V3) that may suggest the presence of this syndrome:

- type 1 (coved type): marked J point and ST segment elevation ≥ 2 mm or 0.2 mV at its peak, followed by a negative T wave, with no isoelectric separation (Fig. 2.2);
- type 2: high early ST segment elevation ST (≥ 2 mm at the J point) giving rise to a gradually descending ST-segment elevation (remaining ≥ 1 mm above the baseline), followed by a positive or biphasic T-wave that results in a saddle-back configuration (Fig. 2.3);
- type 3: ST elevation in the right precordial leads < 1 mm with a saddle-back or coved configuration.

These descriptions are based on the correct placement of the right precordial leads. However, in patients with a high clinical suspicion of Brugada syndrome who have a normal baseline ECG, alternative placement of the right precordial leads in a superior intercostal space (or, in selected cases, rightward displacement) may disclose a Brugada-like pattern. It should be stressed that ST segment alterations are often dynamic, and a typical ECG pattern may be unmasked by several clinical conditions such as a febrile state or pharmacologic agents. Intravenous administration of class I antiarrhythmic agents (sodium channel blockers) such as flecainide, propaphenone and ajmaline may unmask a Brugada pattern, and this is commonly used as a provocative test when a high clinical suspicion of Brugada syndrome is present.

2.2.3 Coronary Artery Diseases

Coronary artery anomalies are a common cause of SCD during exercise in young athletes. ECG alterations include the entire spectrum of ischemic heart disease ECG patterns, from dynamic ST segment and T wave changes to Q waves. On the other hand, since myocardial ischemia is often transient, resting ECG can be completely normal and other diagnostic tests may be necessary.

2.2.4 Ventricular Pre-excitation

ECG is a key tool in the diagnosis of Wolff-Parkinson-White (WPW) syndrome, which is the best known form of ventricular pre-excitation accompanied by tachycardia-related symptoms (Fig. 2.4). Ventricular pre-excitation is defined as:

- PR interval less than 120 ms;
- slurring of the initial part of the QRS complex (also known as delta wave);
- total QRS duration more than 120 ms (due to delta wave);
- secondary repolarization abnormalities, with T wave direction usually opposite as delta wave and QRS.

Patients with ventricular pre-excitation carry a higher risk of developing several types of supraventricular arrhythmias (WPW syndrome) that can degenerate, in rare cases, into ventricular arrhythmias and SCD. People with WPW syndrome experience greater atrial vulnerability, which can lead to atrial flutter and fibrillation; when fast atrioventricular conduction through the accessory pathway is present, an exaggerated ventricular response to atrial arrhythmias may trigger ventricular fibrillation.

2.2.5 The Athlete's Heart

Contrary to what one may expect, a normal ECG in a professional athlete is the exception rather than the rule. The ECG of a professional athlete often mimics overt pathological patterns. Many so-called ECG *abnormalities* may thus not have a real pathological implication, but can be the electrical appearance of structural and functional physiological changes in the cardiovascular system, which are the consequence of increased metabolic requests from the body after constant physical exercise; overall, these adaptations are known as *athlete's heart*. The more common features of the athlete's heart are:

- signs of left ventricular hypertrophy with high QRS voltages (Sokolow-Lyon index > 35 mm);
- ST segment depression and T wave abnormalities;
- ST elevation (early repolarization pattern).

These features, caused by *physiological* hypertrophy in the athlete's heart, are hard to distinguish from the ECG characteristics of pathological hypertrophy, but they are typically reversible after a detraining period (up to 6 months). Prolonged conduction times, sinus bradycardia, incomplete

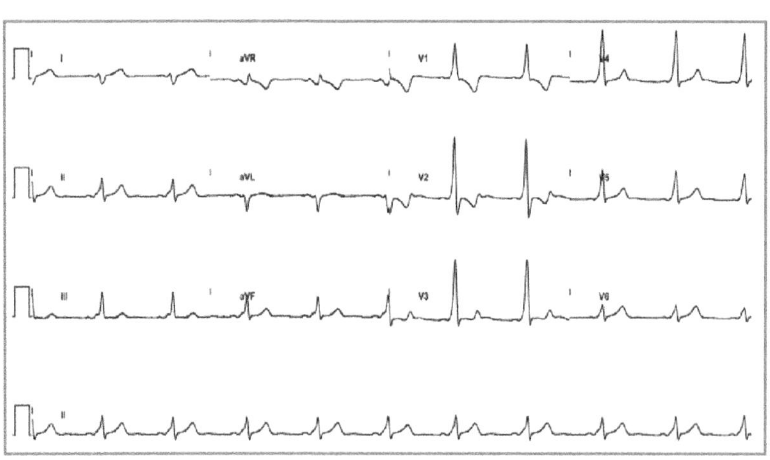

Fig. 2.4 17-year-old athlete with ventricular pre-excitation

Table 2.1 Differential diagnosis between athlete's heart and hypertrophic cardiomyopathy [5]

Hypertrophic cardiomyopathy
- asymmetric left ventricular hypertrophy
- left ventricular end-diastolic diameter (LVDd) < 45 mm
- left atrial enlargement
- left ventricular diastolic dysfunction
- overtly pathological electrocardiographic changes (very high QRS voltages, prominent Q waves, deep negative T waves)
- female gender
- positive family history of hypertrophic cardiomyopathy
- hystology typical for hypertrophic cardiomyopathy
- positive genetic test
Athlete's heart
- left ventricular end-diastolic diameter (LVDd) > 55 mm
- peak oxygen consumption during cardiopulmonary exercise test > 50 ml/kg/min
- no criteria for hypertrophic cardiomyopathy (exclusion diagnosis)
- regression of structural abnormalities after physical deconditioning

right bundle branch block, high amplitude T waves, suggest a physiological adaptation. On the other hand some features, such as high amplitude R waves with RS or Rs morphology in the right precordial leads (V1-V3) or deep Q waves in the lateral (and less frequently inferior) leads, or some T wave inversion patterns, are less common in the *benign* hypertrophy, but not completely absent. Therefore, the diagnostic work-up should include, in addition to 12-lead ECG, an accurate personal and family medical history, physical examination, instrumental exams such as cardiopulmonary stress test and echocardiogram and, whenever necessary, a complete re-evaluation after a detraining period [4]. Table 2.1 shows the proposed criteria to tell these two clinical conditions apart [5].

2.2.6 Other Benign ECG Features

Further *physiological* ECG features are often described in athletes:

- sinus bradycardia: heart rates as low as 25 bpm have been reported (Fig. 2.5);
- various degree atrioventricular (AV) block: first degree and second degree, Mobitz 1, AV block are more common (8%). Second degree, Mobitz 2 and third degree AV block have been described, but they are pretty rare and should be considered pathological. Sinus bradycardia and AV block are caused by a resting autonomic imbalance towards a parasympathetic predominance;
- incomplete right bundle branch block: occurring in 14-31% of athletes, it is often a consequence of the gain in myocardial mass, which causes a slight delay of the conduction time, and it has been shown to be reversible after detraining;
- early repolarization: this has been observed in 50 to 89% of athletes, it may in fact be considered the rule rather than the exception (Fig. 2.4). It is defined as ST elevation in several leads, with an upward concavity in its initial

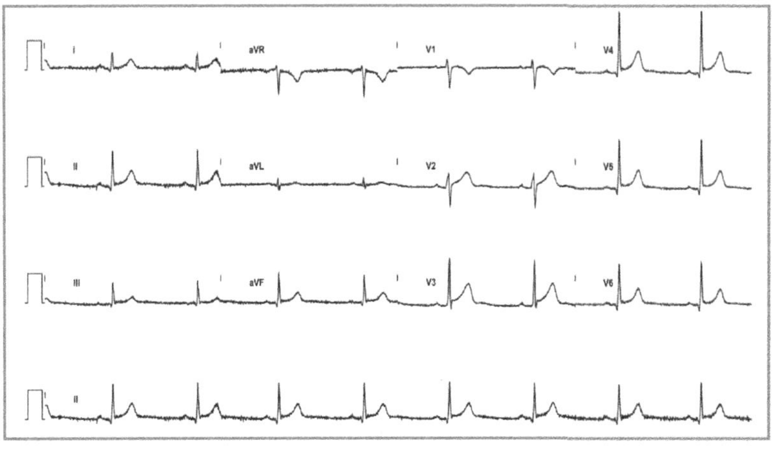

Fig. 2.5 25-year-old athlete with sinus bradycardia and early repolarization

portion and a notching or slurring of the terminal part of QRS, symmetrical and concordant T waves that are of high amplitude and relatively stable over time;
- T wave inversion: reported in approximately 30% of cases. If T wave inversion is dynamic, there is a strong suspicion of coronary artery disease. However, normalization of the T wave during exercise testing or isoproterenol infusion was observed in athletes with subsequent angiographic evidence of normal coronary arteries [6].

2.3 Exercise ECG

Exercise ECG was introduced into clinical practice after the empirical evidence of ST segment depression during angina and the subsequent demonstration that exercise can produce anginal symptoms and/or ST segment depression in patients with ischemic heart disease [7, 8]. Currently this instrumental test met a widespread distribution and its use is no longer restricted to the diagnosis of myocardial ischemia, although this remains its main indication.

Equipment and Protocols

ECG recording is performed using the standard 12-lead ECG, although lateral leads (V5 and V6) alone can detect about 90% of all ST depressions. The two most common systems are the treadmill and cycle ergometer. The exercise protocols allow for a warm-up phase, a gradual increase in the workload with adequate duration at each stage, and a recovery phase; exercise should ideally last about 8-12 minutes. The protocol most commonly used with the treadmill is the *Bruce* protocol, which shows the advantage of having a seventh (final) stage that virtually no one will reach, and it is the most widespread in the scientific literature; its main disadvantage is the significant increase in the workload between one stage and the next, which can make the estimate of maximum oxygen consumption (VO_2max) less accurate and lead some patients to stop earlier. It is important to report the exercise tolerance in metabolic equivalents (METs) rather than minutes of exercise, in order to be able to make comparisons with tests performed with different protocols. A MET is equivalent to an oxygen consumption rate of 3.5 ml/kg/min.

Reliability

The exercise ECG is prescribed in order to select individuals who should undergo further investigations and procedures. Numerous studies have shown a wide range of sensitivity and specificity values for this diagnostic tool, probably because of differences between studies in terms of protocols used and selection of the population; a meta-analysis calculated average sensitivity and specificity of about 66% and 84%, respectively. In individuals with a high probability of false-positive or false-negative results, it is reasonable to use an alternative procedure (myocardial perfusion scintigraphy, exercise or pharmacological stress echocardiography, coronary computed tomography).

Interpretation

The extent of ST segment elevation should be calculated versus baseline (i.e. the PQ junction) or, in case of resting ST segment abnormalities, compared to its original position. In the case of exercise ST depression in a subject with resting ST elevation, the baseline will be referred to. The electrocardiographic pattern considered diagnostic for ischemia (Fig. 2.6) is *horizontal or downsloping ST segment depression ≥ 1 mm at 80 ms after the J point.*

Upsloping ST depression must be interpreted with caution and in the light of other clinical and instrumental data, since its inclusion in the myocardial ischemia criteria can improve sensitivity only at the expense of specificity, it is therefore preferable to consider it to be negative in most cases. When upsloping ST depression is interpreted as positive, it should be at least 1.5 mm below the baseline at 80 ms after point J, with a not very steep slope. ST depression exclusively during the recovery phase has the same meaning and the same predictive power as one that occurs during exercise, which explains why it is important to continue electrocardiographic recording for at least 5 minutes after the end of the exercise.

ST elevation is quite common in patients with previous myocardial infarction, and it is observed almost exclusively in derivations showing Q

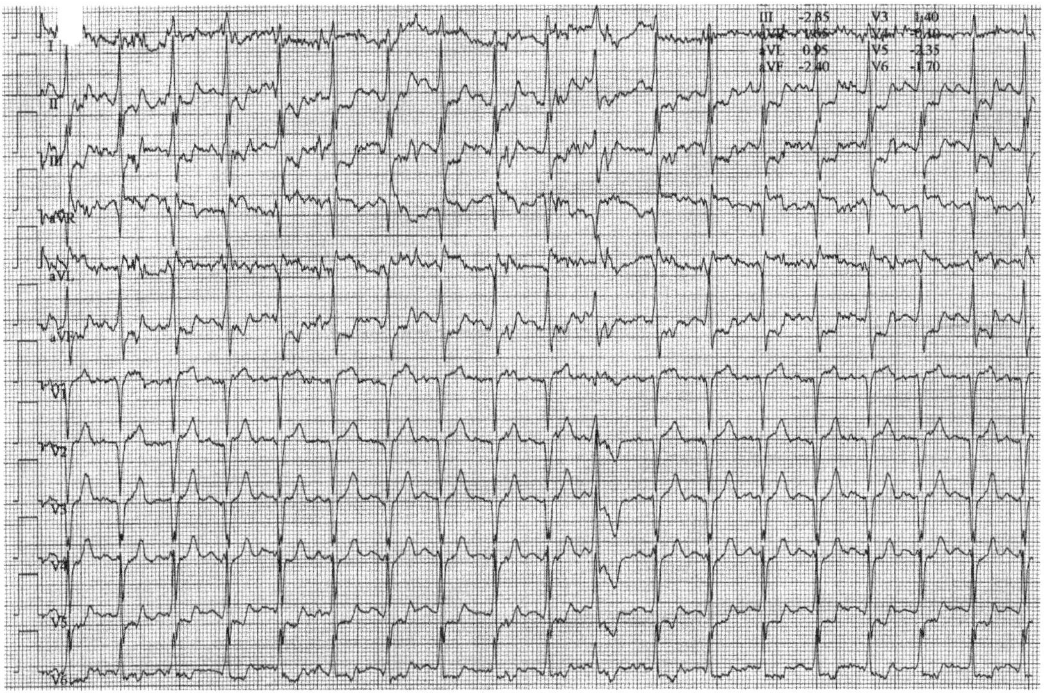

Fig. 2.6 Peak of physical effort during exercise ECG. This ECG is diagnostic of exercise-induced myocardial ischemia (downsloping ST segment depression greater than 1 mm at 80 ms after the J point)

waves; in such cases, the clinical significance of ST elevation is controversial. In contrast, ST elevation in leads other than V1 and aVR in a normal ECG is rare (0.1%) and is a sign of transmural ischemia. The *R wave* has amplitude variations during exercise that have been correlated with ischemic heart disease, but they have not enough predictive power to improve the diagnostic value of the test. Exercise-induced *T-wave inversion* is almost always associated with a significant ST depression and has been identified as an expression of a more severe degree of coronary artery disease, often being related to three-vessel coronary artery disease with high specificity [9].

The appearance of a positive T wave in patients with resting flat or inverted T wave (*T wave pseudonormalization*) was considered a sign of ischemia, but it may be due to other factors and should therefore be interpreted with caution in the absence of further clinical signs.

Another aspect to consider is the onset of *exercise-induced arrhythmias*, such as conduction disorders, supraventricular arrhythmias, and, in particular, ventricular extrasystoles and tachycardias. Ventricular extrasystoles are classified as occasional (< 6/minute) or frequent (> 6/minute), and they can be monomorphous, polymorphous, arranged in pairs or runs of ventricular tachycardia.

Special attention should be paid to the onset of *symptoms*: the combination of typical angina and ST depression provides a 98% probability of significant coronary artery disease.

Contraindications

Even though exercise ECG is considered a non-invasive test, it is not free from risks, the most common being pulmonary edema, hypertensive peaks, ventricular arrhythmias and cardiac arrest. For this reason there is a series of conditions, listed in Table 2.2, where exercise ECG is contraindicated.

Indications for Terminating Exercise Testing

Exercise testing should be terminated according to the patient's level of tiredness. However, it is sometimes necessary to stop it earlier for other reasons (Table 2.3).

Table 2.2 Contraindications to exercise testing

Absolute
- resting ECG alterations suggesting a recent acute cardiac event
- recent acute myocardial infarction
- unstable angina
- uncontrolled cardiac arrhythmias (potentially life-threatening ventricular arrhythmias, atrial arrhythmias with poor pharmacological control causing hemodynamic compromise, high-degree atrioventricular block)
- symptomatic heart failure
- symptomatic severe aortic stenosis
- acute aortic dissection
- acute myocarditis or pericarditis
- recent pulmonary or systemic embolism
Relative
- resting blood pressure > 210/110 mmHg
- moderate stenotic valvular heart disease
- electrolyte disorders
- permanent pacemaker
- frequent or complex ventricular extrasystoles
- ventricular aneurism
- uncontrolled metabolic diseases (diabetes mellitus, thyrotoxicosis, myxedema)
- mental or physical impairment leading to inability to exercise adequately
- hypertrophic cardiomyopathy and other forms of outflow tract obstruction

Table 2.3 Indications for terminating exercise testing

Absolute
- acute myocardial infarction
- moderate to severe angina
- sudden drop in systolic blood pressure of ≥ 10 mmHg from baseline despite an increase in work load, when accompanied by other evidence of ischemia
- significant cardiac arrhythmias (high-degree atrioventricular block, sustained ventricular tachycardia, complex ventricular extrasystole, atrial fibrillation with high ventricular response)
- signs of poor peripheral perfusion (cyanosis, pallor)
- significant dyspnea
- neurological symptoms
Relative
- drop in systolic blood pressure of ≥ 10 mmHg from baseline despite an increase in work load, in the absence of other evidence of ischemia
- horizontal or downsloping ST depression > 2 mm
- ST elevation > 2 mm
- worsening chest pain
- shortness of breath or asthma
- leg pain or claudication
- excessive increase in blood pressure (>250/115 mmHg)
- supraventricular tachycardias
- development of bundle branch block or intraventricular conduction delay that cannot be distinguished from ventricular tachycardia

2.3.1 Exercise Testing with Ventilatory Gas Analysis

Ventilatory gas exchange analysis during exercise testing is a useful additional tool, since it can provide valuable information, such as oxygen consumption (VO_2), carbon dioxide output (VCO_2), minute ventilation and the ventilatory/anaerobic threshold. VO_2 at maximal exercise (VO_2 max) is considered the best index of aerobic capacity and cardiorespiratory function, and it is defined as the point at which no further increase in measured VO_2 occurs despite an increase in work rate. It is an important prognostic index among heart failure patients and it can be referred to for the correct timing of heart transplantation. Moreover, it may help to distinguish a cardiogenic cause from a respiratory cause in cases of dyspnea or functional limitation. It also has a role in the differential diagnosis of athlete's heart and hypertrophic cardiomyopathy: healthy athletes have a significantly higher VO_2 max (> 50 ml/kg/min) than athletes with hypertrophic cardiomyopathy.

2.3.2 Value of Exercise Testing in Athletes

Athletes are a special population because of their *supernormal* physiology, high physical stamina and possible resting ECG variations.

Electrocardiographic assessment during exercise may be required for the evaluation of chest pain when the cause cannot be diagnosed by standard ECG. In subjects older than 35 years the disease to be ruled out is atherosclerotic coronary artery disease. In young athletes other causes of chest pain are more likely, such as coronary artery congenital anomalies.

Although ergometry is mainly used for the evaluation of *myocardial ischemia*, among athletes it is often used to diagnose *arrhythmias*. Several arrhythmias can be triggered by an increase in sympathetic tone and a drop of parasympathetic tone that occurs during exercise. In particular, ventricular arrhythmias have important prognostic implications and are crucial for competitive sports eligibility . There is still substantial disagreement about the significance of ventricular arrhythmias in subjects with normal hearts, and while some groups found an association with increased mortality, others came to completely different conclusions. Ventricular extrasystoles detected with Holter monitoring in normal subjects is usually considered benign [10]. Polymorphous ventricular premature beats (VPB) designate an increased risk only in subjects with left ventricular dysfunction, especially if it is severe. These findings are also applicable to the VPB recorded during exercise testing. In normal subjects, maximal exercise can trigger ventricular arrhythmias in 36-42% of cases, usually at high workloads, while in patients with ischemic heart disease the incidence rises to 50-60%; they occur at relatively lower heart rates and are more reproducible. The suppression of ventricular arrhythmias during exercise is classically considered a criterion of benignity, but a high rate of suppression was also found in patients with ischemic heart disease. Exercise-induced ventricular arrhythmias, even if not sustained, should be considered very seriously and lead to appropriate further investigations, since they can point to severe heart diseases.

An inadequate chronotropic increase during exercise, with an inability to reach 85% of the predicted maximum heart rate (or a heart rate of at least 100 bpm) identifies a *chronotropic incompetence*, which in athletes can be difficult to distinguish from bradycardia due to an increased vagal tone.

Exercise can trigger *supraventricular arrhythmias,* thus providing a diagnosis in patients with a history of palpitations. It should be remembered that, in subjects with WPW, the ST segment is not evaluable for myocardial ischemia, because of basic ST alterations due to the abnormal ventricular depolarization and repolarization sequences; the disappearance of pre-excitation at high heart rates (infrequent finding) could show a low-risk accessory pathway.

Conduction disturbances may be revealed by physical exercise, both in subjects with and without coronary artery disease, while first-degree AV block due to increased vagal tone is typically reduced or even disappears during effort.

Sometimes, patients with *long QT syndrome* have a borderline QT interval at rest, which is markedly prolonged by exercise. Therefore, exercise ECG may be one of the most useful diagnostic tools in these patients.

Amongst athletes with *arterial hypertension* it is of paramount importance to perform a maximal exercise test (that is, with the achievement of maximum workload or at least 85% of the predicted maximum heart rate) with close monitoring of blood pressure to evaluate its trend during exercise for sports participation purposes; current guidelines consider that blood pressure exceeding 240/115 mmHg during exercise and/or not returning to the baseline within 6 minutes of the effort is abnormal.

Because of the wide range of ECG abnormalities in resting athletes, many of them involving the ST segment and T wave, ECG changes during exercise should be interpreted with caution and in light of the overall clinical setting. In there is any doubt, further non-invasive investigations may be useful to detect such abnormalities.

2.4 Signal-Averaged Electrocardiogram (SAECG)

The SAECG (Signal-Averaged Electrocardiogram) is a technique that improves the signal/background noise ratio of an ECG signal when the signal is constant and the noise is random or occasional. By filtering and reducing the background noise, such as myopotentials, this technique allows surface recording of cardiac signals of a few microvolts. The rationale for using high resolution ECG (Fig. 2.7) is the ability to identify low amplitude signals at the end of the QRS complex, known as *late potentials*. The most credited hypothesis is that they represent

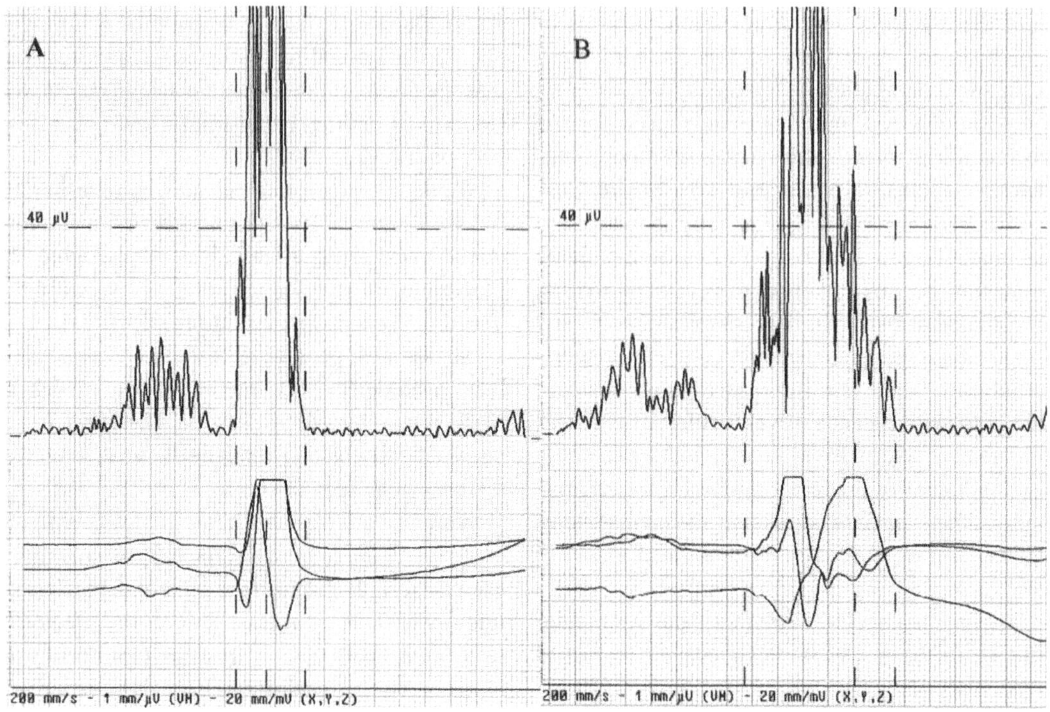

Fig. 2.7 a Negative SAECG; b positive SAECG

delayed local activation of some myocardial regions, and may therefore represent the substrate of some re-entrant arrhythmias. This diastolic activity is more frequently identified in patients with a history of sustained ventricular tachycardia, and was thus correlated with the initiation and perpetuation of re-entrant ventricular tachycardias.

SAECG has therefore been used to identify patients at a higher risk of developing malignant ventricular arrhythmias [11]. At least 300-400 sinus beats with the same morphology should be sampled, and the background noise should be less than 0.3 µV. For 40 Hz high-pass filtering, the test is considered positive in the presence of at least two of the following three criteria:

1. filtered QRS duration (fQRS) > 114 ms;
2. root mean square voltage in the last 40 ms of the fQRS (RMS 40) < 20 µV;
3. low-amplitude signal duration below 40 µV (LAS) > 38 ms.

Late potentials were found in 60 to 90% of survivors of myocardial infarction with a history of sustained ventricular arrhythmias, in 7 to 15% of subjects with previous myocardial infarction but no history of arrhythmias, and in only 0 to 7% of normal subjects. Most clinical studies of late potentials were conducted in patients with previous myocardial infarction, and hence the use of the SAECG in patients at risk of non-ischemic VT and in athletes is currently not well defined. It could be helpful among patients with arrhythmogenic right ventricular cardiomyopathy, for which it constitutes a minor diagnostic criterion. Being a sensitive but non-specific marker of arrhythmic risk, late potentials have an overall limited prognostic value, but the negative predictive value of SAECG, which reaches 89-99%, makes this test a useful tool in order to exclude the presence of an anatomical substrate for the development of ventricular arrhythmias.

2.5 Dynamic ECG (Holter)

Ambulatory ECG recording (Holter) is typically used to detect and characterize abnormal cardiac electrical activity during normal daily activities [12]. It is usually possible to monitor two or three

ECG leads for 24-48 hours, but 12-lead recording is also possible.

Dynamic ECG is not part of the preparticipation screening protocol, but it may be necessary if the baseline 12-lead ECG is not adequate to explain the reported symptoms (usually palpitations or syncope), which may be occasional and not necessarily related to specific triggering events such as physical exercise. However, in the case of very sporadic symptoms, the diagnostic power of a Holter ECG recording can be fairly limited, and in this case it may be necessary to use an external or implantable event recorder or to perform an electrophysiological study.

In healthy asymptomatic young subjects, rhythm disturbances are rather unusual. Nevertheless, particularly in athletes, it is possible to observe a significant number of arrhythmias with no necessarily pathological implication, some of which are caused by excessive vagal tone and therefore more frequent during sleep: marked sinus bradycardia (35-40 bpm), sinus arrhythmia with pauses, sinoatrial exit block, Wenckebach AV block, junctional rhythm, supraventricular and ventricular premature beats. In other cases, ECG Holter monitoring is performed to determine the burden of an arrhythmia that had already been diagnosed with baseline ECG. For example, ventricular extrasystoles can be classified as rare or frequent if they are below or above a certain threshold, respectively. It is also important to assess whether extrasystoles generate complex and potentially life-threatening arrhythmias (non-sustained or sustained ventricular tachycardia).

Repeated Holter ECG recording during follow-up is recommended to assess the clinical response to drug or catheter ablation therapy, to monitor heart rate in the case of atrial fibrillation and to exclude potential side effects of drugs (for example, AV block or pro-arrhythmia). Holter monitoring is also used in the assessment of myocardial ischemia with 12-lead monitoring, because of the possibility of exploring V5 and V6, the most sensitive leads to detect ST segment depression. However, Holter ECG is not a first-line screening tool for asymptomatic subjects who are able to perform physical exercise and have no contraindications to provocative tests. Therefore, patients who are not able to complete physical exercise (for example, patients undergoing peripheral vascular surgery) or with sporadic symptoms such as patients with variant angina, are good candidates for this type of investigation.

2.6 Noninvasive Arrhythmic Risk Stratification Techniques

Large clinical trials have demonstrated the benefits of implantable cardioverter defibrillators (ICD) in terms of mortality in patients with severe left ventricular dysfunction. However, even among high risk populations, only a small number of patients receive appropriate ICD interventions. Moreover, only a small proportion of sudden cardiac deaths occur in this small subgroup of the general population: most sudden deaths occur in subjects deemed as *low risk* or *intermediate risk*, and are therefore completely unexpected. These considerations lay the foundations for the development of novel and more effective tools for the risk stratification of SCD due to malignant ventricular arrhythmias, such as non-invasive arrhythmic markers [13]. The ideal test should be able to identify the majority of subjects who will be affected from VT or VF and to exclude those in whom these events will not occur, and at the same time they should allow the execution of an operation (ICD implantation) that can significantly increase survival in the subgroups with abnormal tests. Since the majority of clinical trials in this field were carried out in survivors of myocardial infarction or heart failure, the use of such tests in the evaluation of athletes is currently not very common.

2.6.1 Heart Rate Variability (HRV)

HRV describes the changes in the heart rate and RR intervals in a variable period of time (for example, 5 minutes or 24 hours) [14]. These variations are almost entirely due to the influence of the autonomic nervous system. Therefore, since it provides a surrogate for autonomic effects on ventricular events, which are thought to play a role in the pathogenesis of VT and VF, HRV has been proposed as a tool for arrhythmic risk stratification. Several studies correlated an HRV reduction (i.e. an altered autonomic function) to increased mortality in patients with myocardial infarction, coronary artery disease or valvular heart disease. Unfortunately, the interpretation of the results of clinical studies is complicated by the large number of different proposed measures. Periodic fluctuations in the heart rate may be represented both in the time and in the frequency domain (Fig. 2.8). The most commonly performed HRV measures in the time domain are:

- SDNN: standard deviation of the normal RR intervals (those measured between consecutive sinus beats);
- SDANN: standard deviation of all the 5-minute normal RR interval means in an entire day;
- SD index: mean of all the 5-minute standard deviations of normal RR intervals during the 24-hour period (this measure is complementary to the SDANN);
- R-MSSD, NN50, pNN50: these other measures are less frequently used. The HRV measures of the frequency domain are usually classified ac-

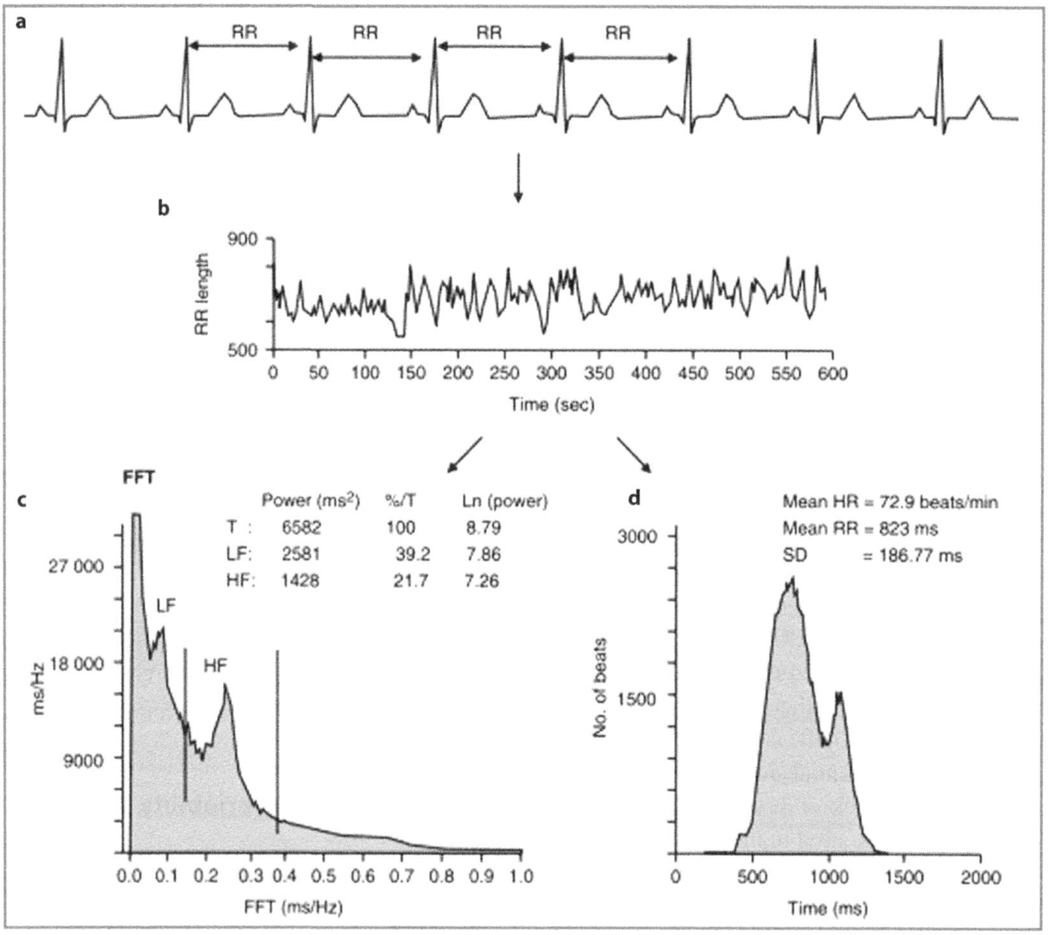

Fig. 2.8 HRV analysis. Analysing consecutive RR intervals on the surface ECG (a), tachograms are obtained (b), which can be analysed in the frequency domain (c) or in the time domain (d). Spectral analysis (c) and the histogram (d) result from a 24-hour Holter ECG recording. The histogram shows 2 peaks: one around 1100 ms, which corresponds to the average heart rate during the night, the other one around 750 ms, which corresponds to the average heart rate during the daylight. *FFT* fast Fourier transformed, *HF* high frequency, *HR* heart rate, *LF* low frequency, *Ln* natural logarithm, *T* total. From: Aubert AE et al. [14], reproduced with the author's kind permission

cording to the range of the analyzed frequencies:
- ULF (ultra-low frequency): < 0.0033 Hz;
- VLF (very low frequency): 0.0033 to 0.04 Hz;
- LF (low frequency): 0.04 to 0.15 Hz;
- HF (high frequency): 0.15 to 0.40 Hz;
- total power.

In general, currently available evidence show that decreased HRV is a powerful predictor of overall mortality in patients with myocardial infarction or heart failure, but there are few data to support a statistically significant correlation of SDNN with an increased risk of sudden death. It is interesting that some drugs that improve survival in heart failure, such as beta-blockers and ACE-inhibitors, can increase HRV. However, since beta-blockers act on the autonomic nervous system, they could reduce the predictive value of HRV after myocardial infarction, especially with regard to sudden death. Despite the theoretical physiological link between a pathological HRV, autonomic tone and arrhythmogenesis, HRV seems to be rather a marker of non-arrhythmic mortality, and is therefore not currently recommended for the risk stratification of sudden cardiac death. Cardiovascular exercise adaptations influence HRV parameters because of changes in the autonomic balance, but due to the scarcity of works about HRV in athletes, it is currently not possible to define its role in this field.

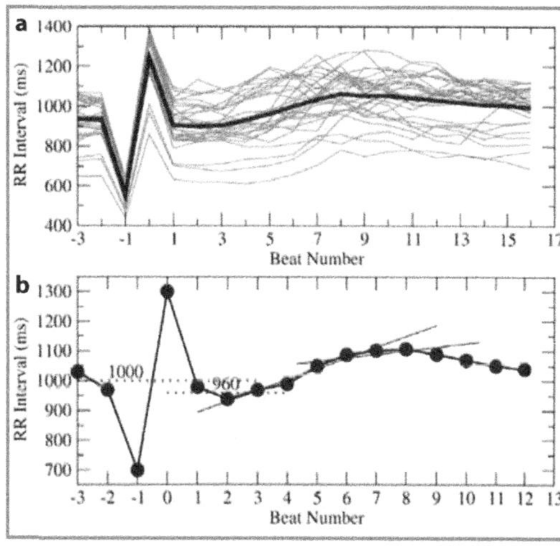

Fig. 2.9 Example of a tachogram and of HRT calculation. **a** The *grey lines* represent RR intervals after the first 25 ventricular premature beats (VPB). The *black line* represents the mean of the tachograms. All the tachograms extrapolated from every VPB in a 24-hour ECG recording are usually used; in this example, only 25 of them are shown. **b** Turbulence onset (TO) quantifies the shortening of the RR interval after the VPB. Turbulence slope (TS) is the steepest slope of the lines extrapolated from 5 consecutive RR intervals. In this case, tachogram, TO = [(960 – 1000) / 1000] x 100 = – 4,0%. The slope of the line extrapolated from beat 2 to beat 6 is greatest at 37.2 ms / beat. Therefore, TS = 37.2. From: Watanabe MA et al [15], reproduced with the author's kind permission

2.6.2 Heart Rate Turbulence (HRT)

HRT describes short-term fluctuations in the cycle length of the 10-15 sinus beats following a ventricular extrasystole with a compensatory pause. Generally, after a PVB the heart rate rises slightly for a few beats and then decreases before returning to the baseline. This phenomenon is displayed in charts called tachograms, which show the beat-to-beat fluctuations of the RR cycle [15] (Fig. 2.9); the chart is aligned so that the compensatory pause corresponds to the RR interval number 0. The measurement of HRT is performed by means of two parameters: *turbulence onset* (TO) and *turbulence slope* (TS).

TO reflects the amount of acceleration after a sinus PVB; it is the percentage difference between the heart rate (RR intervals) immediately following the PVB and the heart rate immediately preceding the PVB. It is calculated using the following equation:

$$\mathrm{TO} = \frac{[(\mathrm{RR1} + \mathrm{RR2}) - (\mathrm{RR\text{-}2} + \mathrm{RR\text{-}1})]}{(\mathrm{RR\text{-}2} + \mathrm{RR\text{-}1})} \cdot 100$$

with RR-2 and RR-1 being the two sinus intervals prior to the PVB while RR1 and RR2 are the two sinus intervals following the PVB. TO is first determined for each PVB, and later the average 24-hour TO value will be calculated. Positive values for TO indicate deceleration of sinus rhythm, while negative values indicate acceleration.

TS reflects the sinus deceleration rate following the previous acceleration, and it corresponds to the steepest slope of the linear regression line for each sequence of five consecutive sinus intervals in local tachogram. The calculations are based on the averaged tachogram and expressed in ms per RR interval.

There is a website (www.h-r-t.org) which provides programs for the calculation of TO and TS and a list of up-to-date publications on HRT. Normal values for HRT are TO < 0% and TS > 2.5 ms/RR interval. In practice, a normal response consists of sinus acceleration followed by a rapid deceleration. This phenomenon is reduced or absent in patients with various heart diseases, and indicating an alteration of the vagal tone. To measure TO and TS it is required a minimum of 5 PVB (preferably 10-15) in 24 hours. HRT cannot be evaluated in patients with arrhythmias or artefacts in the peri-PVB sequences, paced rhythm, or persistent atrial fibrillation. HRT is probably a manifestation of the baroreceptor reflex resulting in complex changes in blood pressure associated with the PVB and the compensatory post-extrasystolic pause.

A pathological HRT is a powerful independent predictor of mortality in patients with coronary artery disease and dilated cardiomyopathy. In some patients it is possible to see an improvement or a normalization of this index during beta-blocker and statin therapy. However, HRT does not seem to predict arrhythmic mortality, but only cardiac mortality, and therefore further studies are needed to establish its clinical utility in the risk stratification of sudden death.

2.3.6 T-Wave Alternans

TWA is defined as a beat-to-beat fluctuation in the amplitude or morphology (or both) of the ST segment and T wave. A TWA visible on the surface ECG is derived from alternation of the myocyte action potential duration. However, a repolarization alternation visible on the surface ECG is quite rare, and therefore the most frequently used marker for this purpose is the T wave variation in the context of microvolts (microvolt T wave alternans, MTWA). *Discordant* alternation (different duration of the repolarization between adjacent myocardial areas) is considered highly arrhythmogenic, since it suggests substantial and heterogeneous repolarization gradients in the myocardium, which can lead to reentry and wavefront fragmentation. Several factors can influence the extent of the TWA, such as sympathetic stimulation, myocardial ischemia and increased heart rate, which enhance it, or vagal stimulation, use of beta-blockers and medullar neurostimulation, which reduce it. TWA analysis should be performed during exercise (exercise test) or atrial pacing in order to achieve a heart rate of 100-120 bpm, with preferably low atrial or ventricular ectopic activity. During exercise several factors coexist, such as an increased sympathetic tone, a reduced vagal tone and an elevated heart rate, which can unmask TWA in the context of a vulnerable substrate.

An increased TWA has been observed in patients with conditions that favour the development of ventricular arrhythmias, such as ischemic heart disease and long QT syndrome, and in subjects with a history of ventricular arrhythmias. The majority of clinical trials performed to date show that MTWA is a powerful marker of arrhythmic mortality. TWA also shows a high negative predictive value (≥ 98%), even among subjects with preserved left ventricular function, thus having the potential to identify patients who may not qualify for ICD implants, but the positive predictive value is as low as 8-10%. The main limitations of MTWA are its dependence on the heart rate, poor reliability in patients with recent myocardial infarction, hypertrophic cardiomyopathy and arrhythmogenic inherited diseases, and the heterogeneity of the cut-off used in various studies.

Before TWA analysis can be included in the clinical management of patients potentially at risk of SCD, it requires additional scientific evidence, a definition of clear boundaries between normal and pathological findings, and further advancements in technical analysis.

Based on these assumptions, TWA may become a routine screening test even in athletes and individuals with high-risk jobs, as well as a prognostic index for patients with left ventricular dysfunction or myocardial infarction.

2.3.7 QT Dispersion (QTD)

The difference between the longest and the shortest QT interval in a 12-lead ECG is an index of the heterogeneity of ventricular repolarization. An abnormally high QTD has been associated with the risk of SCD in different contexts, but so far the evidence of the results extrapolated from the literature is not satisfactory. Furthermore, there are studies in which this correlation has not been demonstrated. There are several techniques for the measurement of this parameter which are difficult to compare between each other, in addition, the test results are influenced by patients' age, body position, time of the day and season in which it is performed. Also, some authors have concluded that QTD is based on an unfounded pathophysiological hypothesis [16]. Alternative markers have been proposed (*T_{peak}-T_{end} interval, T wave nondipolar components, T wave complexity, T wave residuum, T-wave morphology dispersion, etc.*) which should more closely reflect the dispersion of ventricular repolarization, since it is shown by means of T wave morphological changes rather than QT interval alterations. Based on the existing evidence, the use of QTD in the risk stratification of SCD is not recommended.

References

1. Corrado D, Basso C, Pavei A et al (2006) Trends in sudden cardiovascular death in young competitive athletes after implementation of a preparticipation screening program. JAMA 296:1593–1601
2. Marcus FI, McKenna WJ, Sherrill D et al (2010) Diagnosis of arrhythmogenic right ventricular cardiomyopathy/dysplasia: proposed modification of the task force criteria. Circulation 121:1533–1541
3. Gaita F, Giustetto C, Bianchi F et al (2003) Short QT syndrome: a familial cause of sudden death. Circulation 103:965–970
4. Zeppilli P (1988) The athlete's heart: differentiation of training effects from organic heart disease. Practical Cardiol 14:61
5. Maron BJ, Pelliccia A, Spirito P (1995) Cardiac disease in young trained athletes: insights into methods for distinguishing athlete's heart from structural heart disease, with particular emphasis on hypertrophic cardiomyopathy. Circulation 91:1596–1601
6. Zeppilli P, Pirrami MM, Sassara M et al (1980) T wave abnormalities in top ranking athletes: effects of isoproterenol, atropine, and exercise. Am Heart J 100:213–222
7. Bousfield G (1918) Angina pectoris: Changes in electrocardiogram during paroxysm. Lancet 2:457
8. Feil H, Siegel M (1928) Electrocardiographic changes during attacks of angina pectoris. Am J Med Sci 175:225
9. Chikamori, T, Kitaoka H, Matsumura Y et al (1997) Clinical and electrocardiographic profiles producing exercise-induced U-wave inversion in patients with severe narrowing of the left anterior descending coronary artery. Am J Cardiol 80:628–632
10. Buckingham TA (1983) The clinical significance of ventricular arrhythmias in apparently healthy subjects. Pract Cardiol 9:37
11. Breithardt G, Cain ME, el-Sherif N et al (1991) Standards for analysis of ventricular late potentials using high- resolution or signal-averaged electrocardiography. A statement by a Task Force Committee of the European Society of Cardiology, the American Heart Association, and the American College of Cardiology. Circulation 83:1481–1488
12. Kadish AH, Buxton AE, Kennedy HL et al (2001) American College of Cardiology/American Heart Association/American College of Physicians-American Society of Internal Medicine Task Force; International Society for Holter and Noninvasive Electrocardiology. ACC/AHA clinical competence statement on electrocardiography and ambulatory electrocardiography: A report of the ACC/AHA/ACP-ASIM task force on clinical competence (ACC/AHA Committee to develop a clinical competence statement on electrocardiography and ambulatory electrocardiography) endorsed by the International Society for Holter and noninvasive electrocardiology. Circulation 104:3169–3178
13. Goldberger JJ, Cain ME, Hohnloser SH et al (2008) American Heart Association Council on Clinical Cardiology; American Heart Association Council on Epidemiology and Prevention; American College of Cardiology Foundation; Heart Rhythm Society. American Heart Association/American College of Cardiology Foundation/Heart Rhythm Society scientific statement on noninvasive risk stratification techniques for identifying patients at risk for sudden cardiac death: a scientific statement from the American Heart Association Council on Clinical Cardiology Committee on Electrocardiography and Arrhythmias and Council on Epidemiology and Prevention. Heart Rhythm 5:1–21
14. Aubert AE, Seps B, Beckers F (2003) Heart rate variability in athletes. Sports Med 33:889–919
15. Watanabe MA, Schmidt G (2004) Heart rate turbulence: a 5-year review. Heart Rhythm 1:732–738
16. Rautaharju PM (2005) A farewell to QT dispersion. Are the alternatives any better? J Electrocardiol 38:7–9

Echocardiography in Athletes

3

Vittoria Rizzello and Massimo Fioranelli

Two-dimensional and color-Doppler echocardiography is the most widely used imaging method in athletes. In these subjects, echocardiography is a valuable way to diagnose potentially lethal heart diseases. In fact, in the last few years episodes of sudden death associated with physical exercise in competitive athletes have become highly visible events fuelled by new media reports. Often the underlying cause of sudden death in such patients is represented by structural changes to the heart and/or great vessels that may be identified by echocardiography. The existence of heart disease may be an exclusion criterion in competitive sport in order to reduce the risk of sudden death and/or it may justify the implantation of an automatic defibrillator. On the other hand, athletes' hearts, particularly those of well-trained athletes who practise endurance sports (marathons, swimming) or mixed sports (cross-country skiing, cycling, rowing), encounter structural and functional changes that must be identified so that heart disease is not diagnosed incorrectly. The aim of this chapter is to provide a structured guide to cardiac echocardiography in athletes.

3.1 Introduction

Two-dimensional and color-Doppler echocardiography is the most widely used imaging method in athletes. The Italian cardiovascular screening protocol for competitive athletes recommends an echocardiogram for all subjects in whom the medical history, objective examination and/or electrocardiogram yield abnormal findings [1].

In these subjects, echocardiography is a valuable way to diagnose potentially lethal heart diseases. In fact, in the last few years episodes of sudden death associated with physical exercise in competitive athletes have become highly visible events fuelled by new media reports.

Often the underlying cause of sudden death in such patients involves structural changes to the heart and/or great vessels that may be identified by echocardiography. The existence of heart disease may be an exclusion criterion in competitive sport in order to reduce the risk of sudden death and/or it may justify the implantation of an automatic defibrillator. On the other hand, athletes' hearts, particularly those of well-trained athletes who practise endurance sports (marathons, swimming) or mixed sports (cross-country skiing, cycling, rowing), encounter structural and functional changes that must be identified so that heart disease is not diagnosed incorrectly [2].

The aim of this chapter is to provide a structured guide to cardiac echocardiography in athletes.

3.2 Transthoracic Echocardiography

3.2.1 Echocardiographic Windows, Image Planes, and Echocardiographic Views

The *echocardiographic study* of the heart is conducted by placing the transducer in various positions (echocardiographic windows) that enable

V. Rizzello (✉)
"S. Giovanni-Addolorata" Hospital
Rome, Italy

M. Fioranelli and G. Frajese (eds.), *Sports Cardiology*,
DOI: 10.1007/978-88-470-2775-6_3, © Springer-Verlag Italia 2012

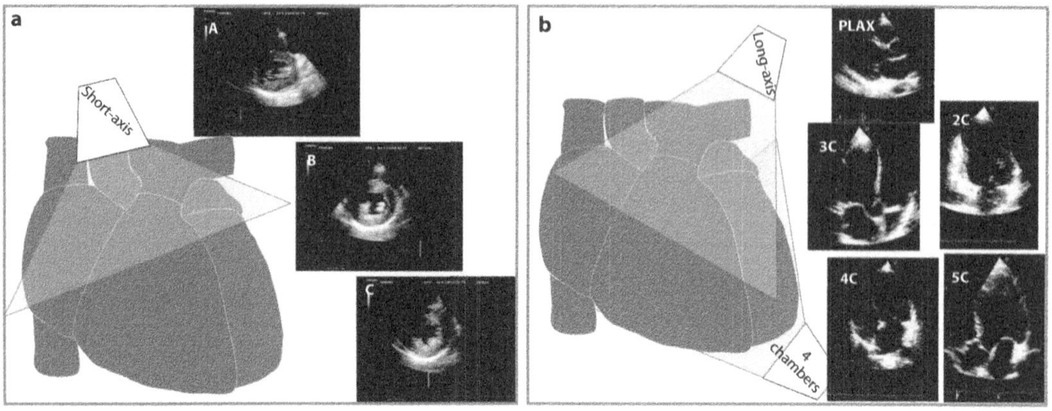

Fig. 3.1 a Short-axis views of the heart at the level of the mitral valve (*A*), papillary muscles (*B*) and apex (*C*). b Echocardiographic views along the long-axis plane of the heart (parasternal long-axis, PLAX; two-chamber, three-chamber) and along the four-chamber plane (four-chamber, five-chamber)

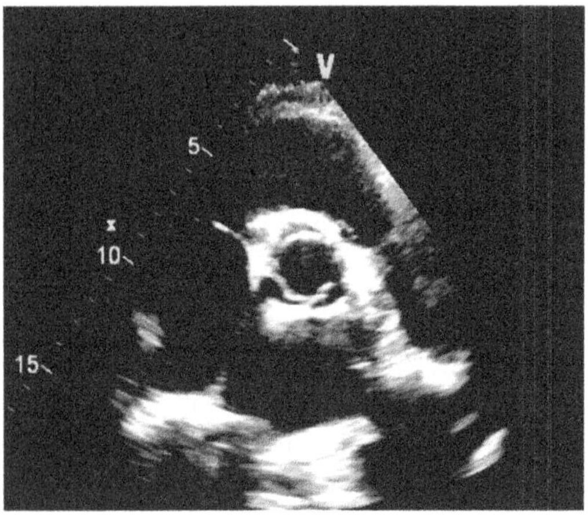

Fig. 3.2 Parasternal short-axis view at the level of the aortic root. In the centre the three aortic cusps can be seen (the right coronary cusp at the top, the left coronary cusp on the right, and the non-coronary cusp at the bottom); to the right of the aorta, the pulmonary valve and the common trunk of the pulmonary artery are seen; to the left of the aorta the tricuspid valve is seen; anteriorly to the aorta, the right ventricle with the outflow tract can be seen; posteriorly to the aorta, the two atria and interatrial septum can be seen

ultrasound beam to slice the heart along its three main axes, providing various views of the heart's structures.

The most common echocardiographic windows for studying the heart are:

- the parasternal window (at the 3rd and 4th intercostal spaces to the left of the sternum);
- the apical window (at the apex of the heart);
- the subxiphoid window (under the xiphoid appendix of the sternum, with the patient in a supine position).

Figure 3.1 shows the three cardiac axes along which the heart scans are made, as well as the corresponding echocardiographic views. The *short-axis plane* cuts the heart transversally, providing a circular view of the left ventricle. The *long-axis plane*, which is perpendicular to the short axis, is parallel to the long-axis of the left ventricle (from the apex to the base) and is defined as an imaginary plane that cuts the left ventricle vertically. The *four-chamber plane* is perpendicular to the long-axis and short-axis planes and is defined as an imaginary plane that cuts the heart horizontally from the apex to the base through either the left ventricle and atrium and right ventricle and atrium.

The echocardiographic views (Fig. 3.1) resulting from cardiac scans along the three main axes of the different echocardiographic windows are:

- the long-axis and short-axis parasternal view of the left ventricle;
- the long-axis (or three-chamber) and two-chamber apical view;

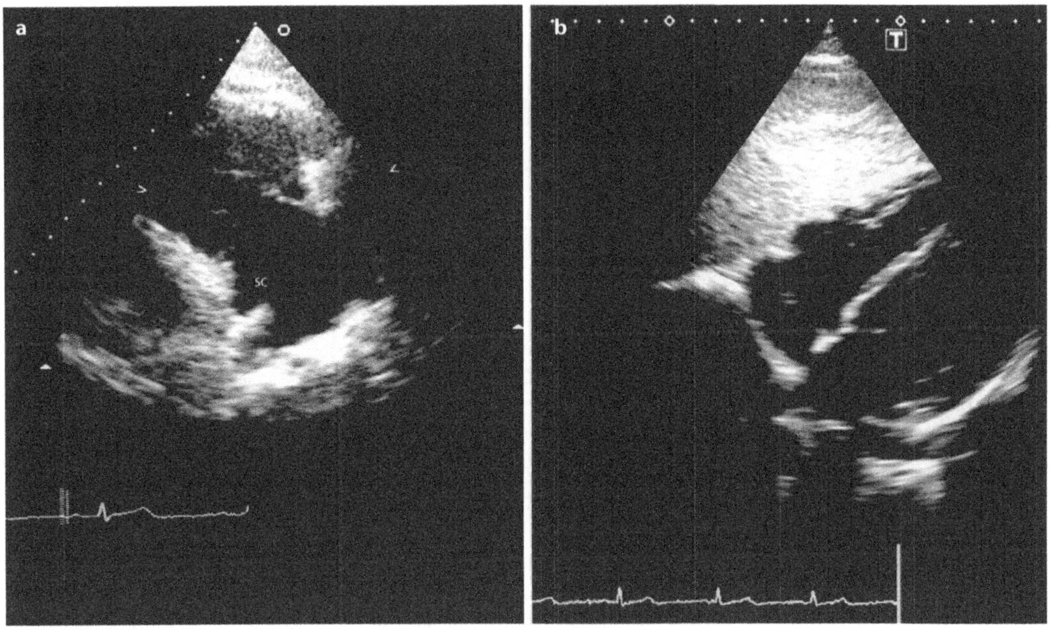

Fig. 3.3 a Parasternal long-axis of the right ventricle in which the right ventricle, the tricuspid valve and the right atrium can be seen. In this view it is also possible to see the coronary sinus entering in the right atrium. b Oblique subcostal view of the right ventricle

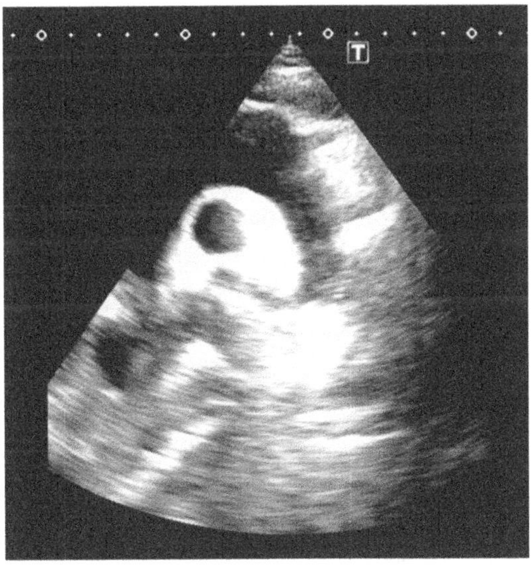

Fig. 3.4 Suprasternal view in which the aortic arch, the origin of the left common carotid artery, the left subclavian artery, the aortic isthmus and the first segment of the descending aorta can be seen. Under the aortic arch a transversal view of the right pulmonary artery is shown

- the four-chamber and five-chamber apical view with the aorta.

There are also three other views in which the great vessels and the structures of the right heart are better visualized:

- the short-axis parasternal view at the base of the heart (Fig. 3.2);
- the long-axis parasternal view of the right ventricle (Fig. 3.3a);
- the oblique subcostal view of the right ventricle (Fig. 3.3b).

Finally, from the suprasternal window, i.e. from the suprasternal notch, the aortic arch and the aortic isthmus are seen (Fig. 3.4). This view is partic-

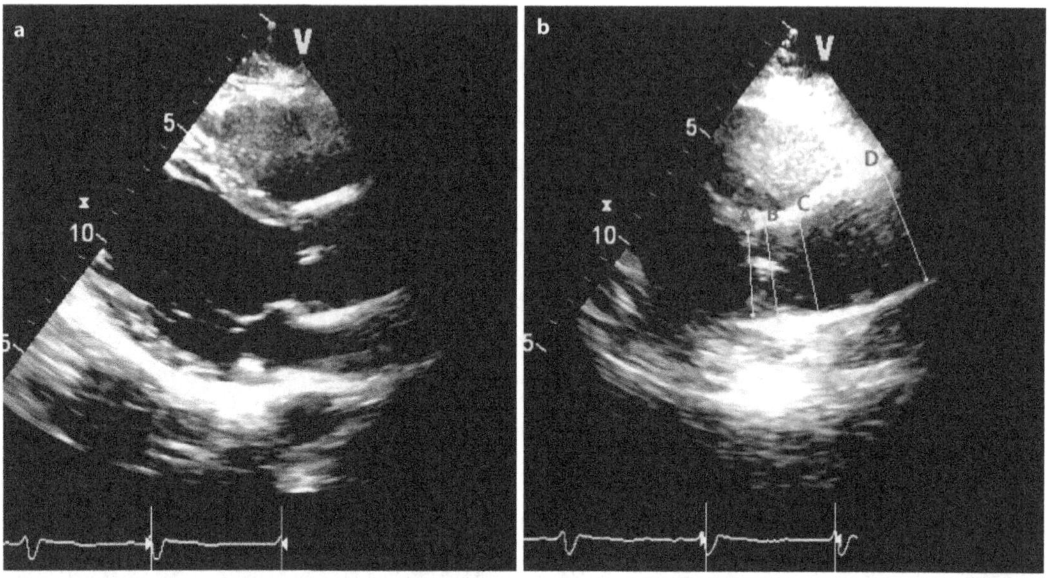

Fig. 3.5 Parasternal long-axis view (a) and high parasternal view for measuring the ascending aorta (b). The points at which measurements of the aorta are taken are shown: *A* left ventricular outflow tract, *B* aortic bulb, *C* sinotubular junction, *D* maximum dilatation of the ascending aorta

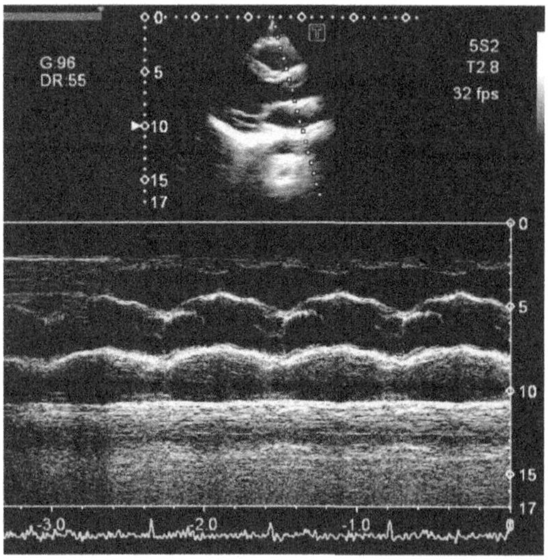

Fig. 3.6 M-mode image of the aortic box in the parasternal long-axis view. Behind the aortic bulb is the left atrium

ularly useful for ruling out coarctation of the aorta or patent ductus arteriosus.

3.2.2 Two-dimensional and M-mode Echocardiography

Although M-mode echocardiography was once the most widely used echocardiographic method, it has now been superseded by the two-dimensional method (2D). M-mode is characterized by the emission of a single ultrasound beam that enables only the structures perpendicular to the scan line to be seen. The main advantage of M-mode is its higher temporal resolution compared to 2D studies, due to a frame rate of 1800/s vs. 30/s for 2D images. M-mode analysis is still used in support of and in addition to 2D analysis, enabling accurate sampling and measurement of rapidly moving structures such as cardiac walls and valves. The use of M-mode in association with 2D imaging makes it possible to align the scan line perpendicular to the structure in question, thus guaranteeing the accuracy of measurements. In the following paragraphs we describe the normal appearance of the heart and great vessels in each echocardigraphic view. In particular, we shall highlight parameters that need special attention in athletes.

3.2.2.1 Parasternal Views

Parasternal Long-axis View

This view is obtained by positioning the transducer at the 3rd or 4th intercostal space to the left side of the sternum, with the transducer marker pointing towards the subject's right shoulder. The parasternal long-axis view enables accurate analysis of the aortic root, the Valsalva sinuses, the sinotubular junction and the proximal 3-4 cm of the ascending aorta (Fig. 3-5a). By moving the transducer 1-2 intercostal spaces higher, it is possible to visualise the other segments of the ascending aorta, enabling the maximum diameter to be measured (Fig. 3.5b). Measuring various segments of the aorta makes it possible to identify subjects with dilated aortas, which is common in patients with Marfan syndrome. M-mode scans of the aorta (Fig. 3.6) at the tip of the cusps enable visualization of the opening of the cusps, which in normal subjects describes the so-called *aortic box*, in which the linear echoes of the right coronary and non-coronary cusps are parallel to each other during the entire duration of systole. If there is a systolic notch on the *aortic box*, the presence of left ventricular outflow obstruction must be suspected. Conversely, fluttering of the linear echoes on the *aortic box* is normal in young subjects (Fig. 3.6).

The left atrium can be seen behind the aorta, and its anteroposterior diameter (in M-mode or 2D) can be measured. The dimensions of the left atrium are typically greater in athletes than in untrained subjects. This increase is benign and is only rarely associated with atrial fibrillation (<1 %) [3].

In the parasternal long-axis view, on the left side of the monitor, is visualized the left ventricle, specifically the interventricular septum and posterior wall, the dimensions of which can be studied using either the 2D or M-mode images. To obtain reliable linear measurements, it is essential to optimise the view in order to obtain the greatest end-diastolic diameter for the left ventricle, in other words the view must include the maximum excursion in the opening of the aortic and mitral valves, in addition to the left ventricle (Fig. 3.7). Normally from the parasternal long-axis view, the apex of the left ventricle cannot be seen. Therefore, the presence in this view of what looks like an apex is the result of an oblique cut through the lateral wall that invalidates the accuracy of the measurements.

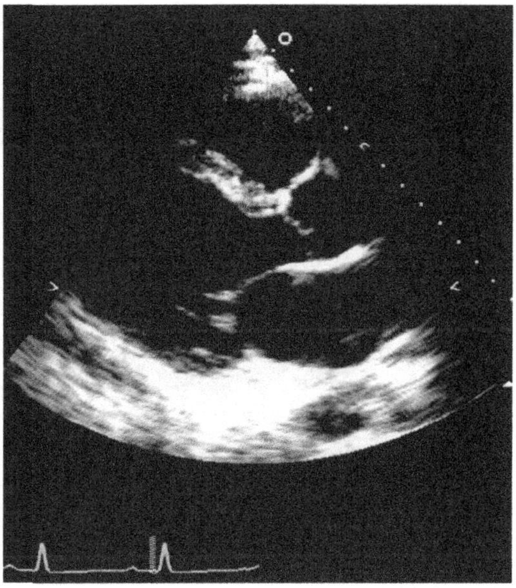

Fig. 3.7 Parasternal long-axis view showing the aortic bulb, the left atrium, the right ventricle, the interventricular septum, the posterior wall of the left ventricle, the right and non-coronary cusp of the aortic valve, and the anterior and posterior leaflets of the mitral valve

The most important structural change in athletes' hearts (particularly for endurance sports) is a variable extent of remodeling, which is represented by an increase in the dimensions and volume of the left (and right) ventricle, while systolic and diastolic function remains normal. A significant increase in the dimensions of the left ventricle (> 60 mm) is present in 15% of high-level athletes [4]. In rare cases, this dilatation can be accompanied by a slight increase in thickness (13-15 mm) [5]. However, there is considerable over-

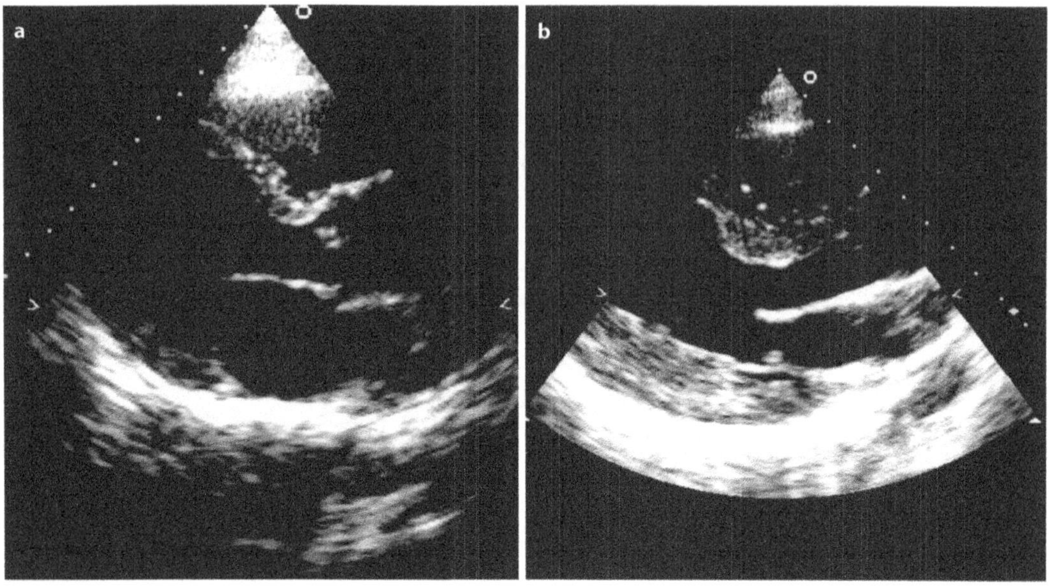

Fig. 3.8 Parasternal long-axis view in a cyclist (a) and in a patient with hypertrophic cardiomyopathy (b). Differential diagnosis between an athlete's heart and hypertrophic cardiomyopathy requires a combination of echocardiographic and clinical factors and the patient's medical history

lap between the cardiac dimensions of athletes and untrained subjects of similar age and sex. In general, there is a 10-20% increase in the thickness and internal dimension of the left ventricle in athletes, but these values usually remain within normal range in each individual athlete [2]. However, in some cases, adaptive remodeling of athletes' hearts, particularly when there is an increase in the thickness of the left ventricle, can imitate hypertrophic cardiomyopathy. It has been reported that about 2% of competitive athletes have left ventricular thickness of 13-15 mm, which is considered a moderate increase, representing a *grey area* overlapping extreme expression of adaptive cardiac remodeling in athletes and mild forms of hypertrophic cardiomyopathy (without marked hypertrophy and/or outflow obstruction) [2]. The echocardiographic criteria that may help in the differential diagnosis between these two conditions are: unusual hypertrophy distributions patterns, reduced intracavity dimensions (< 45 mm) and a change in the relaxation of the left ventricle that are characteristic of cardiomyopathy [6]. Conversely, regression of hypertrophy after deconditioning is typical of an athlete's heart. Finally, it should be remembered that the thickness of the left ventricle is very rarely increased in female athletes, and therefore if left ventricular hypertrophy occurs in a female athlete, a form of hypertrophic cardiomyopathy must always be suspected [6]. Figure 3.8 provides an example of left ventricular hypertrophy in an athlete (cyclist) and a patient with hypertrophic cardiomyopathy.

Certain morphological (and functional) information about the mitral valve can also be obtained using the parasternal long-axis view. Normally the anterior and posterior leaflets of the mitral valves are thin and coapt beneath the mitral annulus, but in subjects with mitral valve prolapse, one or both leaflets may have a redundant appearance (to a varying degree), with the leaflets protruding (to a greater or lesser extent) beyond the mitral annulus (Fig. 3.9). The diagnosis of mitral valve prolapse and the definition of the involvement of both mitral valve leaflets, however, requires the valve to be evaluated in all long-axis views.

Parasternal Short-axis Views

By rotating the transducer clockwise by about 90° from the position used for the parasternal long-axis view, the *parasternal short-axis view of the left ventricle at the level of the mitral valve* is obtained. In

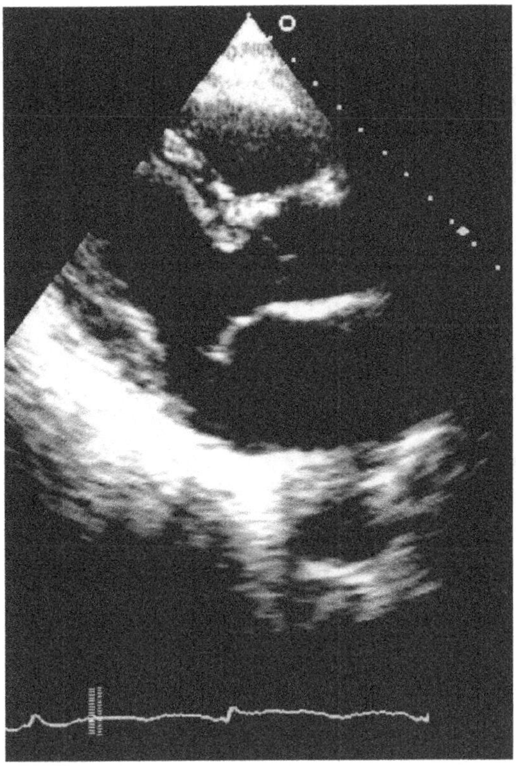

Fig. 3.9 Parasternal long-axis view showing the redundancy and prolapse of the mitral valve leaflets

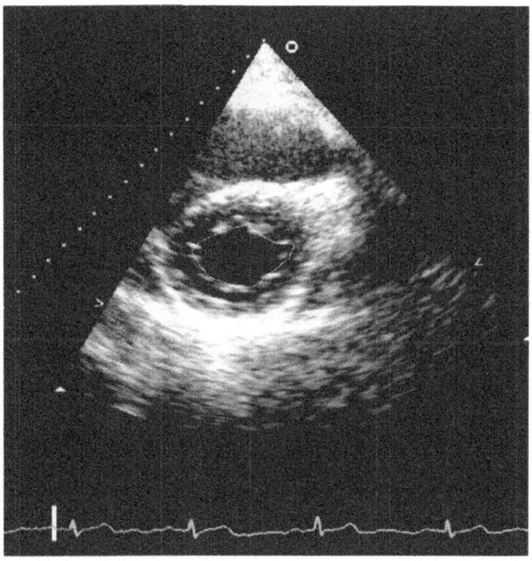

Fig. 3.10 Parasternal short-axis view at the level of the mitral valve. In this view it is possible to see the opening (diastole) and closing (systole) of the mitral valve leaflets and to measure the anatomical area of the mitral orifice (in diastole)

this view it possible to visualise the opening and closing movements of the mitral valve (in diastole and systole, respectively) and measure the anatomical area planimetrically, i.e. by tracing the outline of the internal border of the mitral valve leaflets in diastole. Moreover, the anterolateral and posteromedial commissures (the point at which the anterior and posterior leaflets are joined) of the mitral valve can easily be seen (Fig. 3.10). The right ventricle can be seen in front of the left ventricle, and the thickness of its free wall and its internal diameter can be measured.

By angulating the transducer downwards, a cut of the left ventricle *at the level of the papillary muscles* is obtained, showing one of the muscles located posteromedially and the other anterolaterally. In the short-axis views the left ventricle appears circular, and therefore an oval appearance of the ventricle indicates incorrect alignment that can be corrected if the transducer is moved up slightly and tilted towards the apex. The short-axis view at the level of the papillary muscles enables the thickness and internal dimensions of the left ventricle to be measured accurately in either 2D or M-mode with a scanning beam perpendicular to the short axis, whereas oblique cuts can overestimate the dimensions. By further angulating the transducer downwards, sections of the ventricle closer to the apex can be obtained, whereas moving the transducer slightly sideways and tilting it medially, a short-axis view of the apex can be obtained (Fig. 3.1a).

If the transducer is tilted up from the parasternal short-axis view of the left ventricle at the level of the mitral valve, the *short-axis view at the level of the great vessels* is obtained, in which the aortic bulb, the Valsalva sinuses, the three aortic cusps and the trunk of the pulmonary artery can be seen, along with the pulmonary valve (Fig. 3.2). The two atria and the interatrial septum are behind the aorta, whereas anteriorly to the aorta are visualized the septal and anterior leaflets of the tricuspid valve, the right ventricular inflow and outflow tracts. Analysis of the aortic valve in the short-axis view enables identification of the three aortic cusps: the non-coronary cusp, facing the interatrial septum; the right cusp, facing the right ventricle; and the left, facing the pulmonary artery (Fig. 3.2).

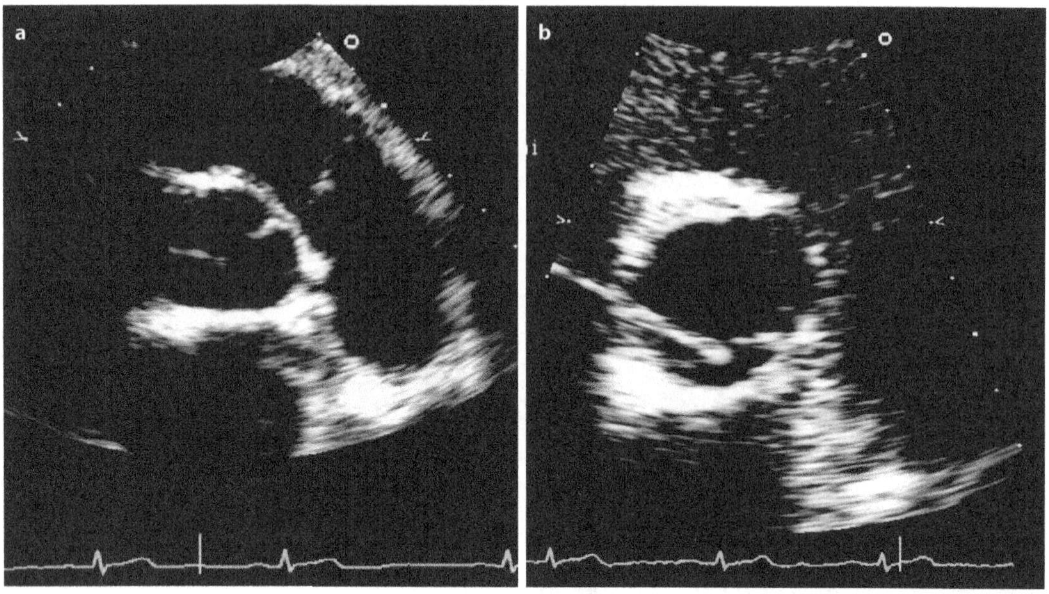

Fig. 3.11 Parasternal short-axis view at the base of the heart showing the three aortic cusps in diastole (a) and systole (b). In a the pulmonary valve can be seen to the right of the aortic valve

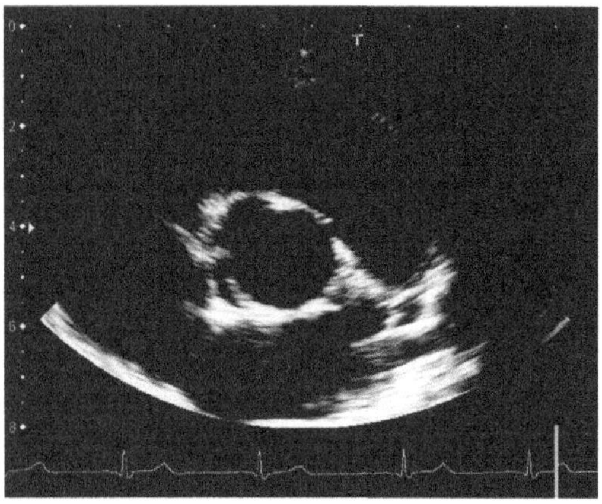

Fig. 3.12 Parasternal short-axis view at the base of the heart showing the typical opening of a bicuspid aortic valve

In systole the three cusps open, forming an almost circular orifice, while in diastole they form a Y-shape in the coaptation line (Fig. 3.11). The aortic cusps are usually thin and have nodular thickening in the middle of the free margin (nodules of Aranzio), which allows the valve to close optimally. Sometimes these nodules increase in size with age. The number of cusps must be identified in systole, since in diastole a raphe (i.e. a fusion cord) in the position of a normal commissure can lead a bicuspid valve to appear trileaflet. Bicuspid valves usually have an oval opening in systole and in most cases there are two cusps of varying dimensions, one in front of the other (Fig. 3.12).

The origin of the coronary arteries can be seen in the short-axis view at the level of the aorta. This moment of diagnosis is essential for the echocardiographic study of athletes due to the higher risk of sudden death from sport in subjects with abnormalities of the origin and course of the coronary arteries. Particularly in endurance athletes and young subjects, some factors, such as a good acoustic window, due to favourable conformation of the chest, increased cardiac and coronary artery dimen-

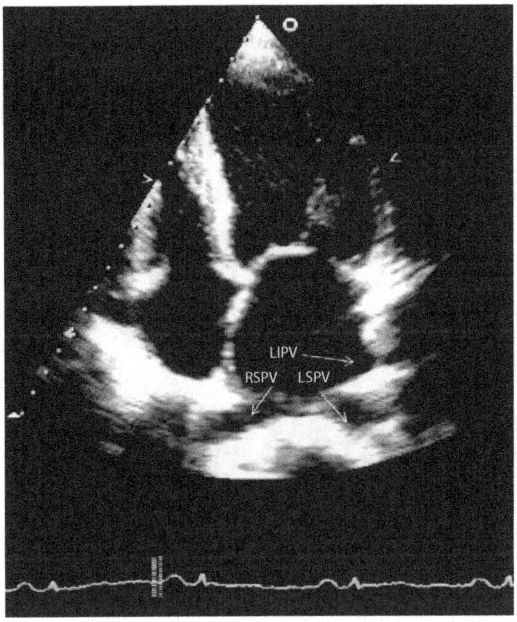

Fig. 3.13 Four-chamber apical view. It is possible to see the lateral wall and the inferior septum of the left ventricle, the right ventricle, the mitral valve, the tricuspid valve, the two atria and the interatrial septum. The left superior pulmonary vein (*LSPV*), the left inferior pulmonary vein (*LIPV*) and the right superior pulmonary vein (*RSPV*) can also be seen

sions, and prolonged duration of the diastole, allow to reliably study both the origin and in part the course of coronary arteries [7]. The ostium and left main of the left coronary artery are visible at their origin at the level of the left coronary cusp and it is also sometimes possible, with small movements of the tranducer, to see the bifurcation of the left main into the anterior descending and circumflex arteries. The ostium and the first part of the right coronary artery are often seen in athletes in front of the right cusp. An even better view can be obtained if the subject in is the right lateral decubitus.

Parasternal Long-axis View of the Right Ventricle

By moving the transducer from the long-axis parasternal view of the left ventricle slightly towards the apex and tilting it medially, the right atrium, the tricuspid valve and the right ventricle can be seen (Fig. 3.2a). In this view, the septal and anterior leaflets of the tricuspid valve are visualized. Sometimes it is possible to see a redundant Eustachian valve at the level the inferior vena cava as it enters in the right atrium. The right ventricle typically has a very trabeculated appearance, particular around the apex, while the outflow area is smoother. In almost all subjects it is possible to see a large trabecula (moderator band) that crosses the apex of the right ventricle obliquely and contains the right branch of the cardiac conduction system. The right atrium and right ventricle are larger in athletes' hearts, without functional and/or structural changes of the ventricular wall.

3.2.2.2 Apical Views

Four-chamber Apical View

The four-chamber apical view is obtained by placing the transducer at the apex of the heart with the marker towards the left harm of the subject. In this view the lateral wall and inferior septum of the left ventricle, the right ventricle with the moderator band, the mitral valve, tricuspid valve, both atria and the interatrial septum (Fig. 3.13) are seen. It is important to find the best position for the transducer in order to visualise the entire length of the left ventricle and to avoid that the real apex of the left ventricle is cut off.

Typically in athletes the left ventricle is rounder than in untrained subjects, with a ratio between the longitudinal diameter (base-to-apex) and transversal diameter (septum-to-lateral wall) of approximately 1.5 [8]. Moreover, it is often possible to see trabeculae, not only in the right but also the left ventricle. These trabeculae can be present at various levels of the ventricle, but are most often found at the apex and are indicated as false tendons. More often the false tendons are stretching from the interventricular septum to the lateral wall of the left ventricle and are very thin, like cords (Fig. 3.14a). Less frequently the false tendons look like muscular trabeculae with a longitudinal course, that are easier to see using non-conventional (*off-axis*) views of the apical or parasternal long-axis views (Fig. 3.14b). In both the cord-like and muscular form, the false tendons have no pathological significance. However, it is particularly important to recognize false tendons and exclude them, especially longitudinal tendons, from the measure of the thickness of the interventricu-

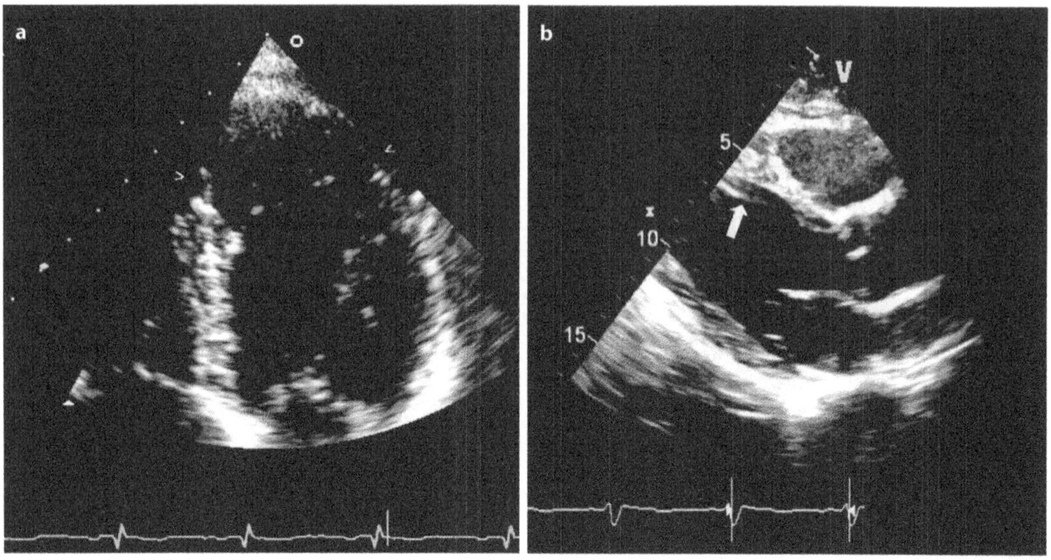

Fig. 3.14 In a it is shown a false tendon between the interventricular septum and the lateral wall, in the four-chamber view. In b it is shown a false tendon running parallel to the interventricular septum, in the parasternal long-axis view

lar septum, to avoid incorrect diagnosis of hypertrophic cardiomyopathy.

In athletes, the good echocardiographic window and the physiological training-induced bradycardia enable adequate visualization of the endocardial border of the left ventricle, a critical prerequisite for accurate measurement of the volumes and ejection fraction of the left ventricle, by tracing the profile of the ventricle in diastole and systole at the level of the interior border of the endocardium, leaving the papillary muscles outside the ventricular cavity. Particularly in endurance athletes, the volumes of the left ventricle may be significantly increased compared with untrained subjects, but no reduction in contractile function is observed, unlike dilated cardiomyopathy.

In the four-chamber view it is possible to visualise the annulus and the anterior leaflet (next to the interventricular septum) and posterior leaflet (next to the lateral wall) of the mitral valve, and to study their morphology as well as the opening and closing movements.

The increased atrial dimensions often seen in athletes also enable easy visualization of two or three pulmonary veins as they enter the left atrium (Fig. 3.13), the left atrial appendage, and the inferior and superior vena cava as they enter the right atrium. It is also often possible to visualise embryonic *remnants* in the right atrium, such as the Eustachian valve in correspondence of the inferior or superior vena cava and the Chiari network. These structures appear as linear, mobile echoes with variable extension into the right atrium.

In the four-chamber view, the posterior leaflet (towards the free wall of the right ventricle) and the septal leaflet (towards the interatrial septum) of the tricuspid valve are visible. The tricuspid valve is located approximately 1 cm nearer the apex than the mitral valve. Displacement of the tricuspid valve towards the apex is characteristic of Ebstein's anomaly.

Finally the right ventricle is triangular in the four-chamber view, but in athletes its shape may be more spherical. The right ventricle is also involved in the remodeling process that is typical of the left ventricle in athletes, but the dimensions of the right ventricle are always less than those of the left.

Analysis of the right ventricle, especially its function and morphology, with special reference to dilatation, wall thinning and possible aneurysms, is of particular importance in athletes due to the possible diagnosis of arrhythmogenic dysplasia of the right ventricle, which is a cause of sudden death in athletes.

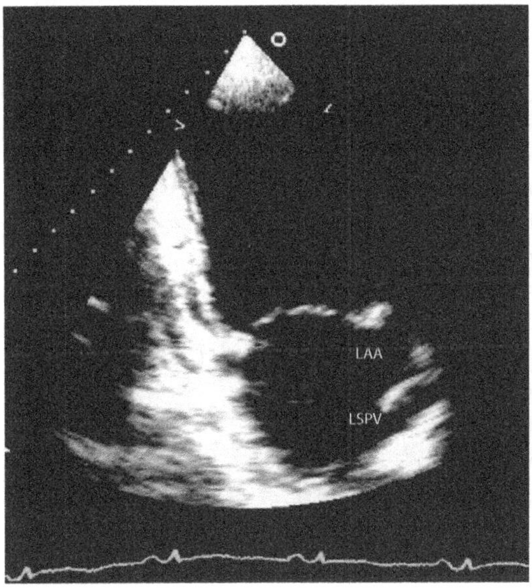

Fig. 3.15 Two-chamber apical view in which it is possible to see the anterior and inferior wall of the left ventricle. The left atrium and the left atrial appendage (*LAA*) are also visible. *LSPV* left superior pulmonary vein

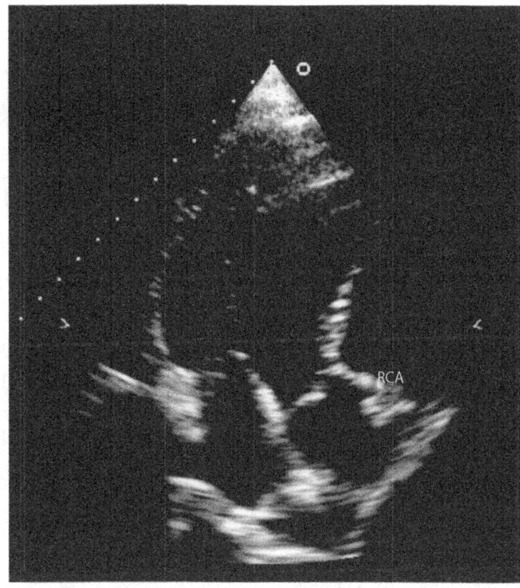

Fig. 3.16 Three-chamber apical view in which the posterolateral wall and the anterior septum of the left ventricle are visible. The first segment of the right coronary artery (*RCA*) can also be seen

Five-chamber Apical View

By angulating the transducer anteriorly from the four-chamber apical view, the five-chamber view, or four-chamber view with aorta, is achieved, in which it is possible also to see the left ventricular outflow tract, the aortic bulb, the right coronary cusp and the non-coronary cusp (Fig. 3.1).

Two-chamber Apical View

By rotating the transducer counter-clockwise by 60°, away from the four-chamber view, the two-chamber view is achieved, in which the left ventricle, the mitral valve and left atrium are visible. In particular, this view shows the anterior wall of the left ventricle (on the right of the monitor) and the inferior wall (on the left). Directing the transducer further back, it is possible to see both papillary muscles. The two-chamber view is used together with the four-chamber to measure the biplane ejection fraction. To accurately measure the volumes, the view must be optimized so that the papillary muscles are not visible. In some subjects it is also possible to see the left atrial appendage near the anterior wall of the left ventricle (Fig. 3.15).

Long-axis or Three-chamber View

By rotating the transducer another 60° from the two-chamber view, the long-axis apical view, or three-chamber view, is achieved, which is very similar to the long-axis parasternal view, enabling visualization of the left ventricle, the outflow tract, the aorta, the aortic bulb, the mitral valve and the left atrium. In particular, the anterior septum (on the right of the monitor) and the posterior wall (on the left of the monitor) can be seen using this view. The aortic cusps seen with this view are the right coronary cusp (facing the right heart) and the non-coronary cusp (facing the left atrium). Sometimes in this view it is possible to see the origin of the right coronary artery (Fig. 3.16).

3.2.2.3 Subcostal View

With the subject in the supine position and the legs bent (to relax the abdominal muscles), placing the transducer under the xiphoid appendix, the subcostal view is obtained, in which all four cardiac chambers are seen (Fig. 3.3b). In particular, the free wall of the right ventricle, the mid portion of the interventricular septum and the posterolateral wall of the left ventricle are seen. This view

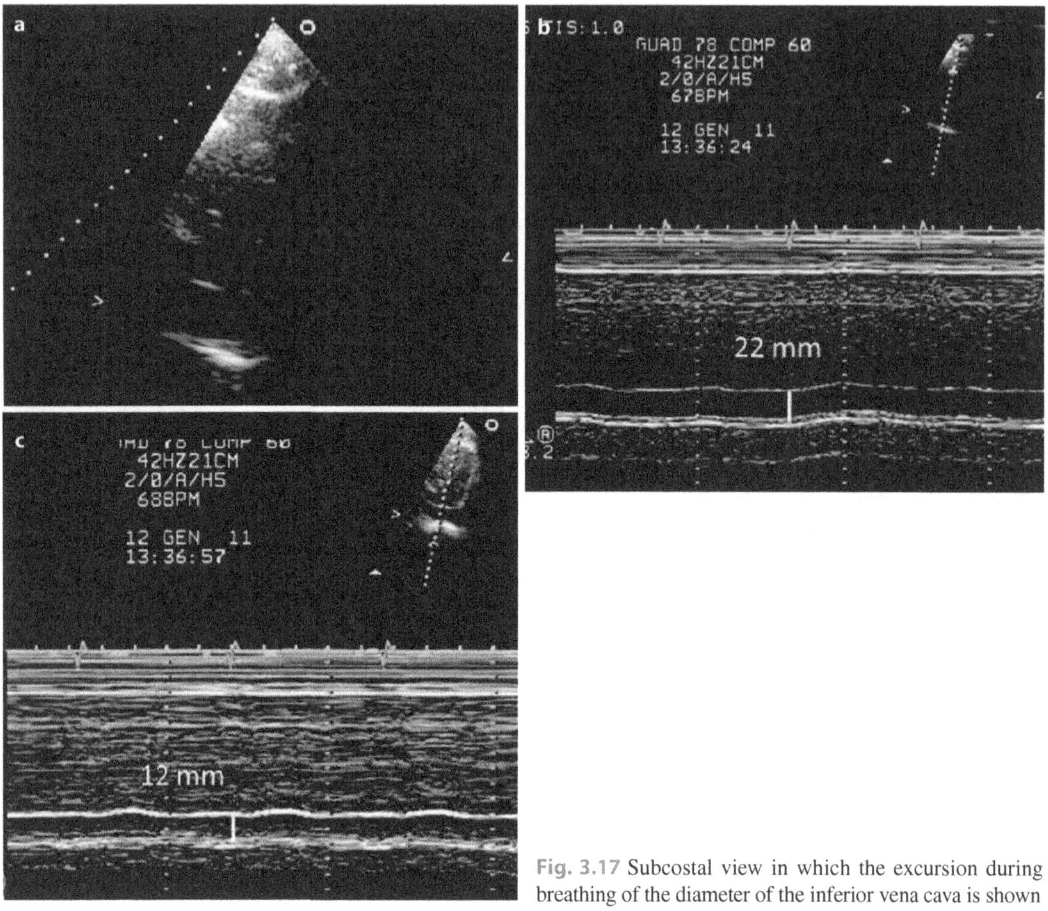

Fig. 3.17 Subcostal view in which the excursion during breathing of the diameter of the inferior vena cava is shown

is ideal for studying the interatrial septum because the septum is perpendicular to the ultrasound beam and can therefore be seen optimally, enabling interatrial defects to be ruled out.

By rotating the transducer down from the four-chamber subcostal view, a longitudinal view of the inferior vena cava is obtained where it enters the right atrium. In this view it is also possible to see the suprahepatic veins. Characteristically in athletes, both the vena cava and the suprahepatic veins may be larger.

Excursions of the inferior vena cava during breathing are useful to determine the pressure in the right atrium and therefore to estimate pulmonary pressure (Fig. 3.17).

3.2.2.4 Suprasternal View

With the subject in the supine position and the neck fully extended, the transducer is placed at the suprasternal notch in order to obtain a view of the aortic arch, both in long-axis and short-axis. In the long-axis view of the aortic arch (Fig. 3.4) the ascending aorta, the aortic arch, the first portion of the descending aorta, the origin of the right brachiocephalic artery, the left common carotid artery and left subclavian artery can be seen. Under the aortic arch, the right pulmonary artery is visible. Beneath the pulmonary artery is visualized the left atrium.

3.2.2.5 Quantitative Analysis of the Cardiac Chambers

Quantification of the Left Ventricle: Diameters, Thickness and Mass

Linear measurements of the thickness and internal dimensions of the left ventricle are obtained in the parasternal long-axis or short-axis views, in both 2D and M-mode (Fig. 3.18), following the leading-

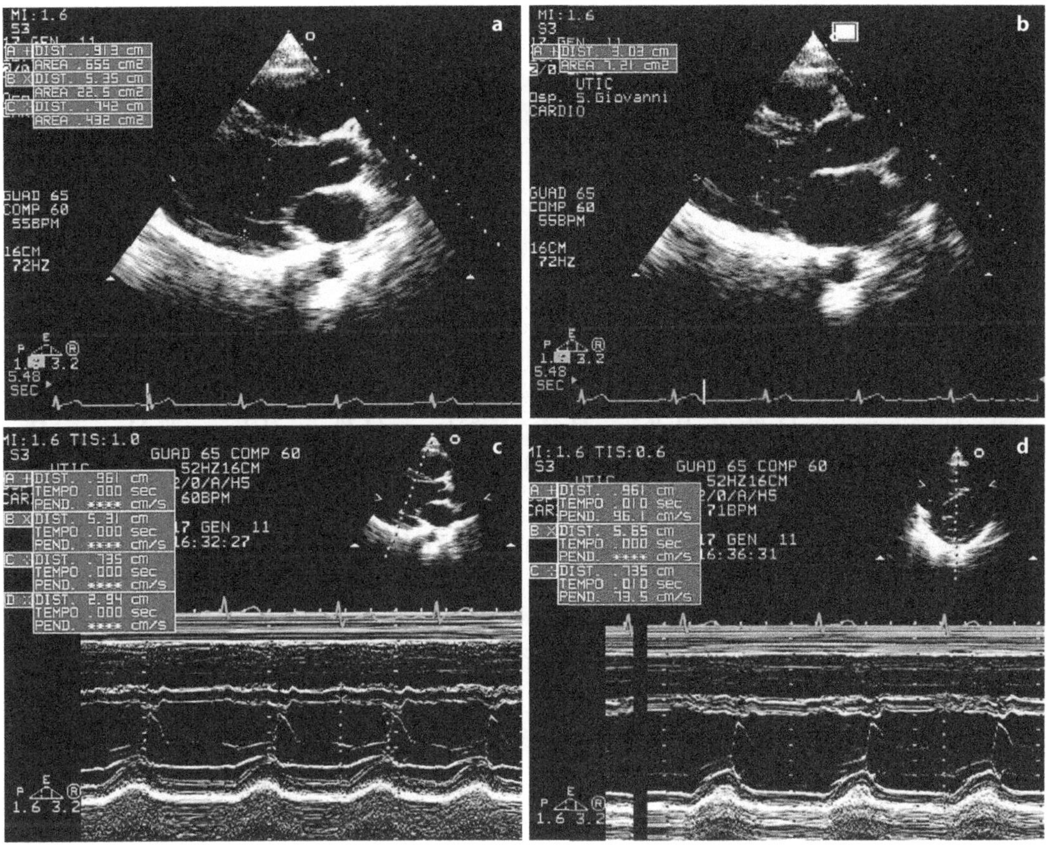

Fig. 3.18 Measurements of the dimensions of the left ventricle in 2D and M-mode imaging in the parasternal long-axis and short-axis views

edge-to-leading-edge rule of the structure in question, according with the recommendations of the American Society of Echocardiography [9,10]. In particular, the diameters must be measured at the shortest axis of the left ventricle, i.e. at the distal border of the mitral valve leaflets [11]. The diameters obtained using the short-axis in M-mode may be slightly larger than those obtained with 2D imaging. Measurements in diastole are made at the onset of the R wave on the ECG, while systolic measurements are taken at the maximum excursion of the endocardium of the posterior wall of the left ventricle (Fig. 3.18). Numerous studies have shown that linear measurements obtained from 2D and M-mode images are highly reproducible with low intra- and inter-operator variability [12].

Table 3.1 shows the normal reference values and corresponding dilatation levels for the left ventricle [11].

From the linear measurements, in 2D or M-mode, it is possible to obtain information on the mass of the left ventricle by applying geometric models.

To estimate left ventricular mass, the American Society of Echocardiography recommends the following formula, validated by necroscopic studies and considering the left ventricle as an ellipsoid:

$$\text{left ventricular mass} = 0.8 \cdot (1.04\,[(\text{LVIDd} + \text{PWTd} + \text{IVSTd})^3 - (\text{LVIDd})^3]) + 0.6\ \text{g}$$

where: LVIDd = left ventricular internal diameter in diastole, PWTd = posterior wall thickness in diastole, IVSTd = interventricular septum thickness in diastole [13]. This formula is indicated in particular for non-deformed ventricles.

Table 3.1 Reference values and levels of left ventricular hypertrophy [11]. The values in bold are recommended and better validated

	Women				Men			
Dilatation	Normal	Mild	Moderate	Severe	Normal	Mild	Moderate	Severe
Dimension								
D dia (cm)	3.9-5.3	5.4-5.7	5.8-6.1	≥6.2	4.2-5.9	6.0-6.3	6.4-6.8	≥6.9
D dia/BSA (cm/m^2)	2.4-3.2	3.3-3.4	3.5-3.7	≥3.8	2.2-3.1	3.2-3.4	3.5-3.6	≥3.7
D dia/h (cm/m)	2.5-2.2	3.3-3.4	3.5-3.6	≥3.7	2.4-3.3	3.4-3.5	3.6-3.7	≥3.8
Volumes								
Vol dia (ml)	56-104	105-117	118-130	≥131	67-155	156-178	179-201	≥202
Vol dia/BSA(ml/m^2)	**35-75**	**76-86**	**87-96**	**≥97**	**35-75**	**76-86**	**87-96**	**≥97**
Vol sist (ml)	18-49	50-59	60-69	≥70	22-58	59-70	71-82	≥83
Vol sist/BSA(ml/m^2)	**12-30**	**31-36**	**37-43**	**≥42**	**12-30**	**31-36**	**37-42**	**≥43**

BSA Body Surface Area, *D* diameter, *dia* diastolic, *h* height, *syst* systolic, *vol* volume.

Table 3.2 Reference values and levels of left ventricular dilatation [11]. The values in bold are recommended and better validated

	Women				Men			
Abnormality	Normal	Mild	Moderate	Severe	Normal	Mild	Moderate	Severe
Linear method								
Mass (g)	67-162	163-186	187-210	≥211	88-224	225-258	259-292	≥293
Mass/BSA (g/m^2)	43-95	96-108	109-121	≥122	49-115	116-131	132-148	≥149
Mass/h (g/m)	41-99	100-115	116-128	≥129	52-126	127-144	145-162	≥163
Mass/h (g/m)$^{2.7}$	18-44	45-51	52-58	≥59	20-48	49-55	56-63	≥64
RWT	0.22-0.42	0.43-0.47	0.48-0.52	≥0.53	0.24-0.42	0.43-0.46	0.47-0.51	≥0.52
IVS thickness (cm)	**0.6-0.9**	**1.0-1.2**	**1.3-1.5**	**≥1.6**	**0.6-1.0**	**1.0-1.3**	**1.4-1.6**	**≥1.7**
PW thickness (cm)	**0.6-0.9**	**1.0-1.2**	**1.3-1.5**	**≥1.6**	**0.6-1.0**	**1.0-1.3**	**1.4-1.6**	**≥1.7**
Volumes								
Mass (g)	66-150	151-171	172-182	≥183	96-200	201-227	228-254	≥255
Mass/BSA	**44-88**	**89-100**	**101-112**	**≥113**	**50-102**	**103-116**	**117-130**	**≥131**

BSA Body Surface Area, *h* height, *PW* posterior wall, *IVS* interventricular septum, *RWT* relative wall thickness.

The calculation of relative wall thickness (RWT) using the formula:

$$\text{RWT} = (2 \cdot \text{PWTd})/\text{LIVDd}$$

allows the categorization of the increase in left ventricular mass as concentric (RWT > 0.42) or eccentric (RWT ≤ 42) and allows concentric remodeling (normal mass with RWT > 0.42) to be identified [11] (Fig. 3.21). Two alternative methods used to evaluate left ventricular mass are based on the area-length formula and the geometric model of the truncated ellipsoid [9].

Both methods are based on the measure of the volume of the myocardium at the level of the papillary muscle, which is obtained by subtracting the volume of the left ventricular cavity from the total volume, included by the pericardium. Using mathematical formulae present into the ultrasound equipment it is possible to quantify left ventricular mass from the areas traced using 2D imaging. The epicardial area is obtained by tracing the epicardial border and that of the ventricular cavity along the border of the endocardium and leaving the papillary muscles outside the traced area. Therefore, for an accurate measurement of the

Table 3.3 Reference values and levels of left ventricular dysfunction [11]. The values in bold are recommended and better validated

	Women				Men			
Dysfunction	Normal	Mild	Moderate	Severe	Normal	Mild	Moderate	Severe
Linear method Fractional shortening %	27-45	22-26	17-21	≤16	25-43	20-24	15-19	≤14
2D method Ejection fraction %	**≥55**	**45-54**	**30-44**	**<30**	**≥55**	**45-54**	**30-44**	**<30**

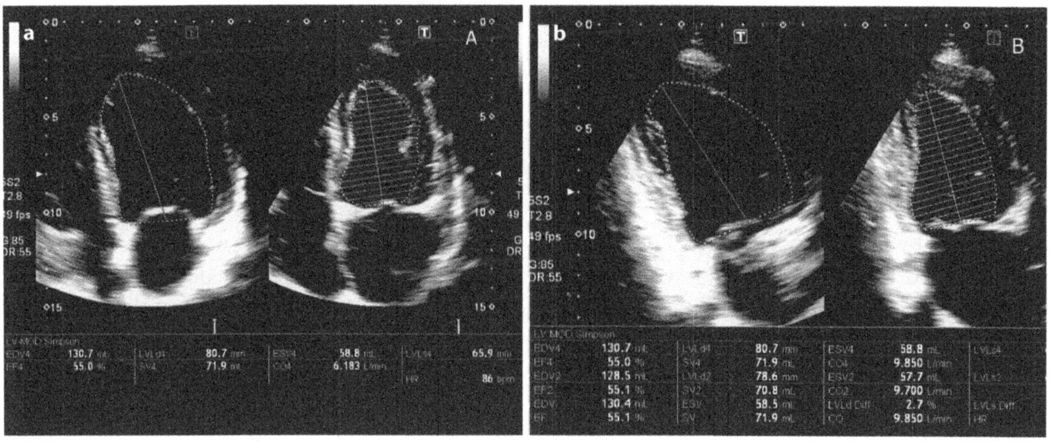

Fig. 3.19 Determination of the left ventricular ejection fraction using the biplane modified Simpson's rule

left ventricular mass, it is necessary to accurately identify the endocardium and the interface between the epicardium and pericardium.

Table 3.2 show the reference values and different levels of abnormality of the left ventricular mass.

Systolic Function of the Left Ventricle: Linear and Volumetric Measurements

The parameters of left ventricular systolic function that can be derived from 2D and M-mode linear measurements are the fractional shortening (FS) and the ejection fraction (EF), which is obtained using methods based on geometric assumptions.

FS is a fairly rough estimate of left ventricular systolic function (normal range: 25-45%) and is calculated as:

$$FS\ (\%) = [LVIDd - LVIDs)/\ LVIDd] \cdot 100$$

where LVIDd = left ventricular internal diameter in diastole, and LVIDs = left ventricular internal diameter in systole [10,14].

From the linear measurement it is possible to calculate diastolic and systolic ventricular volumes, using formulae based on geometric assumptions. The most common methods [10, 14] are the *Teichholz method*, according to which:

$$\text{ventricular volume} = [7.0/2.4 + LVID)] \cdot D^3$$

and the *Zile method*, according to which:

$$\text{diastolic volume (DV)} = 4.5\ (LVIDd)^2$$
$$\text{systolic volume (SV)} = 3.72\ (LVIDs)^2$$

From the ventricular volumes, the left ventricular EF can therefore be derived using the following formula:

$$FE\ (\%) = \frac{VD - VS}{VD} \cdot 100$$

The accuracy of these formulae in estimating left ventricular EF is greatly limited in ventricles undergone geometrical changes, such as patients with previous myocardial infarction. The method rec-

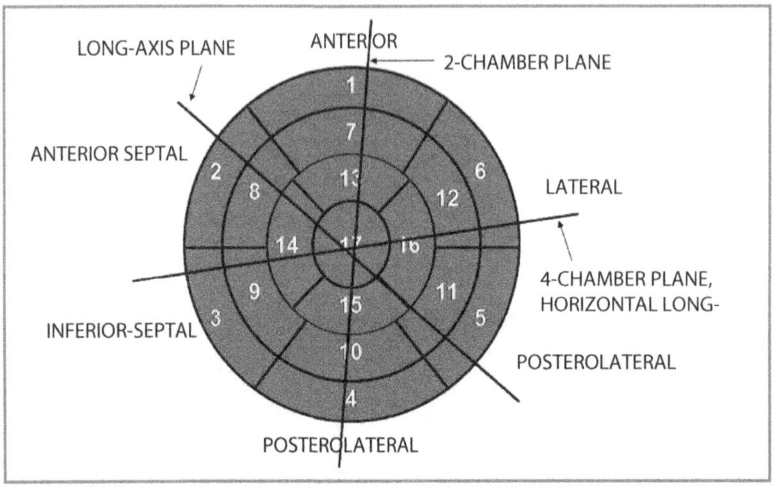

Fig. 3.20 Diagram showing the 17 segments of the left ventricle

ommended by the American Society of Echocardiography to measure ventricular volumes and therefore EF is based on the modified Simpson's biplane rule (Fig. 3.19). This method is based on the principle that the total left ventricular volume is calculated by the sum of a stack of elliptical discs. The height of each disc is calculated as a fraction (usually 1/20) of the long-axis of the left ventricle defined as the longer of the two axes measured in two- or four-chambers. The area of each individual disc is obtained using the two diameters in two- and four-chamber views.

When it is not possible to obtain two orthogonal projections, a monoplane measurement can be used, assuming that the disc is circular. However, monoplane measurement may be inaccurate if large regional kinesis abnormalities are present [9-11, 14]. Table 3.3 shows the normal reference values and corresponding levels of systolic dysfunction of the left ventricle [11]. From the ventricular volumes obtained using the modified Simpson's rule, hemodynamic data such as stroke volume, cardiac output and the cardiac index can be obtained using the following formulae:

- *stroke volume* (SV), ml: diastolic volume – systolic volume;
- *cardiac output* (CO), l/min: SV · heart rate;
- *cardiac index*, l/min/ m^2: CO/body surface area.

Regional Systolic Function of the Left Ventricle

The analysis of the systolic function is usually made by dividing the left ventricle into sixteen segments according to the model recommended by the American Society of Echocardiography [9-11], which states that the left ventricle is divided into six basal segments (anterior septum, inferior septum, inferior, posterolateral, lateral, anterior), six mid-ventricular segments (anterior septum, inferior septum, inferior, posterolateral, lateral, anterior) and four apical segments (septum, lateral, inferior, anterior).

Division of the left ventricle into sixteen segments is a convention that is used exclusively in echocardiography, while other cardiac imaging methods such as magnetic resonance or nuclear imaging use models with more segments, especially for the study of myocardial perfusion. In 2002 in an attempt to standardise segmentation of the left ventricle among the various imaging methods, the American Segmentation Writing Group on Myocardial Segmentation and Registration for Cardiac Imaging proposed a seventeen-segment model (Fig. 3.20), which also includes an apical segment: the apical cap, which is located outside the ventricular cavity and has not endocardium [15]. This seventeen-segment model must be used in studies of myocardial perfusion with contrast echocardiography, while for assessment of left ventricular contraction the traditional sixteen-segment model is indicated, since the seventeenth segment does not contract.

Although there is a large degree of variability in the distribution of the coronary arteries, in the

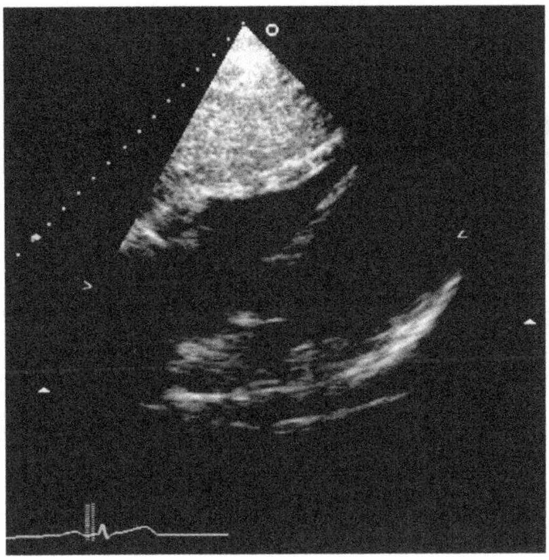

Fig. 3.21 Subcostal view in which the thickness of the free wall of the right ventricle is measured (*measurement in yellow*)

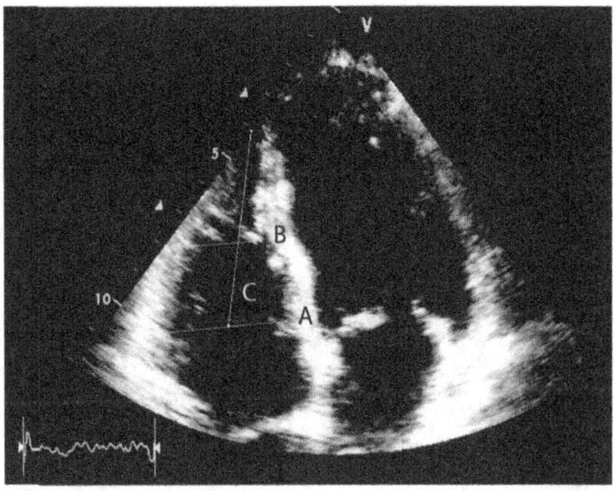

Fig. 3.22 Four-chamber apical view in which are measured the diameter of the right ventricle at the base (*A*) and at level of the moderator band (*B*) and the longitudinal diameter (*C*)

majority of cases the anterior wall, the anterior septum and the apex of the left ventricle are supplied by the left anterior descending artery. The lateral segment of the apex can sometimes be supplied by the circumflex artery, while the mid-ventricular segment of the inferior septum can be supplied by the left anterior descending or the right coronary artery. The basal and mid-ventricular segments of the inferior wall are generally supplied by the right coronary artery, which also supplies the basal segment of the inferior interventricular septum. Finally, the basal and mid-ventricular segments of the lateral wall are supplied by the circumflex artery, while the basal and mid-ventricular posterolateral segments may be supplied by the right coronary or circumflex artery [9-11]. Regional contractile function of the left ventricle is traditionally evaluated with semiquantitative methods by assessing the movement and especially the thickening of each individual segment and determining a score, with points attributed for each ventricular segment. The recommended score for evaluating regional kinesis of the left ventricle uses the following point system [9-11]:

- 1 = normal or hypercontractile;
- 2 = hypokinesia;
- 3 = akinesia;
- 4 = dyskinesia;
- 5 = aneurysm.

By dividing the total number of points for all segments by the number of segments analysed, the wall motion score index is obtained. An essential prerequisite for accurate definition of this value is the optimal visualization of the endocardium, which makes it possible to see the thickening of the segment adequately and to distinguish tethering by normocontractile and hypercontractile segments.

The recent introduction of *tissue Doppler, strain, strain rate* and *speckle tracking* imaging methods makes it possible to carry out quantitative evaluation of the regional contractile function of the left ventricle. However, the wide range of methods used and the lack of standardization makes the use of such methods in clinical daily practice still far.

3.2.2.6 Quantification of the Right Ventricle and the Right Outflow Tract

The right ventricle has a fairly complex geometry, since it develops around the left ventricle, almost enveloping it. The right ventricular inflow tract is located medially in relation to the left ventricle, the body and apex in front and the outflow tract above the left ventricle. It is therefore impossible to see the whole of the right ventricle in a single view and multiple echocardiographic views need to be combined to obtain an accurate evaluation of its shape and function. The thickness of the free wall of the

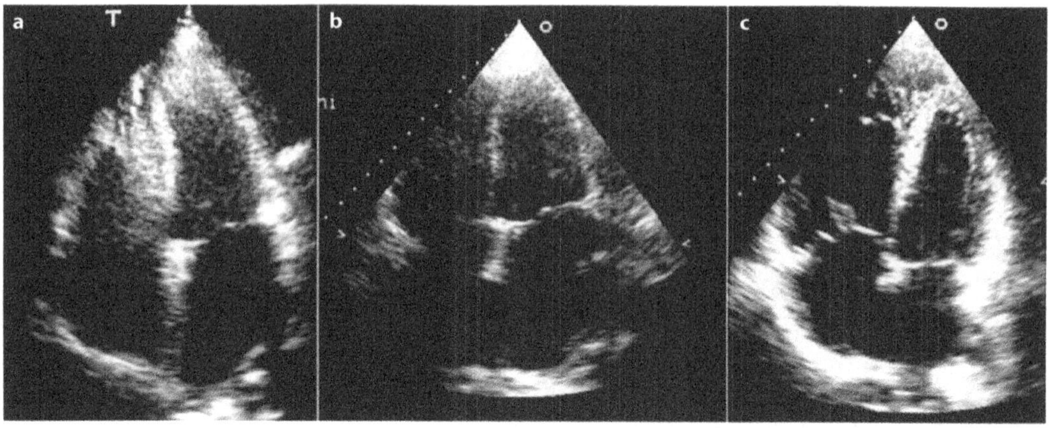

Fig. 3.23 Four-chamber apical view showing a left ventricle with normal dimensions (a), moderately dilated (b) and severely dilated (c)

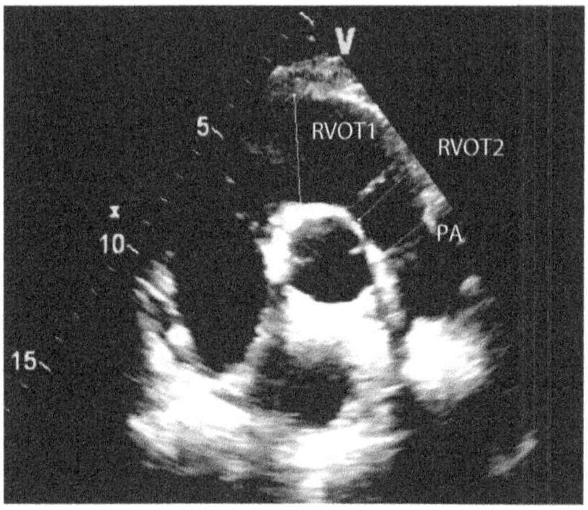

Fig. 3.24 Parasternal short-axis view for measurement of the right ventricular outflow tract (*RVOT1* and *RVOT2*) and the diameter of the pulmonary artery (*PA*)

right ventricle (in M-mode and 2D) can accurately be measured from the subcostal window and is normally < 5 mm [16] (Fig. 3.21). Caution is required so that possible trabeculae and/or pericardial fat deposits are not included in the measurement. The dimensions of the right ventricle are assessed qualitatively using the four-chamber apical view in which it can be seen that in normal conditions the right ventricle is smaller than the left ventricle. If the right ventricle is dilated, its area either equals (moderate dilatation) or exceeds that of the left ventricle, enveloping the apex (severe dilatation) (Fig. 3.23). Quantitative evaluation is carried out by measuring, from the four-chamber apical view, the transverse diameter at the level of the basal and mid-segment of the right ventricle free wall as well as the longitudinal diameter (Fig. 3.22). The normal values and relative dilatation levels are reported in Table 3.4 [11, 17]. A complete investigation of the right ventricle must include measurement of the outflow tract, which extends from the anterosuperior section of the right ventricle to the pulmonary artery. The right outflow tract can be adequately seen in the parasternal short-axis view at the base of the heart, and in this view its dimensions must be measured above the aorta and above the pulmonary valve (Fig. 3.24, Table 3.4). Analysis and measurement of the right ventricular outflow tract is of particular importance in athletes since it is one of the echocardiographic criteria that are useful in the diagnosis of arrhythmogenic right ventricular dysplasia together with global and regional dilatation and dysfunction of the right ventricle [18].

Table 3.4 Reference values, dilatation levels and dysfunction of right ventricle (RV) and the right ventricular outflow tract (RVOT) [11, 17]

	Dilatation			
	Normal	Mild	Moderate	Severe
RV dimensions				
Basal (cm)	2.0-2.8	2.9-3.3	3.4-3.8	≥ 3.9
Mid-ventricular (cm)	2.7-3.3	3.4-3.7	3.8-4.1	≥ 4.2
Longitudinal (cm)	7.1-7.9	8.0-8.5	8.6-9.1	≥ 9.2
RVOT dimensions				
Above aortic valve (RVOT1) (cm)	2.5-2.9	3.0-3.2	3.3-3.5	≥ 3.6
Above pulmonary valve (RVOT2) (cm)	1.7-2.3	2.4-2.7	2.8-3.1	≥ 3.2
Pulmonary artery diameter (cm)	1.5-2.1	2.2-2.5	2.6-2.9	≥ 3.0
	Dysfunction			
	Normal	Mild	Moderate	Severe
Fractional area change (5)	32-60	25-31	18-24	≤ 17

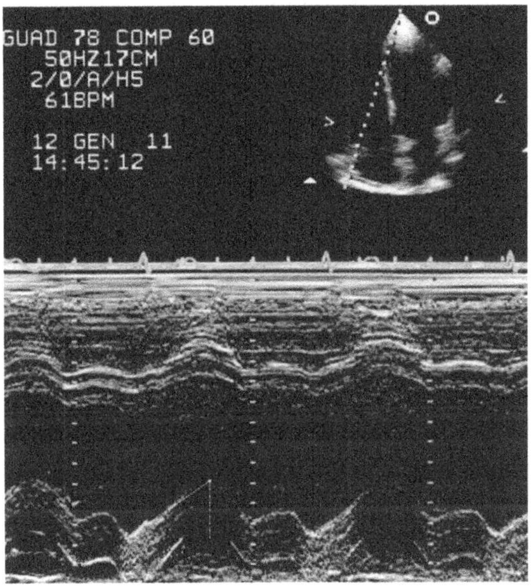

Fig. 3.25 M-mode scan of the free wall of the right ventricle allowing the TAPSE to be seen and measured

Due to the complex geometry of the right ventricle, there are no geometric models for approximating its shape and enabling standardized quantification of its volumes and function, as occurs for the left ventricle. A very simple parameter that allows the evaluation of the right ventricular function is the TAPSE (Tricuspid Annular Plane Systolic Excursion), which is obtained with an M-mode scan of the tricuspid annulus. In systole, the excursion of the tricuspid annulus towards the apex of the right ventricle is 15-20 mm. TAPSE >15 mm indicates normal longitudinal shortening of the right ventricle [11] (Fig. 3.25).

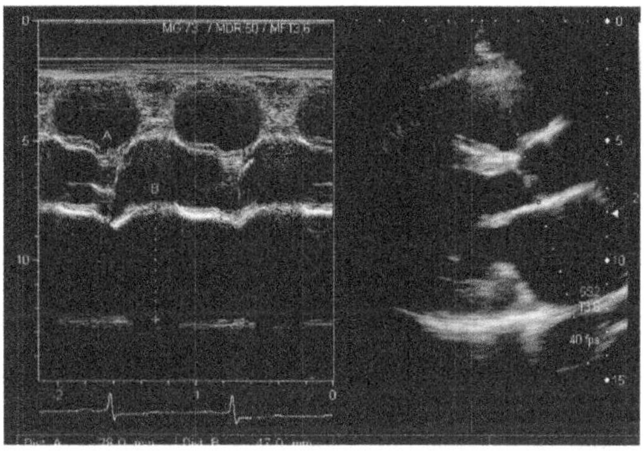
Fig. 3.26 M-mode image in the parasternal long-axis view for measurement of the aortic bulb and the anteroposterior diameter of the left atrium

Another functional parameter is the fractional area change (FAC) of the right ventricle, which is calculated in the four-chamber apical view using this formula:

$$FAC = \frac{(RVEDA - RVESA)}{RVEDA}\%$$

where RVEDA = right ventricular end-diastolic area, RVESA = right ventricular end-systolic area. This parameter correlates well with the EF measured by ventriculography and nuclear magnetic resonance [19].

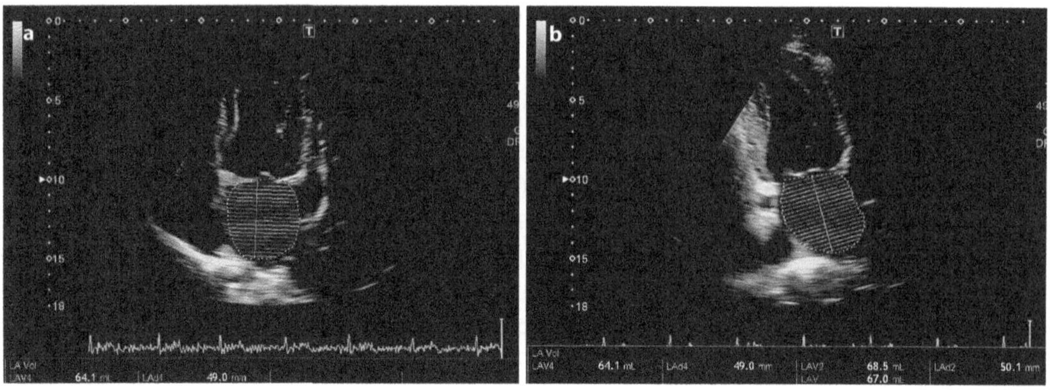

Fig. 3.27 Four-chamber and two-chamber view in which the volume of the left atrium is measured

3.2.2.7 Quantification of the Left and Right Atrium

The left atrium can be seen in multiple echocardiographic views. The long-axis parasternal window enables measurement of the anteroposterior diameter, using both 2D and M-mode images. In the M-mode images, it is a convention to measure the distance between the leading edge of the aortic wall and the leading edge of the posterior wall of the left atrium (Fig. 3.26). Even if this linear measurement is validated with angiographic correlations and is widely used in clinical practice and research, it is in fact a fairly inaccurate representation of the real dimensions of the left atrium, since it is based on the presupposition that all axes of the atrium change all together as the atrium expands, which is often not the truth. It is therefore necessary to measure the volume of the left atrium that allows better quantification of asymmetrical remodeling. The preferable methods for measuring left atrial volume are the area-length method and the Simpson's biplane rule [11]. The normal value for left atrial volume obtained using these methods is equal to 22 ± 6 ml/m^2, as it has been reported in several studies with hundreds of subjects [11]. Some tricks are necessary in order to be measure accurately the left atrial volume:

1. the left atrium must be seen in its total extent, and the top must not be cut off from the image;
2. when tracing the outline of the atrium it is necessary to exclude the pulmonary veins and the left atrial appendage;
3. the lower border must be represented by the annular plane of the mitral valve (Fig. 3.27).

Measurement of the right atrium is less standardized than for the left atrium, as there are few studies that have evaluated the dimensions and volume. From these studies it can be deduced that right atrial volume is similar to that of the left in men (21 ml/m^2) and slightly smaller in women [11].

3.3 Doppler and Color-Doppler Echocardiography

Doppler-echocardiography uses the Doppler effect, which is the change in the frequency of the ultrasound beam when the intercepted object moves towards or away from the transducer. The Doppler effect is described using the following equation:

$$\Delta f = 2 f_t v \cos\theta / c$$

where: Δf = change in Doppler frequency; f_t = transmitted frequency; $\cos\theta$ = cosine of the θ angle between the vector of the moving object and the ultrasound beam; c = constant of the velocity of sound in tissues or blood (1560 m/s); v = velocity of the moving object. From the Doppler effect formula, the velocity of blood can be derived as follows:

$$v, \text{m/s} = \Delta f\, c / 2 f_t \cos\theta$$

A considerable amount of information can be derived based on the blood velocity, such as gradi-

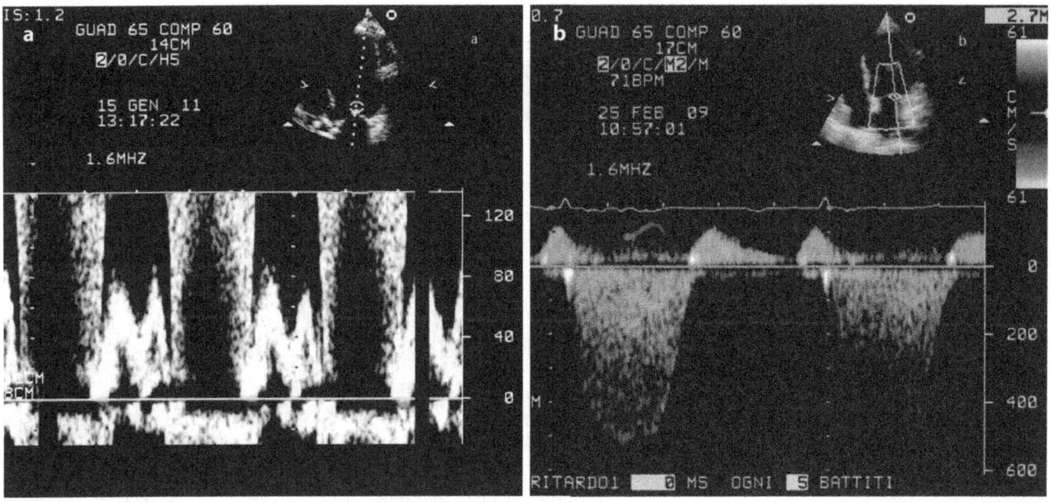

Fig. 3.28 Recording with pulsed-wave Doppler (a) and continuous-wave Doppler (b) of the flow in the presence of mitral valve regurgitation. In the pulsed-wave Doppler recording the aliasing phenomenon can be see, i.e. the regurgitation flow is recorded approaching (above the zero line) instead of moving away from the probe

ents at the level of the cardiac valves, intracardiac pressure, valvular flow and areas.

Pulsed- and continuous-wave Doppler are the two most common forms of spectral Doppler. The flows towards the transducer are usually recorded above the zero line, while flows away from the transducer are recorded below the zero line. Pulsed-wave Doppler enables measurement of blood velocity at the specific point in which the sample volume is positioned. There is, however, a maximum velocity limit (Nyquist limit) beyond which pulsed-wave Doppler recordings cannot be taken, since the aliasing phenomenon occurs, so that the flow appears reversed (Fig. 3.28a).

Pulsed-wave Doppler cannot therefore be used to study the very high velocities that are observed, for example, with aortic stenosis or severe mitral regurgitation. Continuous-wave Doppler, on the other hand, records all velocities along the path of the ultrasound beam, but the velocities of specific sites cannot be distinguished; however, it is not limited by the aliasing phenomenon and therefore makes it possible to record even very high velocities (Fig. 3.28b). Continuous-wave Doppler is therefore used regularly to measure high velocities and transvalvular and intracardiac gradients (ΔP).

Color-Doppler is an evolution of pulsed-wave Doppler, in which more sample volumes are used at the same time, enabling flows to be seen with a color code that usually defines flow towards the transducer in red and flow away from it in blue. Color-Doppler is now an integral part of the echocardiographic examination and enables visualization and semiquantitative quantification of pathological flows such as valve regurgitation, intracardiac shunts or obstructions (Fig. 3.29).

3.3.1 Normal Intracardiac Flows

Normal intracardiac flows can be recorded with either pulsed- or continuous-wave Doppler. To obtain accurate measurements, optimal (parallel) alignment of the ultrasound beam along the evaluated flow is essential.

3.3.1.1 Left Ventricular Outflow

The five-chamber or three-chamber apical view enable parallel alignment of the ultrasound beam with the flow in the left ventricular outflow tract.

By positioning the sample volume of the pulsed-wave Doppler under the aortic valve, in the left ventricular outflow tract, an ejection curve is

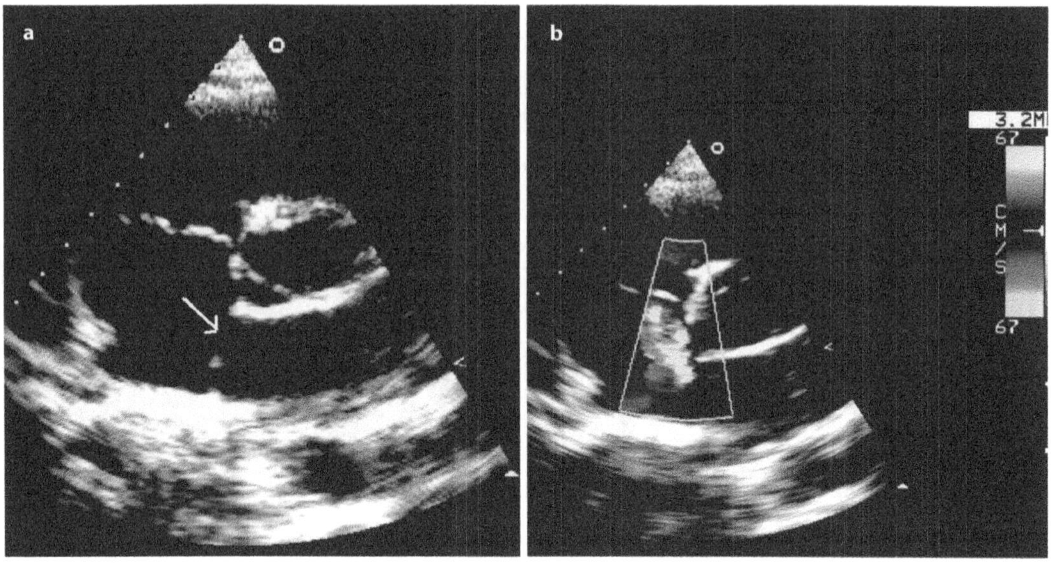

Fig. 3.29 Parasternal short-axis view at the base of the heart. a 2D imaging shows an ostium secundum interatrial septum defect. b The color-Doppler shows a left-to-right shunt

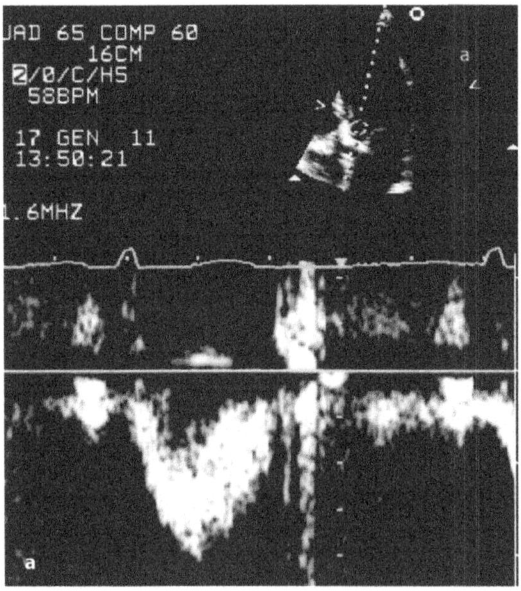

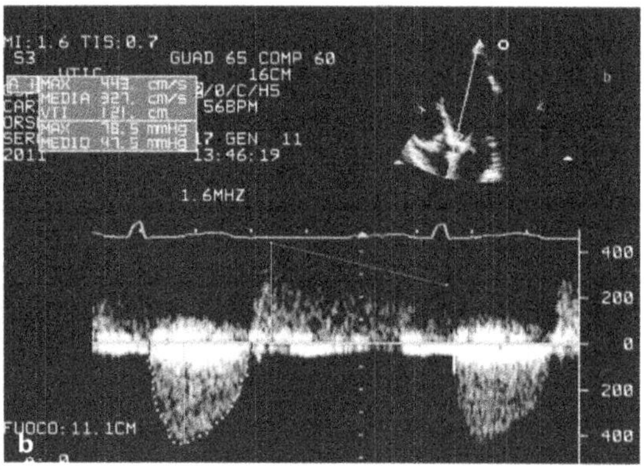

Fig. 3.30 Recording of flow in the left ventricular outflow tract with pulsed Doppler (a) and in the aorta with continuous-wave Doppler in a subject with aortic stenosis (b)

obtained that is characterized by an early velocity peak (Fig. 3.30a) and an area under the curve with no signal, the latter being due to uniform velocity where the sample volume is located. Conversely, by positioning the continuous- wave Doppler along the outflow tract, a complete curve is obtained, in which velocities along the outflow tract and across the aortic valve are recorded (Fig. 3.30b). Maximum velocity across a normal aortic valve is 1-1.2 m/s, while in the outflow tract it is 0.8-1 m/s.

3.3.1.2 Right Ventricular Outflow

The outflow tract of the right ventricle and the pulmonary artery can be studied using the parasternal short-axis view at the base of the heart or the subcostal view modified so that the right ventricular

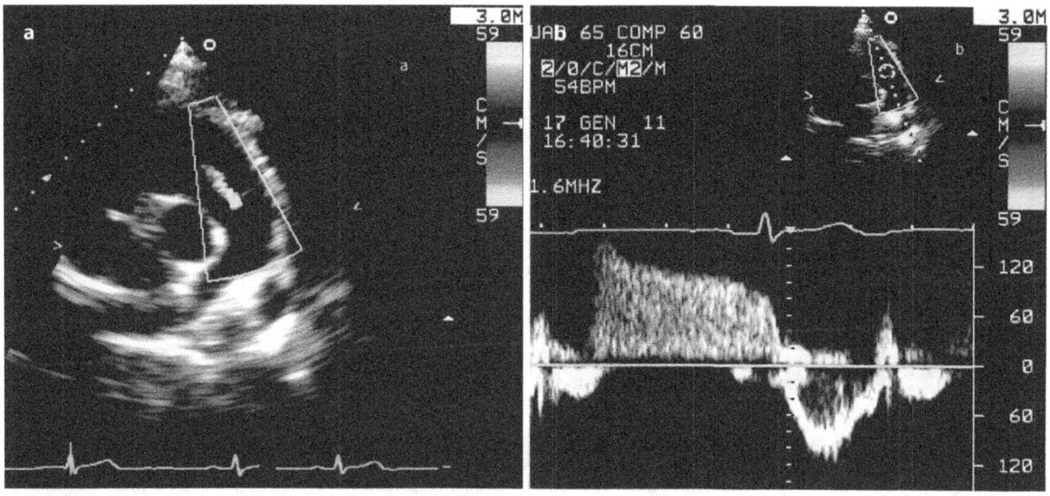

Fig. 3.31 Short-axis view at the base of the heart in which with color-Doppler it is possible to see a slight pulmonary regurgitation jet (a). Descending diastolic velocities are recorded with pulsed Doppler (b)

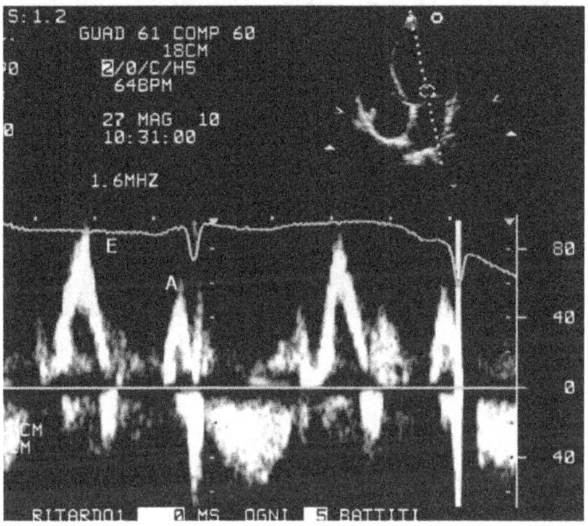

Fig. 3.32 Transmitral flow through the mitral valve. The E/A ratio is equal to 1.8

outflow tract can be seen. Pulsed-wave Doppler located under the pulmonary valve enables visualization of a curve similar to that of the left outflow tract but with a peak velocity that is lower (0.8-1 m/s) and occurs later (mid-systole) (Fig. 3.31). Pulmonary valve regurgitation can be seen in up to 80-100% of athletes. With color-Doppler it is represented as a red flow towards the transducer. With pulsed-wave Doppler, decreasing diastolic velocities are recorded. This regurgitation has no pathological significance.

3.3.1.3 Left Ventricular Inflow

Pulsed-wave Doppler analysis of the transmitral flow makes it possible to evaluate left ventricular filling. Correct sampling of the flow is obtained by positioning the sample volume at the tip of the mitral valve leaflets. The waves described are the E wave, which represents the passive rapid filling phase of the left ventricle, followed by a more or less long phase with no flow, which represents the diastasis, and finally the A wave that represents the late filling of the ventricle, due to atrial contraction (Fig. 3.32). In healthy young subjects, E wave velocity is approximately 1 m/s and A wave velocity is 0.2-0.4 m/s. In older subjects, physiological deterioration of left ventricular filling occurs and is reflected in the gradual reduction of the E wave, prolongation of the deceleration time (DT) of the E wave and accentuation of the A wave, with re-

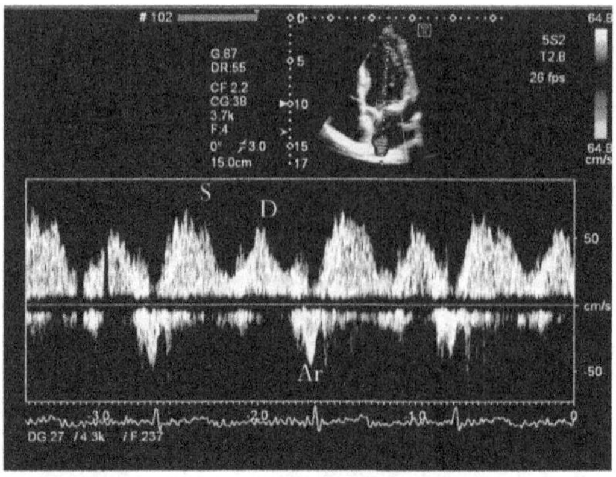

Fig. 3.33 Pulsed Doppler recording the flow in the right superior pulmonary vein

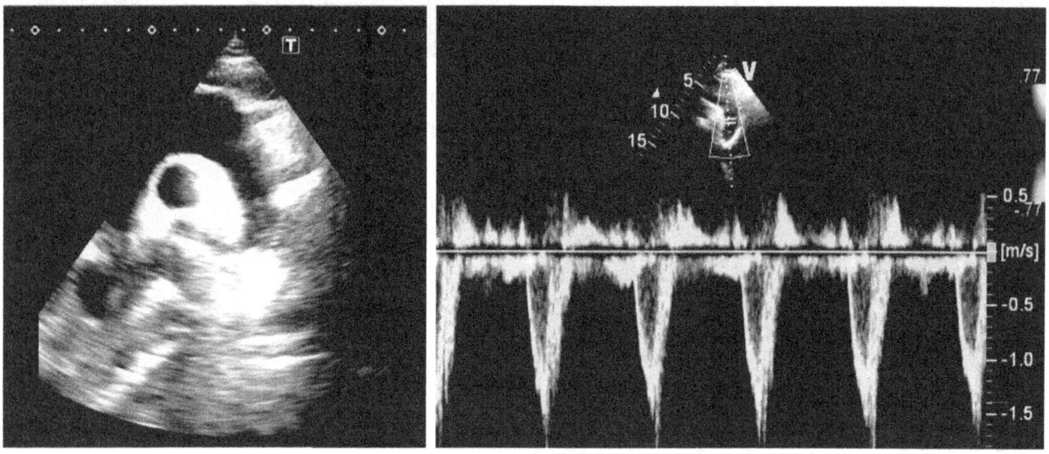

Fig. 3.34 Pulse Doppler recording of flow in the descending aorta

sulting inversion of the E/A ratio that is >1 in young subjects, about 1 in those aged 50-60, and <1 in healthy elderly subjects. In addition to age, the left ventricular filling pattern in healthy individuals is also affected by the preload conditions, heart rate and the PR interval. In athletes, and particularly endurance athletes, frequently it is possible to see a picture of *supernormal* filling of the left ventricle (Fig. 3.32), in which the E wave of early filling is very high , the DT of the E wave is much shorter, and the A wave of atrial filling is very low (due to the minimum contribution of the atrium in ventricular filling, since filling occurs almost exclusively in the early phase).

3.3.1.4 Right Ventricular Inflow

Right ventricular inflow can be measured from the four-chamber apical and the parasternal for the right ventricle views, by placing the pulsed-Doppler sample volume on the tricuspid valve. The aspect is very similar to the transmitral flow, even if the velocities are generally lower. In athletes it is also common to observe mild tricuspid regurgitation (in up to 60-70% of cases), which has no pathological significance. With the color-Doppler a blue flow is observed through the tricuspid valve moving away from the transducer.

3.3.1.5 Pulmonary Venous Flow

Pulmonary venous flow that reflects left atrial filling can be studied by sampling the flow in the right superior pulmonary vein, that is visualized, in the four-chamber apical view, in the point where it enters in the left atrium, next to the interatrial septum. By positioning the sample volume about 1 cm within the vein, the following waves are

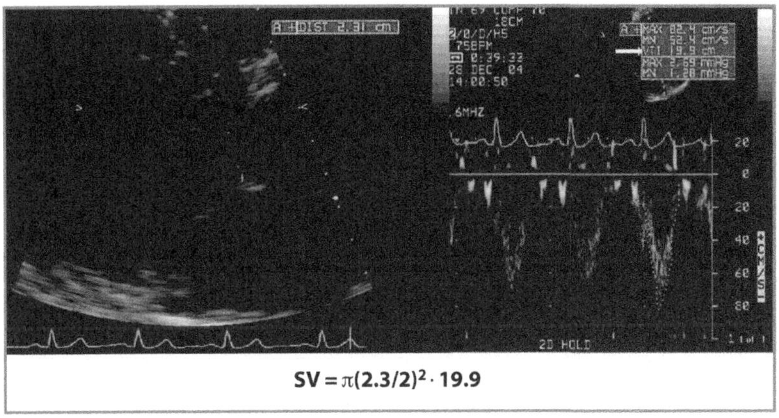

Fig. 3.35 Doppler determination of stroke volume (SV) of the left ventricle. The area of the outflow tract (Alvot) can be calculated using the formula Alvot = $\pi \cdot (d/2)^2$, where d is the diameter of the left ventricular outflow tract. Alvot thus derived is multiplied by the velocity-time integral (VTI) of flow in the outflow tract

seen: the S wave of systolic flow, the diastolic D wave, and the retrograde A wave (Ar), with flow inverted compared with S and D waves, which represents retrograde flow during atrial systole (Fig. 3.33). In athletes it is often possible to see a double component of the S wave, namely S1, which represents atrial relaxation, and S2, which accompanies movement towards the apex of the mitral annulus in systole. The Ar wave is usually rather small in athletes due to poor atrial contribution to left ventricular filling. Dilatation of the left atrium in athletes enables good visualization of two or three pulmonary veins entering the left atrium.

3.3.1.6 Flow in the Descending Aorta

The flow in the descending aorta can be recorded from the suprasternal window by placing the sample volume of pulsed-Doppler in the first portion of the descending aorta, immediately after the origin of the subclavian artery. In normal subjects a systolic anterograde flow is recorded with a maximum velocity of approximately 1 m/s as well as a short proto-diastolic retrograde flow (Fig. 3.34). A similar pattern is also obtained from the subcostal window in the first segment of the abdominal aorta.

3.3.2 Doppler Quantification of Left Ventricular Systolic and Diastolic Function

3.3.2.1 Left Ventricular Systolic Function

Pulsed-Doppler analysis of the flow in the left ventricular outflow tract allows the calculation of left ventricular stroke volume (SV) and therefore cardiac output (SV x heart rate).

SV is obtained by multiplying the area of the left ventricular outflow tract (Alvot) by the velocity-time integral (VTI) of flow in the outflow tract, i.e. by the distance travelled by the blood in each cardiac cycle in centimetres (Fig. 3.35):

$$\text{SV (ml)} = \text{Alvot} \cdot \text{VTI}$$

Alvot, assuming a circular geometry, can be calculated with the following formula:

$$\text{Alvot} = \pi \cdot (d/2)^2$$

where d is the diameter of the left ventricular outflow tract. This measurement of the SV closely relies on the accurate measurement of the left ventricular outflow tract. In fact, since d is squared, small errors in measuring the diameter of the left ventricular outflow tract are amplified when calculating the area.

The diameter of the left ventricular outflow tract must be measured in the long-axis parasternal view, immediately under the aortic valve, in mid-systole, from the septal endocardium to the border of the anterior mitral valve leaflet.

3.3.2.2 Left Ventricular Diastolic Function

Analysis of left ventricular diastolic function involves a combination of multiple Doppler and Tissue Doppler Imaging (see later) parameters.

The first step in assessing diastolic function is the analysis of transmitral flow, which is obtained

Table 3.5 Levels of left ventricular diastolic dysfunction

	Normal	Mild dysfunction (level I)	Moderate dysfunction (level II)	Severe dysfunction (level III)
Transmitral pattern	0.75 > E/A < 1.5 DT > 140 ms	E/A ≤ 0.75	0.75 > E/A < 1.5 DT > 140 ms	E/A > 1.5 DT < 140
E/A ratio during Valsalva manoeuvre	ΔE/A ≤ 0.5	ΔE/A ≤ 0.5	ΔE/A ≥ 0.5	ΔE/A ≥ 0.5
S/D ratio for pulmonary veins	S ≥ D	S > D	S < D	S < D
ARdur-Adur for pulmonary veins	< 0 ms	< 0 ms	> 30 ms	> 30 ms
E/E' ratio	< 8	< 8	≥ 10	≥ 10

Adur duration of mitral A wave, *ARdur* duration of retrograde A wave, *DT* deceleration time [20].

by placing the pulsed-Doppler sample volume at the tip of the mitral leaflet. Normally in subjects aged < 60 years, the E/A ratio is >1. The earliest change in diastolic function is the impaired relaxation (grade I), which is expressed by DT prolongation, reduced E wave velocity, and increased A wave velocity, resulting in an inverted E/A ratio (<1). With the progression of diastolic dysfunction and the increase in left ventricular end-diastolic pressure, there is a renewed tendency for early acceleration of filling that leads to *pseudo-normalization* of the E/A ratio to >1 (grade II). In the severe (grade III) diastolic dysfunction with a severe reduction in left ventricular compliance and a severe increase in filling pressure, there is a restrictive pattern with very early filling of the left ventricle, extreme reduction in DT, and a near absence of late atrial filling, so that the E/A ratio becomes ≥1.5.

The second step when investigating diastolic function is to study the pulmonary veins. In normal subjects, the S and D waves are almost equal. If there is mild diastolic dysfunction, the D wave is reduced. As dysfunction progresses, the S wave become smaller, with an S/D ratio of < 1 and an increase in the velocity and duration of the Ar wave. The third step is a TDI study of the mitral annulus and the definition of the E/E' ratio, i.e. the ratio between the velocity of the mitral valve E wave and the velocity of the mitral annulus E' wave in TDI. This ratio correlates with invasive left ventricular end-diastolic pressure and an E/E' value of ≥10 is a sign of increased invasive left ventricular filling pressure [20]. In athletes the supernormal transmitral pattern can sometimes imitate level II or III of diastolic dysfunction, but integration of a pulmonary vein investigation and an E/E' ratio enables the normal picture for an athlete to be distinguished from moderate and severe levels of diastolic dysfunction. Additionally diastolic dysfunction is usually associated with structural and functional changes to the left ventricle that are generally absent in healthy athletes. Table 3.5 shows a schematic representation of the changes in mitral flow, pulmonary veins and mitral annulus TDI patterns as diastolic dysfunction progresses [20].

3.3.3 Doppler Evaluation of Cardiac Valves

Doppler-echocardiography allows the quantification of the pressure gradient (maximum and mean) across cardiac valves, and the calculation of valvular areas and regurgitant volumes. The principle applied when measuring transvalvular and intracardiac gradients is the modified Bernoulli equation, according to which the gradient across a stenosis or between two cardiac chambers can be calculated as:

$$\Delta P = 4(V2^2 - V1^2)$$

where V1 is the proximal velocity, V2 is the velocity across the orifice or between two chambers. However, since V1 is normally much lower than V2, V1 can be omitted and therefore $\Delta P = 4V^2$ [10,14].

3.3.3.1 Determination of dP/dt

When mitral regurgitation occurs, the curve of continuous-wave Doppler representing mitral regurgitation can be used to determine dP/dt

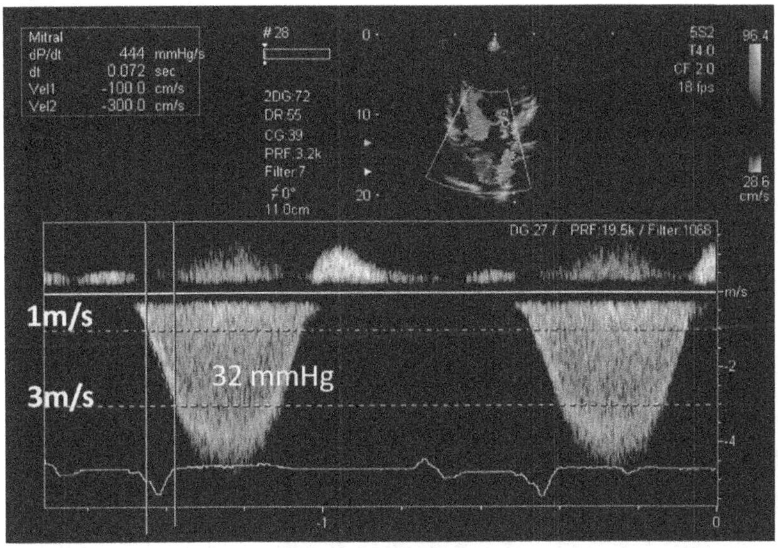

Fig. 3.36 Determination of the dP/dt ratio

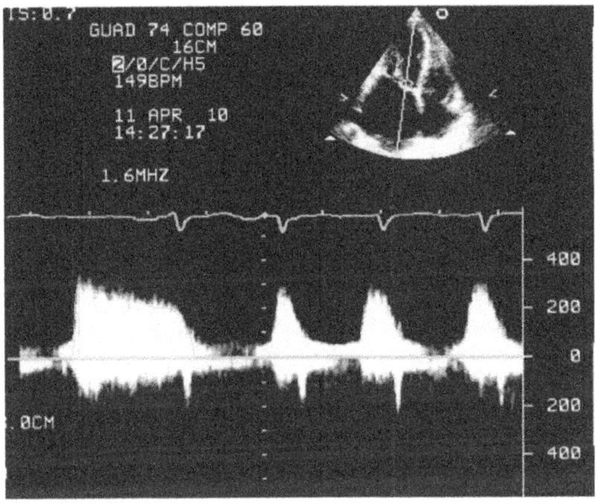

Fig. 3.37 Measurement of the gradient through a mitral stenosis (maximum 38 mmHg, mean 21 mmHg)

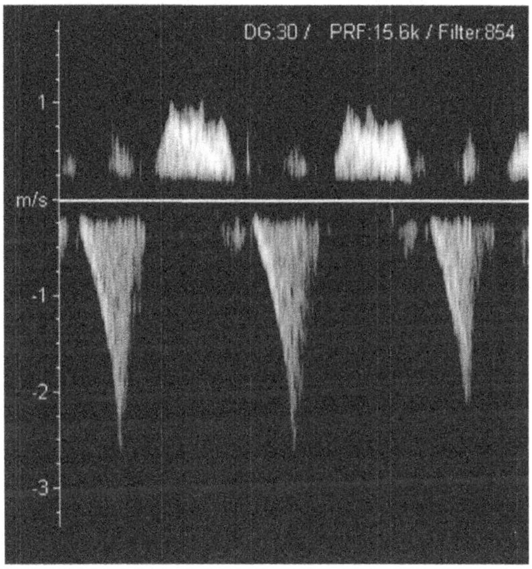

Fig. 3.38 Typical shape of an intraventricular gradient in a patient with obstructive hypertrophic cardiomyopathy

(mmHg/s), which is a measure of left ventricular systolic function. This method uses the time required for the regurgitant flow to pass from a velocity of 1 m/s to 3 m/s and therefore, according to the Bernoulli equation, to develop a gradient of 32 mmHg. Normally this interval is ≤ 32 ms and therefore dP/dt is ≥ 1,000 mmHg/s. With left ventricular dysfunction the time interval required to develop a gradient of 32 mmHg is longer, and therefore the dP/dt is reduced (Fig. 3.36).

3.3.3.2 Determination of Transvalvular and Intracardiac Gradients

Measurement of the pressure gradient that develops through a stenotic valve is the method to determine its severity. The maximum gradient is determined using the modified Bernoulli equation by measuring the peak transvalvular flow velocity, while the mean gradient is calculated by tracing the envelope of the transvalvular flow. Figure 3.30b provides an example of aortic stenosis with

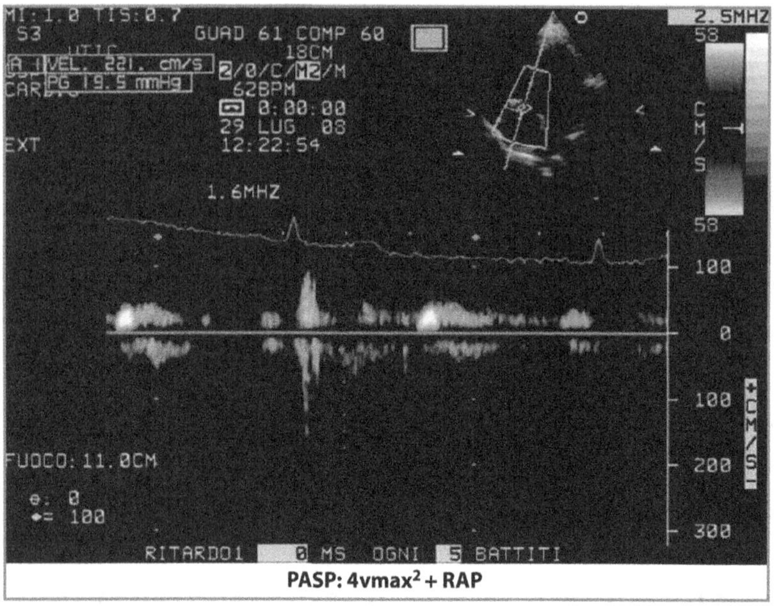

Fig. 3.39 Determination of pulmonary artery systolic pressure (PASP). Tricuspid regurgitation flow is used to determine the gradient between the right atrium and right ventricle. This gradient must be added with the value of the estimated right atrial pressure (*RAP*), obtained by studying the inferior vena cava

Table 3.6 Estimation of right atrial pressure

Inferior vena cava	Change with breathing	Estimated right atrial pressure
Small (< 1.5 cm)	Collapse	0-5 mmHg
Normal (1.5-2.5 cm)	Reduction > 50%	5-10 mmHg
Normal (1.5-2.5 cm)	Reduction < 50%	10-15 mmHg
Dilated (> 2.5 cm)	Reduction < 50%	15-20 mmHg
Dilated with suprahepatic veins also dilated	No change	> 20 mmHg

a maximum gradient of 78 mmHg and a mean gradient of 47 mmHg. Figure 3.37 shows an example of mitral stenosis. In this way it is also possible to measure the intraventricular gradient which can develop in subjects with interventricular defects or obstructive hypertrophic cardiomyopathy. The intraventricular gradient that develops in subjects with obstructive hypertrophic cardiomyopathy typically has an end-systolic peak that distinguishes it from the rounder profile of the aortic stenosis (Fig. 3.38).

3.3.3.3 Determination of Pulmonary Artery Pressure

To measure systolic pressure in the pulmonary artery, the pressure gradient between the right ventricle and right atrium is used, which can be measured in the presence of tricuspid regurgitation. The gradient is calculated using the modified Bernoulli equation in which the maximum velocity of the tricuspid regurgitation flow is inserted as V2 (Fig. 3.39). An estimate of the right atrial pressure is added to the gradient obtained between the atrium and the right ventricle to obtain pulmonary systolic pressure. Table 3.6 summarises the estimate of right atrial pressure in relation to the dimensions of the inferior vena cava and its changes during respiration [14].

To estimate diastolic pressure of the pulmonary artery, the V2 of the modified Bernoulli equation is represented by the end-diastolic velocity on the pulmonary valve regurgitation profile. An estimate of right atrial pressure is added to the obtained gradient [14].

3.3.3.4 Determination of Valvular Areas

The area of a valvular orifice can be calculated using the *continuity equation*, which is based on the

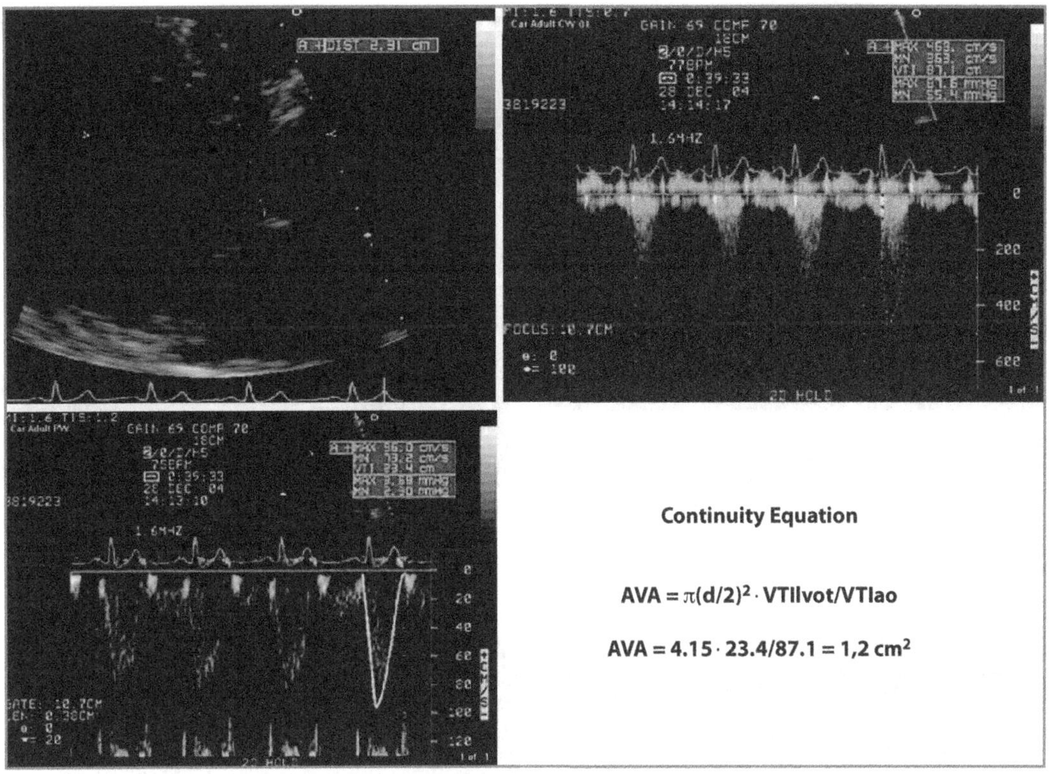

Fig. 3.40 Example of calculation of the aortic valve area (AVA) using the continuity equation

principle of conservation of mass by which proximal and distal flow at an orifice must be equal to the flow inside it. The continuity equation that enables a valvular area to be calculated is as follows:

$$A_1 \cdot VTI_1 = A_2 \cdot VTI_2$$

where A_1 = proximal area, A_2 = area across the valvular orifice, and VTI = velocity-time integral of the flow in the corresponding location. From this equation it can be determined that

$$A_2\ (cm^2) = A_1 \cdot (VTI_1/VTI_2)$$

The continuity equation can be used to calculate the areas of all cardiac valves, however, usually it is used for calculation of the area of the aortic valve, for which A_1 and VTI_1 are represented by the area and VTI of the left ventricular outflow tract (Fig. 3.40). An aortic area of $\leq 1\ cm^2$ indicates severe aortic stenosis [21].

On the contrary, the Doppler calculation of the mitral valve area (MVA) is most commonly carried out using the pressure half time (PHT) method, with the following equation:

$$MVA\ (cm^2) = 220/PHT$$

where 220 is an empirically derived constant equal to a MVA of approximately 1 cm^2. PHT represents the time taken by the pressure gradient through the valve to halve and is measured by tracing the slope of early-diastolic flow through the mitral valve (Fig. 3.41). A mitral area of $\leq 1\ cm^2$ indicates severe stenosis [21].

3.3.3.5 Quantification of Valvular Regurgitation

Color-Doppler is the most common method of qualitative or semiqualitative evaluation of valvular regurgitation. The parameter generally used is the regurgitant jet area that is measured by tracing the jet profile, but this parameter tends to underestimate regurgitation in the presence of eccentric jets (Fig. 3.42).

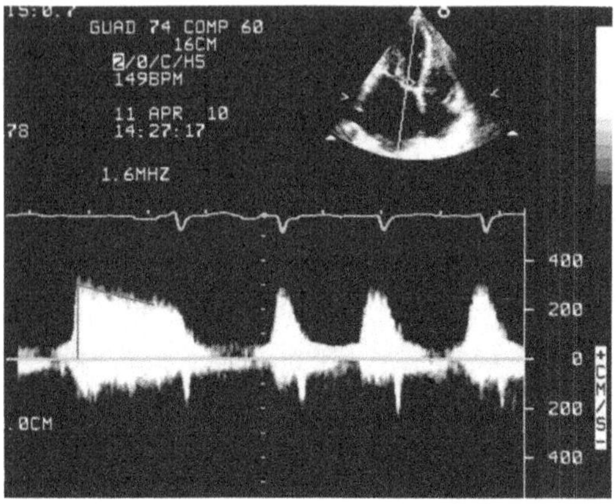

Fig. 3.41 Doppler determination of the mitral valve area. PHT measured using continuous-wave Doppler is 305 ms, corresponding to an area of 0.7 cm^2

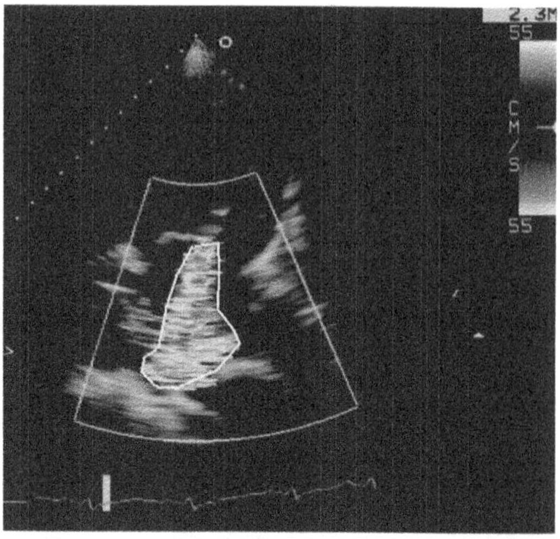

Fig. 3.42 Determination of the jet area and jet area/left atrial area ratio in a subject with severe mitral valve regurgitation

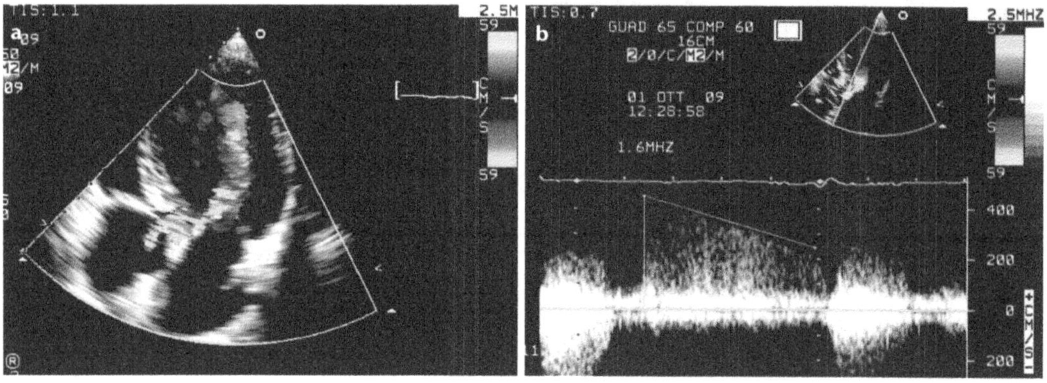

Fig. 3.43 Color-Doppler in a subject with severe aortic regurgitation. With continuous-wave Doppler, decreasing diastolic velocities can be seen, with a PHT equal to 128 ms (a). The steep slope of the regurgitant jet is another parameter of severe aortic regurgitation (b)

In the quantification of aortic regurgitation, the PHT method is commonly used in addition to the jet area (Fig. 3.43). A PHT of less than 200 ms indicates severe aortic regurgitation.

Conversely, in the quantification of mitral valve regurgitation, the recommended method is the Proximal Isovelocity Surface Area (PISA) method, which is a modified continuity equation using the property of flow convergence when a fluid approaches a restricted orifice. According to this method, the blood that approaches an orifice forms concentric isovelocity hemispheres, in which velocity becomes higher as the area of the hemisphere becomes smaller. With color-Doppler, by changing the aliasing velocity of the flow approaching the regurgitant orifice, it is possible to see the hemisphere proximal to the orifice, the radius of which, and therefore the area, can be measured. Flow through the proximal isovelocity area is equal to the flow across the regurgitant orifice (according to the principle of conservation of mass). By calculating regurgitant volume in the proximal isovelocity area and knowing the maximum regurgitant velocity through the regurgitant orifice, it is possible to determine the effective regurgitant orifice (ERO)

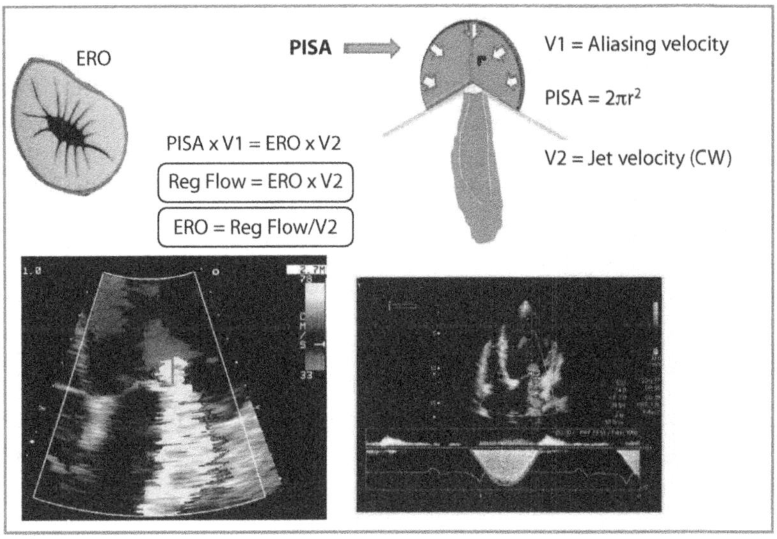

Fig. 3.44 Example of the PISA method (Proximal Isovelocity Surface Area) for determining the effective regurgitant orifice (*ERO*) area in mitral valve regurgitation. Regurgitant flow (*Reg Flow*) can be calculated by multiplying the isovelocity area (derived using the formula $2\pi r^2$) by the aliasing velocity. With the continuity equation, the regurgitant flow is divided by the velocity of the regurgitant jet and the ERO is obtained. An ERO of 0.40 cm2 indicates severe mitral valve regurgitation

area by applying the continuity equation (Fig. 3.44). The PISA method has also been applied to evaluations of aortic and tricuspid valve insufficiency, even if in this context it is less widely validated or recommended.

3.3.3.6 Determination of the Hemodynamic Significance of Left-right Shunts

The hemodynamic significance of intracardiac shunts is calculated using the ratio between the pulmonary flow and the systemic flow (Qp/Qs). This ratio is obtained by dividing the SV in the pulmonary artery by the SV in the aorta according to the formula:

$$Qp/Qs = Apa \cdot VTIpa/Alvot \cdot VTIlvot$$

where Apa is the pulmonary artery area, Alvot is the left ventricular outflow tract area, and VTIap and VTIlvot are the velocity-time integral in the pulmonary artery and the left ventricular outflow tract, respectively. Assuming that the pulmonary artery and left ventricular outflow tract areas are circular, they can be calculated with this formula:

$$A = \pi \cdot (d/2)^2$$

A Qp/Qs ratio of ≥ 1.5 indicates a significant hemodynamic shunt.

3.4 Transesophageal Echocardiography

The indications for transesophageal echocardiography (TOE) in athletes are limited to cases (which in reality are very rare) in which the transthoracic echocardiographic window is not suitable, as well as cases in which the transthoracic examination has not been conclusive in the diagnosis of certain diseases and/or in the differential diagnosis between embryonic remnants and intracardiac masses.

The following will be described in the next paragraphs:

- the protocol and risks of TOE;
- the main transesophageal views with reference to the visualized cardiac structures;
- the main applications of TOE in sports cardiology.

3.4.1 Protocol and Risks

TOE must be conducted by an expert on transthoracic echocardiography. The investigation is usually carried out with mild sedation, in association with a local aaesthesia of the pharynx to reduce patient discomfort and to make the examination more tolerable. When the examination is performed under sedation, the vital parameters must be monitored continuously. The risks relating to

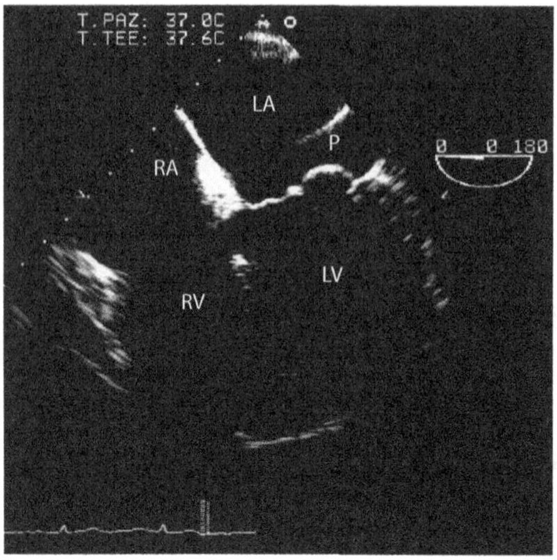

Fig. 3.45 4-chamber transesophageal view in which the prolapse (*P*) of the posterior leaflet of the mitral valve can be seen. *RA* right atrium, *LA* left atrium, *RV* right ventricle, *LV* left ventricle

TOE are very low and include oesophageal perforation, dental damage, bleeding, aspiration of secretions or food (related to the introduction of the probe into the esophagus), hypotension, respiratory depression, arrhythmias, bronchospasm (in relation to sedation).

The risk of aspiration is reduced by conducting the examination in fasting subject, in a left lateral decubitus position and having the subject continue to fast until recovery of the local aaesthesia. In subjects with a history of oesophageal diseases and swallowing disorders it is necessary to carry out a pre-procedure barium swallow. Organic oesophageal diseases (stenosis, diverticulum) are a contraindication for TOE. Prophylaxis for endocarditis is not required before TOE in any subjects.

3.4.2 Transesophageal Views

TOE is currently performed with multiplane probes that scan the heart on multiple planes. Images obtained during TOE, although standardized, can vary widely according to the relative position of the esophagus, heart and diaphragm in each subject. Therefore, instructions related to rotation (from 0° to 180°), angulation (up or down), turning and tilting (lateral movement on the same plane) of the transesophageal probe must be taken only as an indication and be adapted to suit each subject.

Transesophageal views are defined as transesophageal (obtained with the probe in the esophagus) or transgastric (with the probe in the stomach).

3.4.2.1 Transesophageal Four-chamber View

By advancing the probe into the esophagus until it is behind the left atrium (usually in a high oesophageal position), with the tip tilted towards the apex of the heart, at 0° rotation, the oesophageal four-chamber view is obtained (Fig. 3.45), in which it is possible to see the left atrium, right atrium, left ventricle as far as the apex (inferior septum on the left and lateral wall on the right of the monitor) and the right ventricle (free wall on the left of the monitor). In addition, the following structures are visualized: the mitral leaflets (anterior leaflet towards the septum and posterior leaflet towards the lateral wall), the septal and anterior leaflets of the tricuspid valve, and the interatrial septum with the fossa ovalis. With posterior angulation of the probe, the coronary sinus can be seen, while anterior angulation visualises the left ventricular outflow tract and the aorta (transesophageal five-chamber view).

3.4.2.2 Transesophageal Two-chamber View

By continuing the rotation up to 60°, the two-chamber view is obtained in which it is possible to visualise the left atrium, the left ventricle (inferior wall to the left and anterior wall to the right of the monitor) and the two mitral valve commissures (posteromedial on the left and anterolateral on the right of the monitor). A further rotation up to 90° enables visualization of the left atrial appendage, while by slightly withdrawing and turning the probe laterally, the left superior pulmonary vein can be seen entering the left atrium, above the left atrial appendage.

3.4.2.3 Transesophageal Long-axis View

By continuing the rotation up to 120°, the long-axis view of the left ventricle is obtained, showing

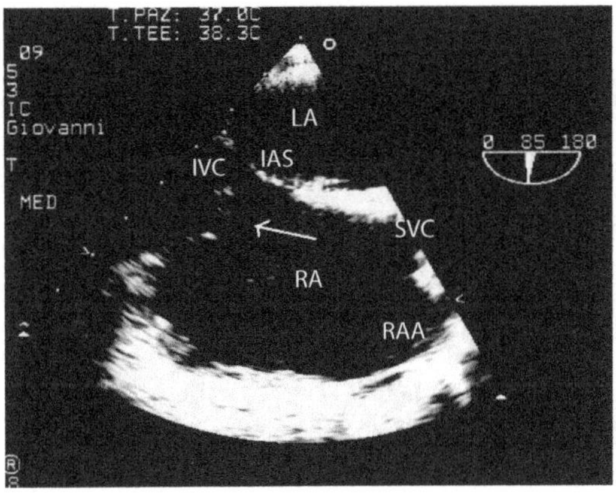

Fig. 3.46 Bicaval transesophageal view in which a prominent Eustachian valve is seen (*arrow*). *LA* left atrium, *RA* right atrium, *RAA* right atrial appendage, *IAS* interatrial septum, *IVC* inferior vena cava, *SVC* superior vena cava

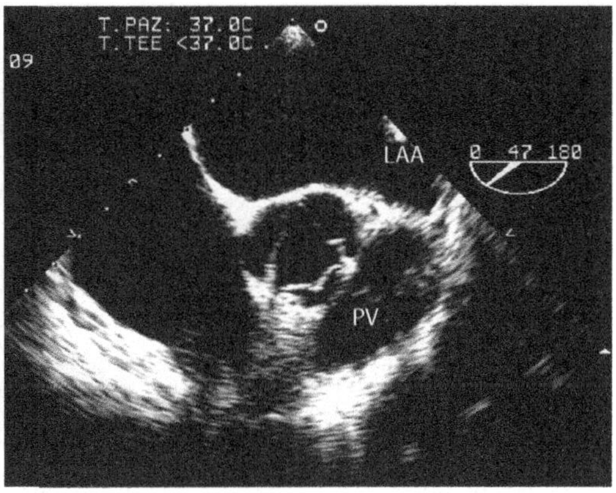

Fig. 3.47 Short-axis transesophageal view in which the left atrial appendage (*LAA*) can be seen. In the centre of the image the aortic valve is visible. In front of the aorta the pulmonary valve (*PV*) can sometimes be seen

the left atrium (on the left), the left ventricle (posterolateral wall on the left), the anterior septum (on the right), the left ventricular outflow tract (on the right), and the aortic valve (non-coronary cusp on the left and right coronary cusp on the right) together with the aortic bulb. Finally, there is a view along the long axis of the two mitral valve leaflets. With the probe at 90° rotation, by turning it toward the left side of the subject, the long-axis view of the right ventricular outflow tract, the pulmonary valve, and sometimes the pulmonary artery trunk are visualized. On the contrary, with the probe at 90° rotation, by turning it toward the right side of the subject, the bicaval view is obtained, in which the left atrium (at the top, near the probe), the interatrial septum, the right atrium (at the bottom), the right atrial appendage (at the bottom on the right), the superior vena cava (to the right of the interatrial septum) and inferior vena cava (to the left of the interatrial septum) are seen. An optimal view of the Eustachian valve and/or the Chiari network (Fig. 3.46) can also be obtained. Finally, by moving the probe backwards and to the right side of the subject, the right pulmonary veins can be seen, whereas turning the probe to the left side of the subject shows the left pulmonary veins.

Transesophageal Short-axis View

The short-axis scan of the base of the heart is obtained at 30-45°, with a slight withdrawal of the probe from the high esophagus in order to obtain an optimal view of the aortic valve with its three cusps (the non-coronary cusp facing the interatrial septum, the left coronary cusp on the right of the monitor, and the right coronary cusp near the right ventricle). Often it is also possible to see the origin of the first portion of the coronary arteries. In this view the two atria, the interatrial septum, the tricuspid valve and the inflow tract of the right ventricle are also visible (Fig. 3.47).

By turning the probe laterally and angulating superiorly from the 0° position, it is possible to see the left atrial appendage and its trabeculae as well as the left superior pulmonary vein. Sometimes the prominence separating the left atrial appendage from the left superior pulmonary vein can be very prominent, mimicking a thrombus. By advancing the probe further into the esophagus and angulating it inferiorly, the inferior left pulmonary vein can also be seen. The right pulmonary veins are visible when the probe is turned medially and withdrawn (for the right superior pulmonary vein) or angulated downwards (for the right inferior pulmonary vein).

3.4.2.5 Transgastric Views

By advancing the probe further into the esophagus and crossing the gastro-oesophageal junction, the stomach is reached. Angulating the probe superiorly, at 0° rotation, the short-axis view of the left

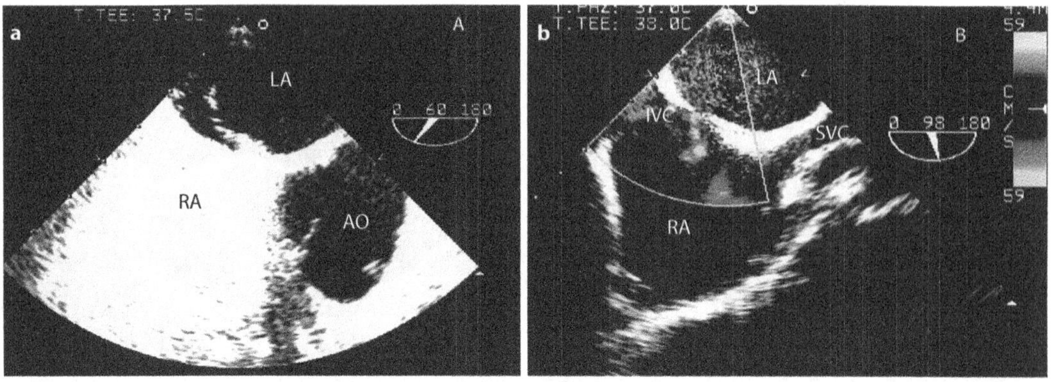

Fig. 3.48 a Short-axis transesophageal view showing the wide passage of a bubble from the right atrium (*RA*) to the left atrium (*LA*) during the Valsalva manoeuvre in a patient with a patent foramen ovale. *AO* aorta. b Bicaval oesophageal view in which it is possible to see a small basal left-to-right shunt with color-Doppler. *IVC* inferior vena cava, *SVC* superior vena cava

ventricle is obtained at the level of the papillary muscles. By withdrawing the probe slightly towards the esophagus, the mitral valve leaflets (anterior leaflet to the left and posterior leaflet to the right) are seen. Continuing the rotation up to 90°, a transgastric two-chamber view of the left ventricle is obtained, and by moving the probe towards the right side of the subject, the right ventricle and the right atrium are seen. Finally, by advancing the probe all the way into the stomach, at 0° rotation, a transgastric four-chamber view is obtained, whereas angulating the probe anteriorly the left ventricular outflow tract and the aorta are also seen in a transgastric five-chamber view, which is ideal for studying the transaortic flow. With further rotation to 120°, in some patients, a transgastric long-axis view is obtained, in which it is possible to obtain optimal alignment with the flow in the left ventricular outflow tract and the aorta.

3.4.2.6 Views of the Descending Aorta

Both in the transesophageal and transgastric views, the descending aorta can be seen by turning the probe backwards, with a 0° rotation for the short-axis view and a 90° rotation for the long-axis view. By withdrawing the probe from the transgastric position towards the esophagus it is possible to see the entire course of the aorta. At the level of the aortic arch the probe must be angulated inferiorly and turned medially to obtain an adequate view of the aortic arch.

3.4.3 TOE Applications in Sports Cardiology

3.4.3.1 Patent Foramen Ovale and Interatrial Septal Aneurysm

Patent foramen ovale (PFO) is a congenital abnormality found during autopsies in 25-35% of the general population. It has acquired particular clinical relevance in sports cardiology after the demonstration of a probable relationship between PFO and the risk of decompression sickness during diving. PFO can be diagnosed by transthoracic echocardiography with injection in a right antecubital vein of a saline echo contrast to observe the passage of bubbles from right to left, in resting conditions or, more frequently, during the Valsalva manoeuvre. However, TOE is more sensitive in the diagnosis of PFO and also enables identification of unusual characteristics of the interatrial septum that are associated with a higher risk of embolism, such as the tunnel-like appearance of the PFO, the extreme mobility of the membrane, a large detachment of the valve, and the presence of an interatrial septum aneurysm. PFO is diagnosed when, after injection of a saline echo contrast in a right antecubital vein during the Valsalva manoeuvre, the passage of bubbles from the right atrium to the left atrium is observed. This passage must occur between 1-3 beats from the visualization of the echo contrast on the right atrium (Fig. 3.48a). Echo contrast signals seen later on the left atrium are due to intrapulmonary arteriovenous

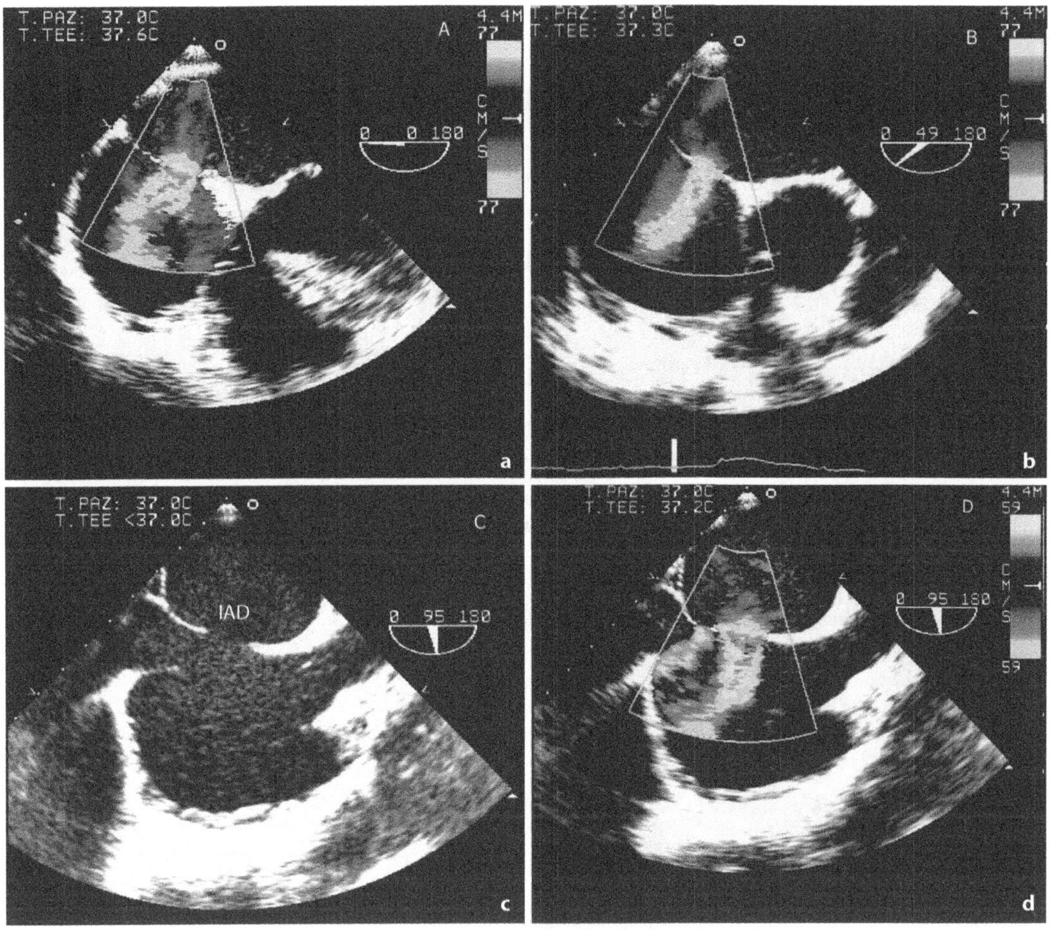

Fig. 3.49 4-chamber (a), short-axis (b), and bicaval (c and d) transesophageal views in which it is possible to see an ostium secundum interatrial septum defect (*IAD*) with a wide left-to-right shunt with color-Doppler

communication. The use of echo contrast during the Valsalva manoeuvre enables visualization of PFO in about 25% of the population. Spontaneous passage during the injection of echo contrast occurs in only 5% of the population and can sometimes be seen also with color-Doppler (Fig. 3.48b).

Interatrial septum aneurysm is defined as a transient bulging of the fossa ovalis during systole and diastole, towards both the right and left atrium, with a total excursion of the plane of the interatrial septum of ≥ 15 mm, and no signs of increased pressure on the right or left atrium. In 90% of cases, the aneurysm is associated with small fenestrations, i.e. PFO. According to some autopsies, the incidence is 1% of the general population.

The transesophageal views that allow both PFO and possible interatrial septum aneurysm to be seen are the short-axis view with aorta and the bicaval view.

3.4.3.2 Interatrial Septal Defects and Persistent Left Superior Vena Cava

Interatrial septum defects are the most common form of congenital heart disease in adults. They often occur asymptomatically and are found by transthoracic echocardiography carried out for another reason. TOE has a greater diagnostic accuracy than transthoracic echocardiography, particularly for sinus venosus defects. Therefore, in the

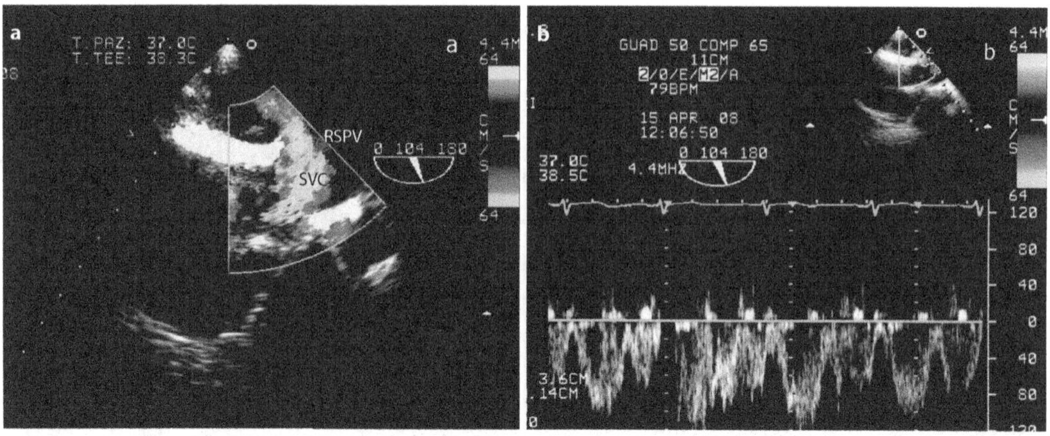

Fig. 3.50 Bicaval transesophageal view in which it is possible to see a sinus venosus type of interatrial defect associated with anomalous venous return of the right superior pulmonary vein (*RSPV*) in the superior vena cava (*SVC*). With color-Doppler ultrasound a wide left-to-right shunt (**a**) is visible with inversion of pulmonary venous flow (**b**)

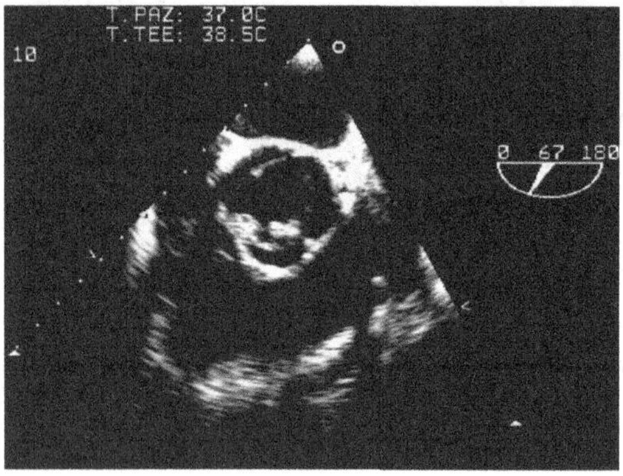

Fig. 3.51 Short-axis transesophageal view showing a bicuspid aortic valve. Partial calcification of the anterolateral cusp with a medial raphe is visible

event of unexplained dilatation of right sections, interatrial defects must always be suspected and TOE performed.

The transesophageal views that enable visualization of interatrial defects are the short-axis view with aorta at 45° rotation, the four-chamber view at 0°, and the bicaval view at 90° (Fig. 3.49). The sinus venosus defect is often associated with partial anomalus pulmonary venous return. In the bicaval view it is possible to see the right pulmonary vein, crossing the superior vena cava and draining directly into the right atrium instead of the left (Fig. 3.50). The sinus venosus defect is also associated with the persistence of the left superior vena cava, which drains into the coronary sinus. This abnormality, which in rare cases (0.3-0.5% of the general population) can also be isolated, is suspected in the presence of dilatation of the coronary sinus at transthoracic echocardiography (Fig. 3.51). The confirmation of persistent left superior vena cava is obtained by injecting a saline echo contrast into a left antecubital vein and visualising it first in the coronary sinus and then in the right sections. With TOE the dilated coronary sinus can be seen in its the long-axis with the four-chamber view at 0° rotation, by angulating the probe backwards. The left superior vena cava can be seen between the left atrial appendage and the left superior pulmonary vein in the two-chamber view between 70° and 90° rotation.

3.4.3.3 Bicuspid Aortic Valve, Aortic Coarctation and Aortic Dilatation

A *bicuspid aorta valve* is the most common form of congenital heart disease, reported in 1-2% of the general population. The clinical relevance of the bi-

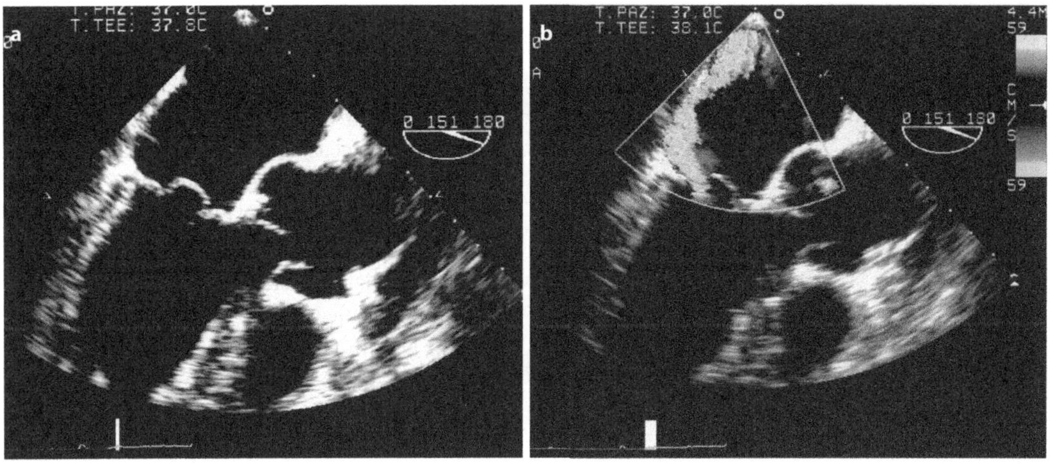

Fig. 3.52 Long-axis transesophageal view in which a prolapse of the anterior leaflet of the mitral valve (a) is visible with an eccentric regurgitation jet (b)

cuspid aortic valve in sports cardiology is justified by its association with sudden death. In athletes, given the good echocardiographic window, bicuspid aortic valve can already be diagnosed using transthoracic echocardiography, but sometimes it is necessary to confirm it with TOE. Short-axis view between 30° and 45° rotation enables adequate visualization of the cusps (Fig. 3.51). The two cusps usually have different dimensions, one larger than the other, and an oval opening. Generally the coronary arteries originate from the largest cusp. In the long-axis transesophageal views at 120° rotation, it is sometimes possible to see the prolapse of one of the cusps.

In 10% of subjects, bicuspid aortic valve is associated with aortic coarctation. Therefore in subjects with bicuspid aortic valve it is also necessary to explore the aortic isthmus, i.e. the point of passage between the aortic arch and the descending aorta, in order to rule out aortic coarctation. Aortic coarctation is a constriction of the aorta, of variable extension, associated, at the Doppler study, with the acceleration of the systolic anterograde flow that persists also in diastole, if restriction is severe. The view that best enables investigation of aortic coarctation is the transthoracic suprasternal view and the very high transesophageal view by turning the probe back to visualise the aorta.

Additionally, the bicuspid aortic valve is often associated with *dilatation of the sinus of Valsalva and the ascending aorta*, which in subjects with Marfan syndrome usually involves even the sinotubular junction. In the 120° transesophageal view, TOE allows measurement of the diameters at the level of the annulus, bulb, junction and ascending aorta with greater accuracy than transthoracic echocardiography. Measuring the diameters of the aorta is of particular clinical importance since the risk of aortic dissection is proportionally related to the level of the aortic dilatation.

3.4.3.4 Subaortic Valvular Stenosis

Subaortic stenosis may be studied adequately with transthoracic echocardiography (long-axis parasternal and apical views), but if the images are not optimal, TOE, in the transesophageal view at 120° rotation, enables optimal visualization of the anatomy of the stenosis. The anatomical appearance varies from thin, small membrane to a fibromuscular structure, which is sometimes provided with a mobile membrane. The color-Doppler study shows the presence of subvalvular flow acceleration. Often aortic valve regurgitation is also associated due to continuous exposure of the valve to high flow velocities that lead to fibrocalcific degeneration.

3.4.3.5 Mitral Valve Prolapse

Mitral valve prolapse is very common in athletes and has been recognized as the only abnormality in some cases of sudden death in athletes. How-

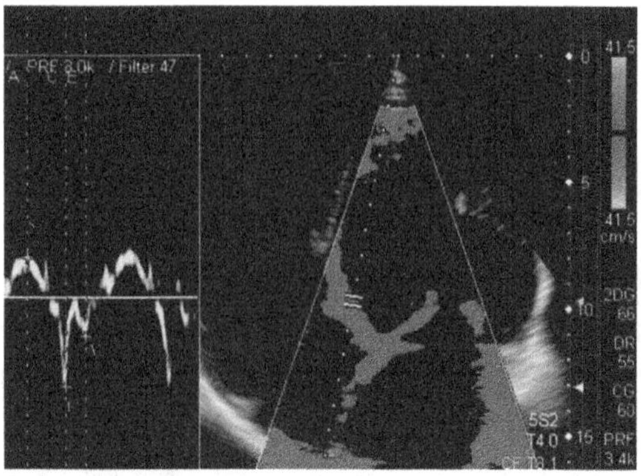

Fig. 3.53 Pulsed-wave TDI at the basal segment of the interventricular septum

ever, the relationship between mitral valve prolapse and sudden death is somewhat controversial.

TOE is indicated in the evaluation of mitral valve prolapse in cases in which transthoracic images are inadequate, when cord rupture and valve flail are suspected, and in perioperative evaluations of subjects with severe mitral valve regurgitation in whom mitral repair is indicated. TOE makes it possible to study the valve anatomy with greater accuracy, to determine thickening and redundancy of the leaflets, as well as prolongation of the chordae tendineae, and to identify valve scallops involved in the prolapse and the origin of the corresponding regurgitation (Fig. 3.52).

3.5 Tissue Doppler Imaging and Deformation Imaging

Tissue Doppler Imaging (TDI) is a progression of conventional Doppler than makes it possible, through opportune changes to the filters and internal algorithms of the machine, to study the velocity and deformation of the cardiac muscle. Unlike conventional Doppler, which is characterized by high-velocity and low amplitude signals from the blood flow, TDI has low-velocity (rarely more than ± 20 cm/s) and high amplitude signals (approximately 40 dB more than conventional Doppler signals). Modern echocardiographic machines are commonly equipped with TDI software, enabling routine TDI analysis to quantify systolic and diastolic function of the left and right ventricles.

Three different TDI methods are available: spectral pulsed-wave TDI, 2D color-TDI and M-mode color-TDI [23].

Spectral pulse TDI has a great advantage of enabling on-line measurement of myocardial velocities and time intervals with a high time resolution (8 ms). Pulsed-wave TDI is obtained by placing the pulsed-Doppler sample volume at the centre of each myocardial segment to study regional function. It is important that during acquisition the patient holds its breath. The waves described are shown in Figure 3.53. The S wave represents systolic velocity, the E' wave represents the relaxation velocity for the myocardial segment during the rapid filling phase, and the A' wave is a passive movement due to atrial contraction. From the pulsed-wave TDI analysis, time intervals can also be measured, i.e. isovolumetric contraction time (between the start of the Q wave on the ECG to the start of the S wave) and isovolumetric relaxation time (between the end of the S wave and the start of the E' wave). In the apical views, longitudinal shortening and lengthening of all visualized left ventricular segments (even if the velocities are much lower and harder to study at the apex) and that of the free wall of the right ventricle can be analysed. By positioning the sample volume at the mitral or tricuspid annulus, it is obtained a wave profile similar to the TDI at myocardial level. Pulsed-wave TDI at mitral and tricuspid annulus represent overall left and right ventricular function, respectively.

With *2D color- and M-mode color-TDI*, the TDI color code shows velocities approaching the transducer in red and those travelling away from it in blue. Different levels of intensity are attributed proportionally to the increase in velocity, for which faster segments appear more intense that less rapid segments. Unlike pulsed-wave TDI analysis, velocities can only be quantified off-line. The advantage of color-TDI is the possibility of measuring the subendocardial velocities and subepicardial velocities separately, enabling the normal velocity gradient from the endocardium to the epicardium to be identified. The M-mode color-TDI also has an increased time resolution (5-10 ms). In the 2D color-TDI , two-dimensional images are represented in movements according to the conventional color code, but with low frame rates. Reducing the scan-

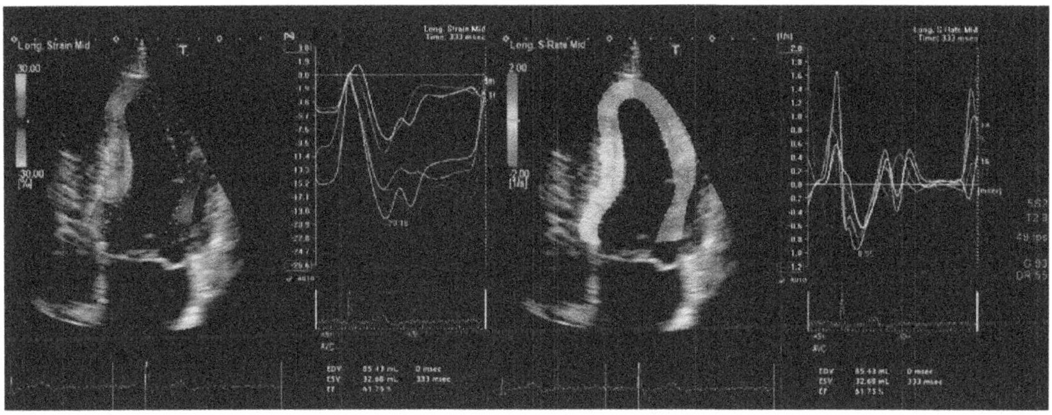

Fig. 3.54 Analysis of strain and strain-rate derived from speckle tracking

ning sector to analyse one wall at a time allows higher frame rates to be obtained, so that a greater proportion of cardiac events can be evaluated (with a time resolution of 10-100 ms) [23].

Strain, Strain Rate and Speckle Tracking

Investigation of the velocities of the myocardium with the TDI methods has significant limitations represented by the dependence of the velocity from the angle, the translation of the heart and the tethering of a segment from the adjacent segments, which may invalidate the accuracy of myocardial velocity measurements. These limitations can be overcome (at least in part) by studying myocardial deformations with the strain rate and strain derived from TDI. The strain rate is the velocity of deformation of the myocardium and the first deformation parameter that is obtained by TDI. Strain is the time derivative of strain rate and is a measure of the quantity of deformation [23] (Fig. 3.54). When the ventricle contracts, the heart muscle shortens longitudinally and circumferentially (negative strain) and thickens or lengthens radially (positive strain).

In addition to TDI-derived strain and strain rate, myocardial deformation can be analysed with the speckle tracking method, based on the possibility to tag along the deformation of each single myocardial *speckle* in all directions during the cardiac cycle. From this analysis it is possible to derive curves that enable velocity, strain and strain rate to be measured in each myocardial segment. Information obtained with this method is not derived from Doppler and therefore it is not affected by the angle dependence [24].

3.5.1 TDI in Athletes

Various authors have shown that TDI in athletes shows *supernormal* systolic and diastolic velocities, i.e. higher than those of untrained subjects, both in the left and right ventricle [25]. Other studies have shown that with TDI and strain analysis it is possible to distinguish between normal hypertrophy in athletes and abnormal hypertrophy.

In the study by Palka et al. [26], M-mode color-TDI was used to show that athletes have a significantly higher myocardial velocity gradient than subjects with hypertrophic cardiomyopathy or arterial hypertension. In the study by Vinereanu et al. [27], the cut-off point of <9 cm/s for the S wave, measured at the basal segment of the inferior wall of the left ventricle, had a sensitivity of 87% and a specificity of 97% in the identification of patients with hypertrophic cardiomyopathy. Similar results have been reported with the new method of speckle tracking [28].

Nevertheless, although these data are still very promising and suggest the potential usefulness of velocity and myocardial deformation assessment when evaluating athletes' heart so far these methods are only used by dedicated experts and specialized laboratories.

References

1. AA.VV. (2010) Protocolli cardiologici per il giudizio di idoneità allo sport agonistico 2009. Medicina dello sport 63:5–137
2. Marron BJ, Pelliccia A (2006) The heart of trained athletes. Cardiac remodeling and risks of sports, including sudden death. Circulation 114:1633–1644
3. Pelliccia A, Maron BJ, Di Paolo FM et al (2005) Prevalence and clinical significance of left atrial remodeling in competitive athletes. J Am Coll Cardiol 46: 690–696
4. Pelliccia A, Culasso F, Di Paolo F et al (1999) Physiologic left ventricular cavity dilatation on elite athlete. Ann Intern Med 130:23–31
5. Pelliccia A, Maron BJ, Spataro A et al (1991) The upper limit of physiologic cardiac hypertrophy in highly trained elite athletes. N Engl J Med 324: 295–301
6. Marron BJ, Pelliccia A, Spirito P (2005) Cardiovascular disease in young trained athletes. Insights into methods for distinguishing athlete's heart from structural heart disease, with particular emphasis on hypertrophic cardiomyopathy. Circulation 91:1596–1601
7. Zeppilli P, Dello Russo A, Santini C et al (1998) In vivo detection of coronary artery anomalies in asymptomatic athletes by echocardiographic screening. Chest 114:89–93
8. Maron BJ (1986) Structural features of the athletes heart as defined by echocardiography. J Am Coll Cardiol 7:190–203
9. Schiller NB, Shah PM, Crawford M et al (1989) Recommendations for quantitation of the left ventricle by two-dimensional echocardiography. American Society of Echocardiography Committee on Standards, Subcommittee on Quantitation of Two-Dimensional Echocardiograms. J Am Soc Echocardiogr 2:358–367
10. Feigenbaum H, Armstrong W, Ryan T. (2005) Feigenbaum's echocardiography,6th edn. Lippincott, Williams and Wilkins, Philadelphia
11. Lang RM, Bierig M, Devereux RB et al (2006) Recommendation for chambers quantification. Eur J Echocardiography 7:79–108
12. Palmieri V, Dahlof B, DeQuattro V et al (1999) Reliability of echocardiographic assessment of left ventricular structure and function: the PRESERVE study: Prospective Randomized Study Evaluating Regression of Ventricular Enlargement. J Am Coll Cardiol 34:1625–1632
13. Devereux RB, Alonso DR, Lutas EM et al (1986) Echocardiographic assessment of left ventricular hypertrophy: comparison to necropsy findings. Am J Cardiol 57:450–458
14. Otto CM, Aurigemma GP, Bartel T et al (2007) The practice of clinical echocardiography, 3th ed. Saunders Elsevier, Philadelphia
15. Cerqueira MD, Weissman NJ, Dilsizian V et al (2002) Standardized myocardial segmentation and nomenclature for tomographic imaging of the heart: a statement for healthcare professionals from the Cardiac Imaging Committee of the Council on Clinical Cardiology of the American Heart Association. Circulation 105: 539–542
16. Matsukubo H, Matsuura T, Endo N et al (1977) Echocardiographic measurement of right ventricular wall thickness. A new application of subxiphoid echocardiography. Circulation 56:278-284
17. Foale R, Nihoyannopoulos P, McKenna W et al (1986) Echocardiographic measurement of the normal adult right ventricle. Br Heart J 56:33–44
18. Marcus FI, McKenna WJ, Sherril D et al (2010) Diagnosis of arrhythmogenic right ventricular cardiomyopathy/dysplasia proposed modification of the task force Criteria. Circulation 121:1533-1541
19. Weyman A (1994) Practices and principles of echocardiography, 2nd edn. Lippincott Williams and Wilkins, Philadelphia
20. Redfield MM, Jacobsen SJ, Burnett Jr JC et al (2003) Burden of systolic and diastolic ventricular dysfunction in the community: Appreciating the scope of the heart failure epidemic. JAMA 289:194– 202
21. Baumgartner H, Hung J, Bermejo J et al (2009) Echocardiographic assessment of valve stenosis: EAE/ASE recommendations for clinical practice. JASE 22:1–23
22. Lancellotti P, Moura L, Pierard LA (2010) European Association of Echocardiography Recommendations for the assessment of valvular regurgitation. Part 2: mitral and tricuspid regurgitation (native valve disease). Eur J Echocardiogr 11:307–332
23. Marwick TH (2006) Measurement of strain and strain rate by echocardiography Ready for prime time? J Am Coll Cardiol 47:1313–1327
24. Mondillo S, Galderisi M, Mele D et al (2011) Speckle tracking echocardiography: a new technique for assessing myocardial function. J Ultrasound Med 30: 71–83
25. Caso P, D'Andrea A, Galderisi M et al (2000) Pulsed Doppler Tissue imaging in endurance athletes: Relation between left ventricular preload and myocardial regional diastolic function. Am J Cardiol 85:1131–1136
26. Palka P, Lange A, Fleming AD, Donnelly JE, Dutka DP, Starkey IR, Shaw TR, Sutherland GR, Fox KA. Differences in myocardial velocity gradient measured throughout the cardiac cycle in patients with hypertrophic cardiomyopathy, athletes and patients with left ventricular hypertrophy due to hypertension. J Am Coll Cardiol. 1997;30:760–8.
27. Vinereanu D, Florescu N, Schulthorpe N et al (2001) Differentiation between pathologic and physiologic left ventricular hypertrophy by tissue Doppler assessment of long axis function in patients with hypertrophic cardiomyopathy or systemic hypertension and in athletes. Am J Cardiol 88:53-58
28. Galderisi M, Lomoriello VS, Santoro A et al (2010) Differences of myocardial systolic deformation and correlates of diastolic function in competitive rowers and young hypertensives: a speckle-tracking echocardiography study. J Am Soc Echocardiogr 23:1190–1198

Vascular Ultrasound

4

Ombretta Martinelli, Luigi Irace and Paolo Gozzo

Athletes rarely complain of signs or symptoms suggestive of vascular disease; it may therefore be undiagnosed for a long time, with severe consequences for the competitors [1]. Vascular diseases should be considered when athletes experience symptoms that cannot be related to musculoskeletal injuries.

Therefore, physical examination should always include provocative tests specific to vascular disorders in order to simulate the sport-specific positions and effort levels during vascular testing.

The appropriate use of instrumental diagnostic techniques may confirm the clinical diagnosis and enable prompt and appropriate treatment of the vascular disorders in athletes.

Traditionally, intra-arterial digital subtraction angiography (DSA) is considered the diagnostic standard in the evaluation of vascular diseases. However, DSA is invasive and may be associated with well-documented limitations that make this method unsuitable for screening or follow-up examinations.

For these reasons, less invasive methods, including vascular ultrasound imaging (US) multi-detector computed tomography angiography (CTA) and magnetic resonance angiography (MRA), have been devized to detect vascular diseases.

For athletes, an ultrasound examination should be considered as part of the diagnostic investigations carried out at the beginning of a sport, especially if it is competitive, and during following periodic medical visits, in order to rule out anomalies, anatomic variants and/or vascular injuries. Although musculoskeletal injury is the most frequent cause of pain and dysfunction in athletes, similar symptoms due to vascular damage of the lower or upper limbs may occur in a similar way and be detected by means of an US study during both basic and dynamic manoeuvres. US studies provide reliable data on the location, extent and severity of a vascular injury [2].

Color and power Doppler systems provide simultaneous real-time acquisition of the image in relation to the anatomical structures and the Doppler signal relative to the blood flow pattern. More recently, three-dimensional and multiplanar reconstruction of ultrasound data make it possible to determine the relative position of structures and the location of the vessels within the volume examined from different perspectives. The use of amplifiers for the ultrasound signal has led to a further improvement in the definition of ultrasound imaging (US imaging).

All these technological innovations contribute to the accuracy of US imaging as the first-line noninvasive instrumental test for the evaluation of both venous and arterial disease in athletes.

Venous duplex ultrasonography is a readily available test for the reliable diagnosis of venous thrombosis in the extremities, with a specificity ranging from 88% to 100%, and sensitivity of between 78% and 100% [3]. The prompt recognition of venous thrombosis in an extremity, such as spontaneous, effort-induced thrombosis of the axillary or subclavian vein in Paget-Schroetter syndrome, can be obtained using ultrasound, and also

O. Martinelli (✉)
Department of General Surgery
University of Rome "La Sapienza"
Rome, Italy

M. Fioranelli and G. Frajese (eds.), *Sports Cardiology*,
DOI: 10.1007/978-88-470-2775-6_4, © Springer-Verlag Italia 2012

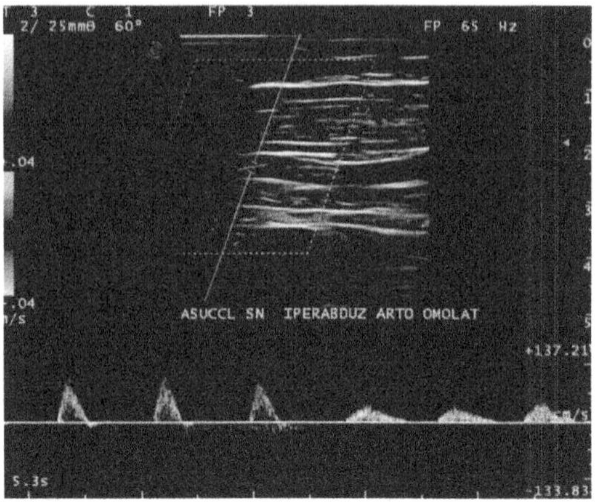

Fig. 4.1 Color-Doppler imaging shows progressive reduction of the subclavian artery flow during abduction of left upper limb in a 22-year-old weight-lifter

provides reliable data for the appropriate therapy and prevention of post-thrombotic chronic insufficiency in these predominantly young patients [4]. US imaging also provides precious information about the *age* of the thrombus based on its different echogenic pattern, which is related to the risk of pulmonary embolism. Once venous thrombosis has been identified, US imaging is used electively to monitor the course in response to medical therapy.

CTA or MRA are indicated to confirm the proximal extension ofiliac-caval thrombosis as detected by US or in the case of suspected pelvic vein thrombosis.

Hemodynamic studies using US imaging are also indicated to evaluate superficial venous insufficiency in the athletes who may suffer from chronic swollen limbs or varicose veins.

US imaging is particularly suitable for investigating peripheral arteries in order to detect steno-obstructive disease that is often related to extrinsic compression in thoracic outlet syndrome (TOS), vascular aneurysms and generally post-traumatic dissections. US examinations also provide data on the arterial anatomy and hemodynamics of the peripheral vessels during dynamic manoeuvres (abduction of the ipsilateral upper limb and anteropulsione-retropulsion of the ipsilateral upper limb), which make it possible to identify the presence and location of extrinsic vascular compression where it cannot be detected in basal conditions (Fig. 4.1). Ankle brachial pressure index measurements by continuous-wave (CW) Doppler and color/power Doppler imaging are complementary investigations following physical examination for both the aorto-iliac and femoro-distal tract [5]. Some studies have yielded different results in terms of diagnostic accuracy for arterial segments above and below the knee. The median sensitivity and specificity of DU are 88% and 95% above the knee and 84% and 93% below the knee [6]. Published diagnostic criteria concerning color-Doppler imaging in peripheral arteries of the extremities have sensitivity and specificity levels exceeding 90% for the detection of significant stenosis or occlusion [7]. The high negative predictive value of this technique (93%) means that normal DU reliably rules out significant occlusive or aneurysmal disease. When used appropriately, color-Doppler technology provides most of the essential anatomic information in addition to hemodynamic data for extensive peripheral arterial mapping, and makes it possible to distinguish between tight stenosis and occlusion, to determine the corresponding level [8].

US evaluations provide accurate data on the structural features of the arterial wall lesion, and it is important to determine the nature of the arterial stenosis, such as iliac endofibrosis (Fig. 4.2).

In athletes requiring surgical intervention, secondary diagnostic imaging is indicated in order to confirm the indication and treatment and to plan surgical or endovascular revascularization for the vascular diseases detected by US [9].

At present three-dimensional CTA or three-dimensional MRA are accurate techniques for complete visualization of the vascular tree and the gathering of information on surrounding anatomical structures, such as the presence of a cervical rib, in order to perform simultaneous resection of the contributing anomalous musculotendinous or skeletal structures, as well as vascular reconstruction, if indicated.

Due to the development of multi-detector CTA scanners, CTA provides increasingly high volumetric coverage, good separation of different vascular phases, improved z-axis resolution, and short acquisition times for visualising the entire

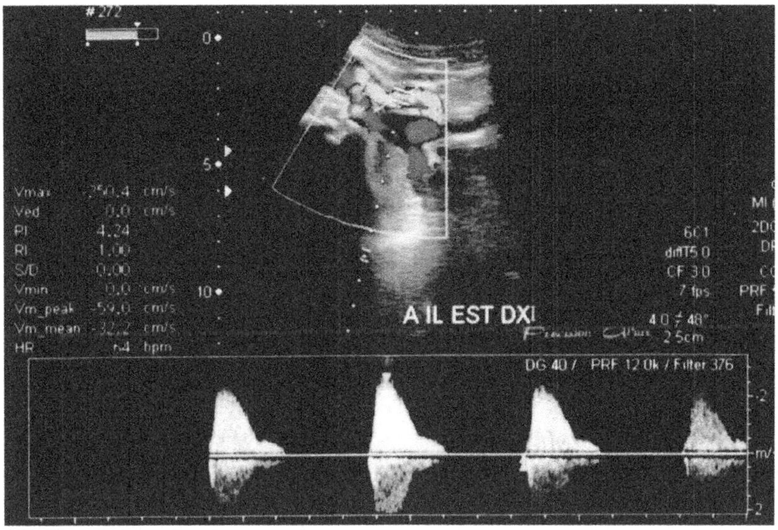

Fig. 4.2 Color-Doppler study showing a tight stenosis of the left external iliac artery in a 36-year-old cyclist

vascular tree during a limited period [10]. Furthermore, CTA provides more post-procedural imaging processing and rotation of three-dimensional images to any angle. Recent CTA reports indicate sensitivity and specificity rates of around 98% for detecting vascular disorders [11]. Major drawbacks of the frequent use of multi-detector CTA may be the administration of potentially nephrotoxic or allergenic iodinate contrast agents and exposure to ionizing radiation. MRA should therefore be considered as an alternative to CTA since its diagnostic accuracy seems to be comparable to CTA, with a specificity of 96% and a sensitivity level of 98% [12].

Due to their relative invasiveness, higher cost and reduced availability compared to US, CTA and MRA should be borne in mind for secondary diagnosis when suggested by an initial ultrasound or when US imaging is inconclusive. The use of US and tomographic techniques has greatly reduced the use for DSA, which is currently performed for endovascular procedures.

When clinical data lead to the suspicion of sport-related vascular disease, several reliable instrumental techniques are currently available to confirm the diagnosis, which should be formulated as early as possible for the most suitable treatment. Prompt and effective intervention to correct vascular disease can enable the athlete to return to optimal activity in his/her chosen sport.

References

1. Doraiwamy VA, Giri J, Mohler E (2009) Premature peripheral arterial disease – difficult diagnosis in very early presentation. Int Angiol 18(9): 45–47
2. Moneta GL, Strandness DE Jr (1987) Peripheral arterial duplex scanning. J Clin Ultrasound 15:645–51
3. Baarslag HJ, van Beek EJ, Koopman MM (2002) Prospective study of color duplex ultrasography compared with contrast venography inpatients suspected of having deep vein thrombosis of the upper extremities. Ann Intern Med 136:865–72
4. Molina JF, Hunter DW, Dietz CA (2007) Paget-Schroetter syndrome treated with throbolytic and immediate surgery. J Vasc Surg 45:328–34
5. Kohler TR et al (1987) Duplex scanning for diagnosis of aorto-iliac and femoro-popliteal disease. Circulation 76:1074–79
6. Pemberton M, London NJ (1997) Color flow duplex imaging of occlusive arterial disease of the lower limb. Br J Surg 84:912–9
7. Collins R, Burch J, Cranny G, Aguiar-Ibanez R, Craig D, Wright K, Berry E, Gough M, Kleijnen J, Westwood M (2007) Duplex ultrasonography, magnetic resonance angiography, and computed tomography angiography for diagnosis and assessment of symptomatic, lower limb peripheral arterial disease. BMJ 16:1257–1273
8. Zierler RE, Zierler BK (2007) Duplex sonography of the lower extremity arteries; Semin. Ultrasound CT MR. 1997;18:39
9. Elsman BH, Legemate DA, Van der Heijden FH, de Vos HJ, Mali WP, Eikelboon BC (1995) Impact of the ultrasonographic duplex scanning on the therapeutic decision making in lower-limb arterial disease. Br J Surg 82: 630–3
10. Laswed T, Rizzo E, Guntern D et al (2008) Assessment

of occlusive disease of abdominal aorta and lower extremities arteries: value of CT angiography using an adaptative acquisition method. Eur Radiol 18(2):263–72
11. Schernthaner R, Standler A, Lomoschitz F et al (2008) Multidetector CT angiography in the assessment of the lower peripheral arterial occlusive disease: accuracy in detecting the severity, number, and length of stenosis. Eur Radiol 18(4):665–671
12. Collins R, Cranny G, Burch J, Aguiar-Ibanez R, Craig D, Wright K et al (2007) A systematic review of duplex scanning ultrasound, magnetic resonance angiography and computed tomography angiography for the diagnosis and assessment of symptomatic, lower limb peripheral arterial disease. Health Technol Assess 11:191–202
13. Lujan S, Criado E, Puras E, Irquierdo LM (2002) Duplex scanning or arteriography for preoperative planning of the lower limb revascularization. Eur J Vasc Endovasc Surg 24:31–6

CT of the Coronary Arteries: Identification and Characterization of the Atherosclerotic Plaque

5

Ilaria D'Angeli and Paolo Pavone

5.1 Introduction

CT coronary imaging is the most advanced and fastest technique that involves the use of multislice computed tomography to *freeze*, with detailed imaging, cardiac motion, providing a static image of the heart and blood vessels. As a technique that uses electromagnetic radiations, CT scan is based on the principle that, when an X-ray beam passes through a part of the human body, some photons pass through it, some are absorbed and others are dispersed (*scattered*). The total quantity of photons that leaves the irradiated body part is therefore less than the total quantity emitted by the source. This phenomenon is called *attenuation*: it depends on both the atomic composition of the irradiated section, i.e. the density of the organ or tissue, and the energy of the photons. The X-ray beam, after passing through the section of the body under examination, is detected by the detectors on the opposite side with respect to the beam source and converted from photons to electrical signals. The intensity of the electrical signal is proportional to the magnitude of the attenuation. Therefore, the advantage of CT is to create static images of the organ that is physiologically in motion and produce *slices* of tissue (CT images) in which individual structures are directly viewed side by side without overlapping. During the acquisition of a *slice*, the X-ray tube and the detectors, which pick the X-rays themselves, rotate around the patient, who is lying on a bed (Fig. 5.1); each image is, therefore, the product of the processing of a large amount of data obtained with the tube-detector system positioned in different directions of the space with respect to the subject examined.

The older scanners required 18-20 seconds to perform a single rotation of the tube around the patient; today, we have the *multislice* CT (MSCT) (Fig. 5.2), in which the rotation of the tube takes up to 0.3 seconds with contemporary acquisition, in spiral mode, up to 128 detectors.

There are also CT scanners with double X-ray tube, in which the two tubes, perpendicular to each other, emit radiations at the same time and the data are detected by two separate groups of detectors. The acquisition time for a single rotation, therefore, is reduced by half (less than 0.15 seconds) (Fig. 5.3).

In conclusion, CT is a technique with increasingly higher spatial and temporal resolution; a

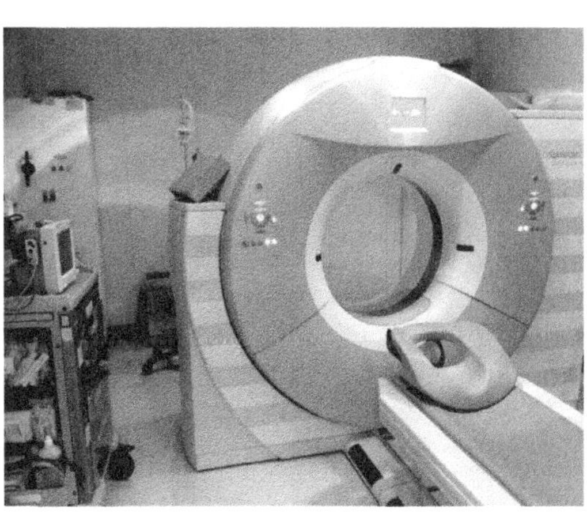

Fig. 5.1 CT equipment

P. Pavone (✉)
Radiology Department
Casa di Cura Mater Dei
Rome, Italy

M. Fioranelli and G. Frajese (eds.), *Sports Cardiology*,
DOI: 10.1007/978-88-470-2775-6_5, © Springer-Verlag Italia 2012

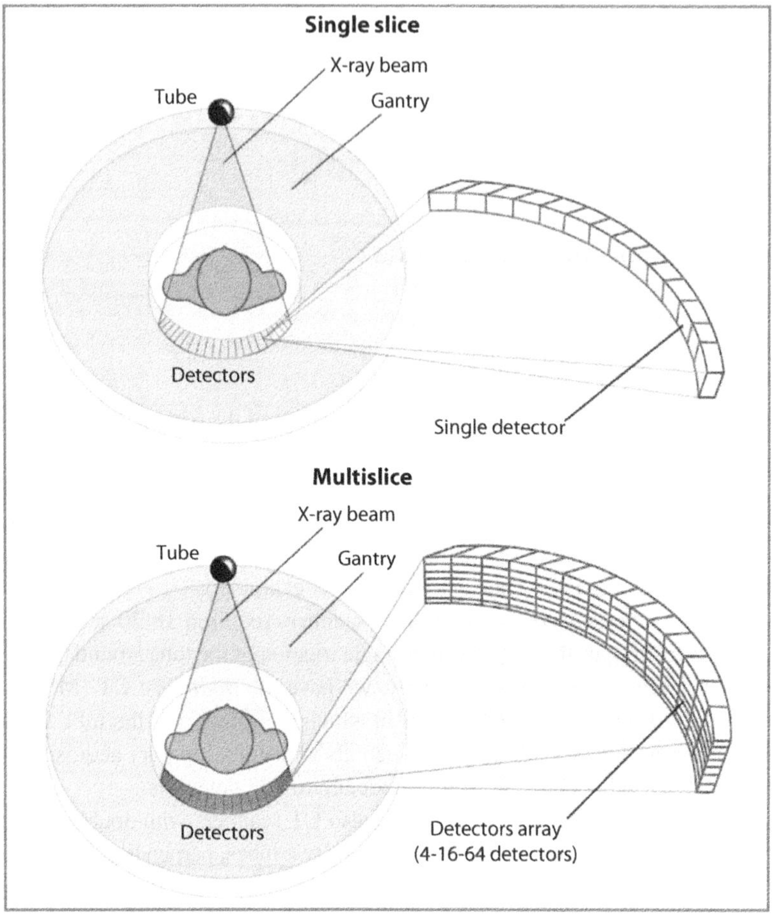

Fig. 5.2 Diagram showing single slice and multislice detectors

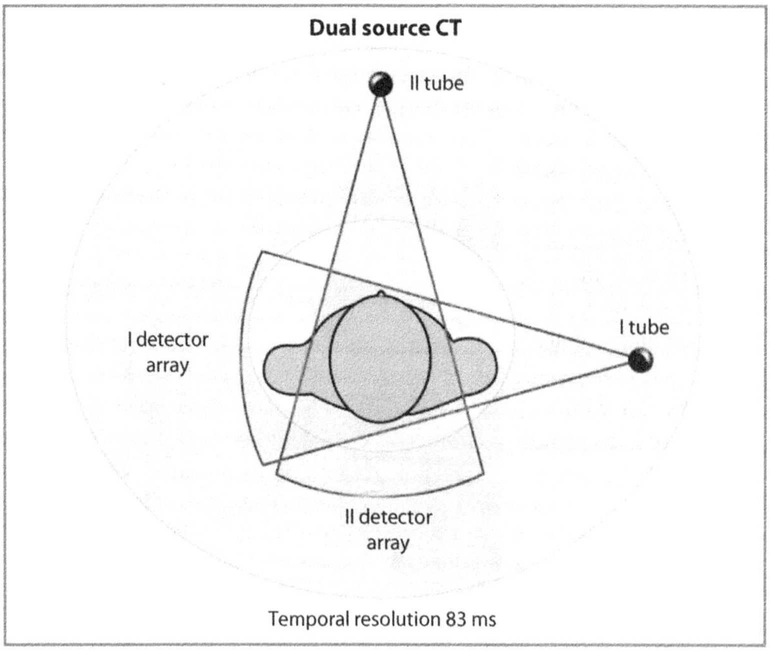

Fig. 5.3 CT scanner with double X-ray tube. The two tubes, mounted perpendicularly on the gantry, emit radiation simultaneously. Data are obtained from two separate groups of detectors. The acquisition time for data in a single rotation, therefore, is halved

great advantage over the high temporal resolution of the technique is the possibility to study patients with higher baseline heart rate (HR up to 75 bpm) maintaining a good quality of the images.

5.2 How to Achieve a High Diagnostic Quality of CT Examinations

When we perform a CT scan of the coronary arteries, we should achieve some objectives: first, obtaining images of the cardiac structures as quickly as possible; specific scanner protocols are used to study the coronary arteries: one of them is called *heart rate synchronization* which allows us to obtain images in a very short time.

The second purpose is to make sure that during the rapid and dynamic acquisition of the images, there is high contrast liquid concentration in the coronary lumen.

In fact, the high internal density of the vascular structure, allows us to perfectly view the coronary artery, its lumen and to evaluate the presence of possible atherosclerotic pathology of the vessel wall. A third objective is to obtain an effective reduction of the heart rate (bradycardia), often a fundamental measure for the success of the exam.

5.2.1 Bradycardia

Reducing the heart rate promotes filling of the coronary lumen by lengthening the diastolic phase; the ideal heart rate is between 50 and 65 bpm. To achieve optimal heart rates, beta-blockers such as atenolol, metoprolol and bisopropol are administered orally or intravenously. In our experience, we prefer the oral preparation, giving the patient a beta-blocker tablet about 45-60 minutes before the examination. In other cases, we inject, via an antecubital vein, a rate-short duration action beta-blocker (esmolol). As soon as the rate decreases to the desired value, we run a scan. In some cases, we can also administer an anti-anxiety drug if the patient experiences a sensation of discomfort that could lead to a related increase in heart rate.

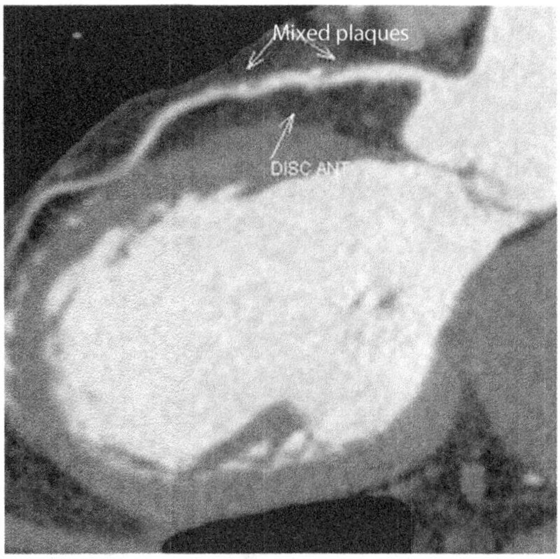

Fig. 5.4 High concentrations of contrast media in the left heart cavity, which appears clear; the *washed* cavities of the bolus of normal saline solution appear hypodense, i.e. darker

5.2.2 Injection of the Contrast Medium

The contrast medium, by filling the coronary arteries, increases the difference in attenuation between the lumen and the wall of the vessel and enables a precise analysis of the size of the lumen and of any stenosis. This is made possible by increasing the density of the contained blood, or blood mixed with contrast medium; in fact, we pass from a value of density of the blood of 40-50 Hounsfield units to a value of 300-500 units during the passage of contrast medium (0 units Hounsfield for the density of water, 1000 for the compact bone, -1000 for the air). The greater the density of the contents of the coronary arteries during the acquisition of images, the higher their quality (Fig. 5.4). The contrast medium, with a high concentration of iodine (about 70-80 ml for 64-slice and 45-55 ml for 128-slice CT), is injected intravenously, followed by a bolus of saline solution (about 50-70 ml). The contrast is administered using an automatic, double-head injector in which the two syringes containing contrast and saline solution respectively are connected together using a Y connector, equipped with a one-way valve to prevent reflux. The injection of the contrast liquid can be performed at different flow rates: normally the injection rate varies from 3 to 5 ml per second.

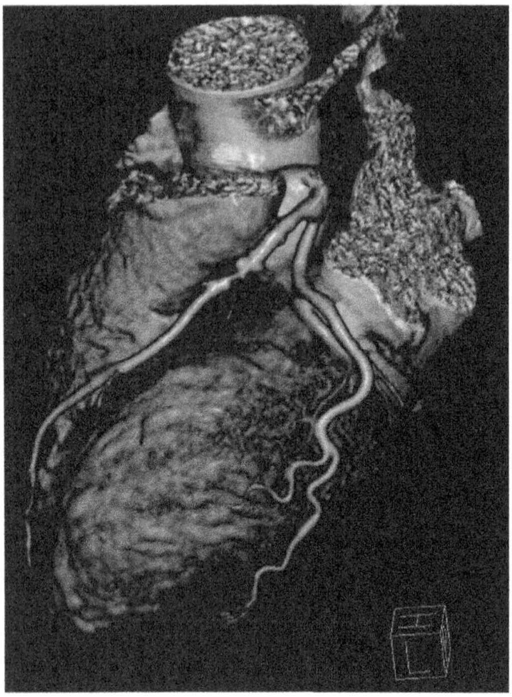

Fig. 5.5 CT image of the coronary arteries is a three-dimensional imaging technique

5.2.3 Heart Rate Synchronization

Data acquisition is carried out by the scanner during the transit of the contrast medium at the level of the coronary arteries. These data, which are processed for the reconstruction of images at the end of the acquisition, are acquired with the technique of *heart rate synchronization*. In other words, the CT scanner acquires the radiological data and the electrocardiogram of the patient simultaneously. At the end of the examination, the computer reconstructs the images, processing them only in a specific phase of the cardiac cycle, the end-diastole, when the coronary arteries are considerably filled with contrast medium. For the 128-slice CT scanner, the end-diastolic volume of each phase is approximately 4 cm: for a complete acquisition, we need data that roughly correspond to 4-5 end-diastolic phases to obtain the entire heart volume; in other words, the complete picture of the heart corresponds to the addition of many individual images and individual volumes that each correspond to a different end-diastolic phase. To obtain images only in a specific phase of the cardiac cycle is necessary, however, that there is a temporal *coherence*. In other words, the same structure must be acquired in different cardiac cycles, at the same instant. To do this, we require an electrocardiographic gating to synchronise image acquisition with the QRS complex. In addition, with the electrocardiographic signal, we can modulate, in the acquisition phase, the dose of radiation for the patient, by increasing the dose itself in late diastole and decreasing it in systole: in this way we obtain a better signal-noise ratio where necessary, applying the principles radiation protection.

5.3 Three-dimensional Images

Computed tomography of the coronary arteries is a three-dimensional imaging technique (Fig. 5.5). Information obtained during the acquisition is processed by the operator at the console: they are the result of different spatial planes, the coronary arteries and all the structures analysed.

5.3.1 Planimetric Techniques

As soon as the scanner acquires data corresponding to the anatomical heart shadow, the first display that appears is a series of axial images of 1 mm thickness or less, contiguous to each other.

5.3.1.1 Multiplanar Reformatting (MPR)

From the volume obtained with the scanning is possible to reconstruct the image in different spatial planes (Fig. 5.6). The more often used plans are the axial (head-foot), the coronal (sternum-vertebral) and the sagittal plan (right-left). Thus, we have the possibility of obtaining, in the same plan, structures which in reality are not anatomically located in a same plan, such as the vessels that, in their course, go through several floors. This mode is called *curved MPR* and is exceptionally useful in the study of the coronary arteries. This is achieved by pointing the cursor at the beginning of a structure (for example, an artery), displayed on the axial, coronal or sagittal plan, and follows its course within a volumetric image, positioning the cursor

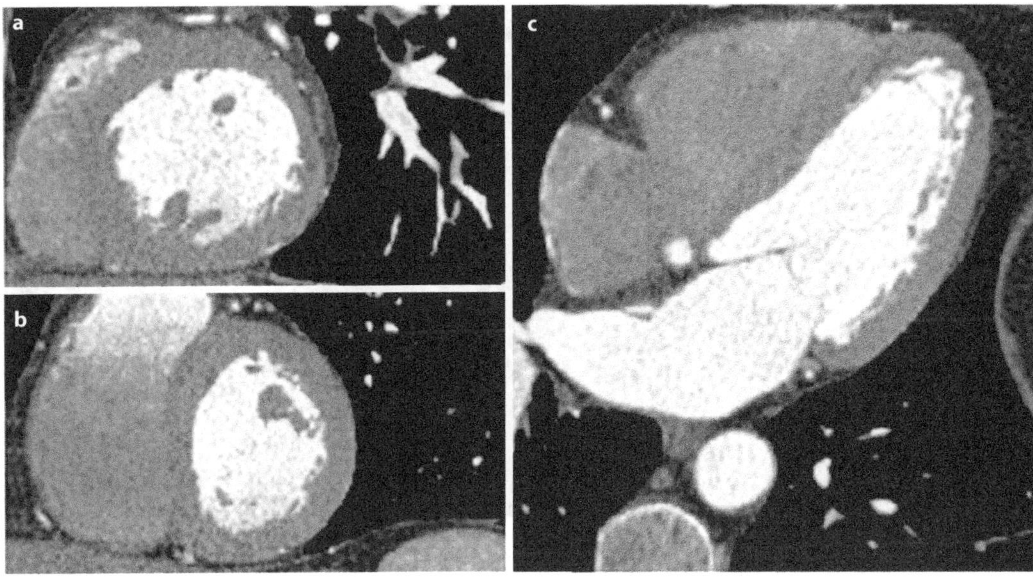

Fig. 5.6 Planimetric analysis (multiplanar reformatting, MPR). Reconstruction of images along the three planes of the space. a,b short-axis sagittal and coronary plane; c long-axis axial plane

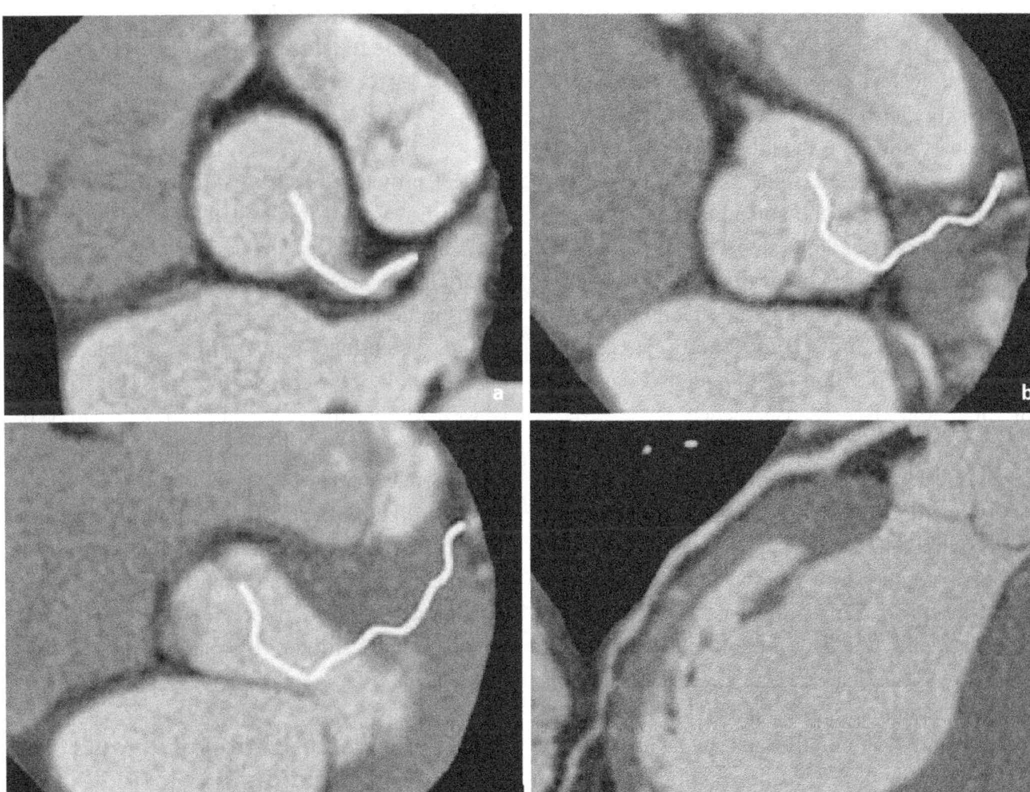

Fig. 5.7 Reconstruction of the image of a coronary artery on a curved plane; a-c each section is evaluated and the cursor is positioned at the centre of the vessel, being visualized since it is opacified from the contrast medium; d the combination of all sections is reconstituted as a curved planar image that contains the vessel in the interior

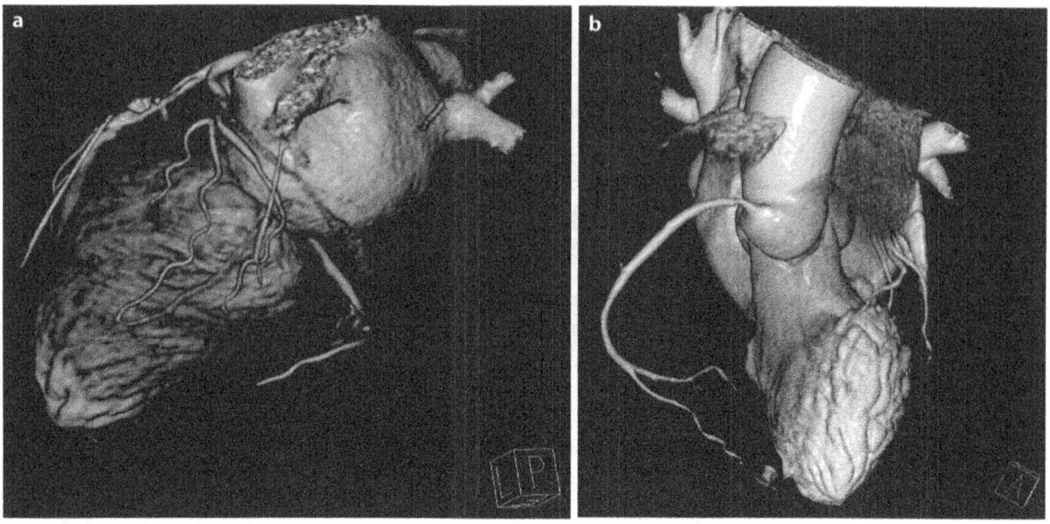

Fig. 5.8 a,b Volume rendering. 3D model in which all structures are visualized separately (arteries, veins, heart)

in the centre of the vessel and moving from section to section, on a plane in cranio-caudal direction (Fig. 5.7). The image that is obtained is a flat image, rectilinear, of a structure which in reality is curved (Fig. 5.7d). This planimetric image of single coronary arteries is the most important in defining the vascular lumen (light, as opacified by contrast medium) from the surrounding fatty tissue (dark, because the low density) and the myocardium (intermediate density). In addition you may better see the vascular wall that appears even more evident if affected by atherosclerotic disease, both with fibrolipidic (hypodense, dark) and calcific plaque (hyperdense, clear).

5.3.1.2 Volume Rendering (VR)

Using this mode of representation, each piece of data acquired has an assigned color, brilliance and transparency depending on the density and its location in space. This allows us to create a 3D model in which the different structures (arteries, veins, myocardium) can be viewed individually, separated from each other in a spatially coherent structure and similar to the anatomical image (Fig. 5.8 a,b). This method of reconstruction is very useful to get an overall picture of the coronary tree, particularly in patients with aorto-coronary bypass: it allow us to precisely define the number and location of the grafts (Fig. 5.9 a,b).

5.4 Coronary Arteries CT: Identification and Characterization of Atherosclerotic Plaque

The CT provides, for the first time in the history of the cardiovascular imaging, the opportunity to acquire anatomical data concerning the coronary artery in a non-invasive way and with high diagnostic resolution. The invasive coronary angiography, in fact, is a luminogram and it is not able to evaluate the wall of the coronary arteries (Fig. 5.10). It is well known that even large plaques may develop within the vessel wall without protruding into the lumen, because of the so-called *positive remodeling*. Unlike the coronary angiography, the CT is able to detect even subclinical plaques and wall lesions which do not protrude into the lumen and are asymptomatic. Furthermore, CT is able to differentiate the composition of the plaques.

5.4.1 Characterization of Plaque: Fibrolipidic and Calcified Plaque

The direct visualization of atherosclerotic plaque allows us to characterize it in relation to the different density taking its components. We can differ-

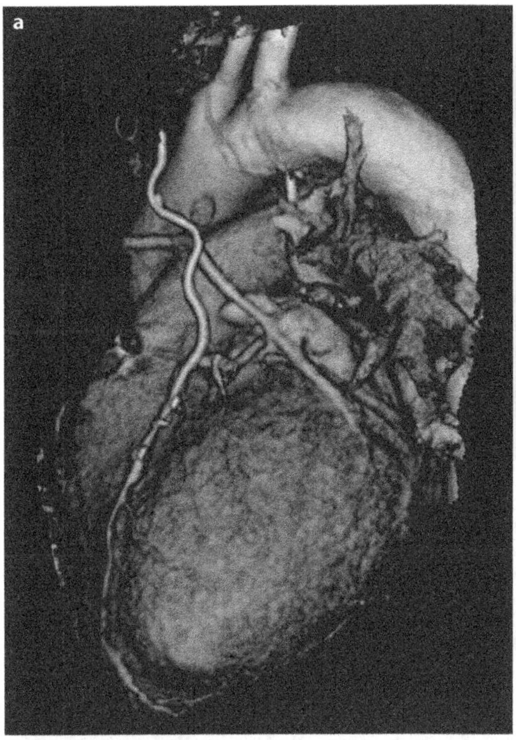

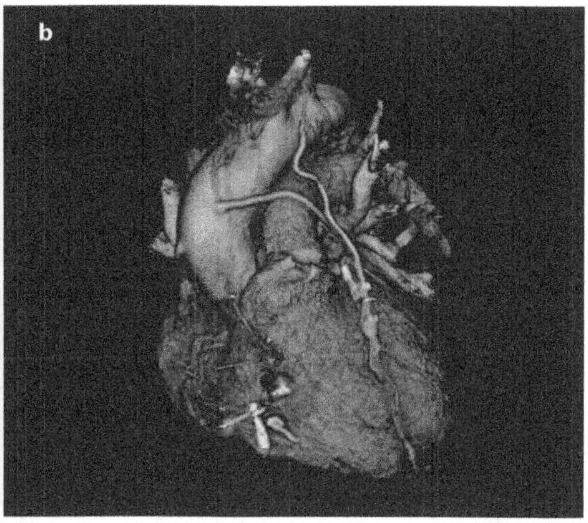

Fig. 5.9 a,b Patient with aorto-coronary by-pass. The volume rendering technique is very useful to obtain information on the number and position of venous artery grafts (a) and venous grafts (b)

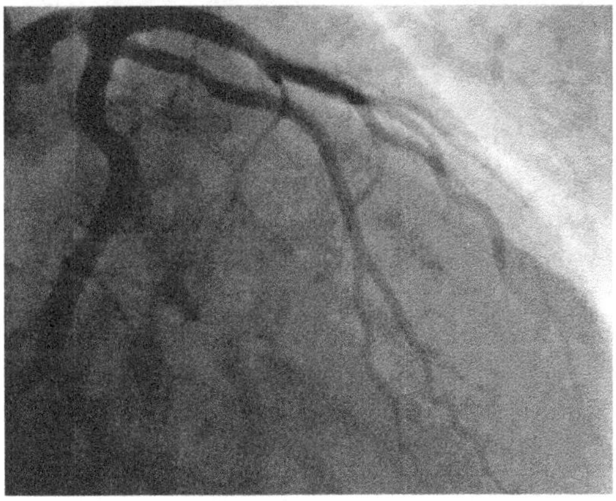

Fig. 5.10 Coronagraphy is a luminogram in which it is not possible to visualise the artery walls but only the internal lumen filled with the contrast medium

entiate atherosclerotic plaques in fat (very low density, less than 0 Hounsfield units), predominantly fibrous plaques (medium-density low, around 20-30 Hounsfield units) and calcified plaques, with very high density, clearly hyperdense and light (density greater than 300-500 Hounsfield units) (Fig. 5.11 a-d).

The atherosclerotic disease has a progressive course and includes inflammatory processes of the wall leading to activation of several molecules in the blood stream. In general, the formation of calcium occurs when the atheromatous plaque is already formed and consequently is found in the more advanced and stabilized lesions. It is often displayed as parietal calcified nodules, eccentric, often almost extraluminal (Fig. 5.12). On the other hand, the presence of a fibrolipidic plaque can mean that the atherosclerotic process is still in progress and the presence of *vulnerable plaques* can lead to the onset of myocardial infarction (Fig. 5.13). Coronary CT, therefore, has the task to view and characterize this type of plaque to prevent with pharmacological and/or invasive (angioplasty) interventions the occurrence of acute events. Finally, there are *mixed* plaques, with a calcified component, more often central, with a shell, or a fibrolipidic cap, which represents the component of active arteriosclerotic disease. This type of plaque can fit in the group of vulnerable plaques, because their fibrolipidic cap could become thinner and thinner until the rupture, resulting in an acute coronary event.

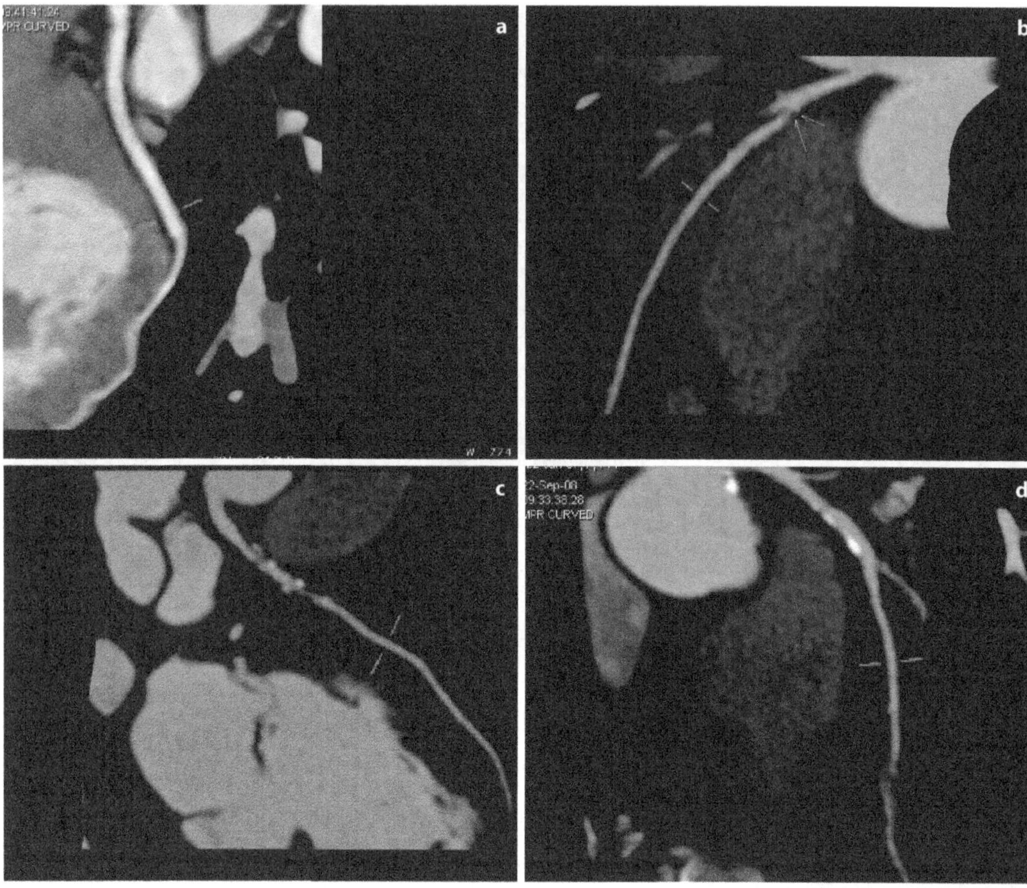

Fig. 5.11 a Coronary artery with no stenosis; b lipidic plaque at the ostium of the anterior descending artery; c fibrolipidic or mixed plaque in the proximal tract of the anterior descending artery; d calcific plaque in the medium tract of the circumflex artery

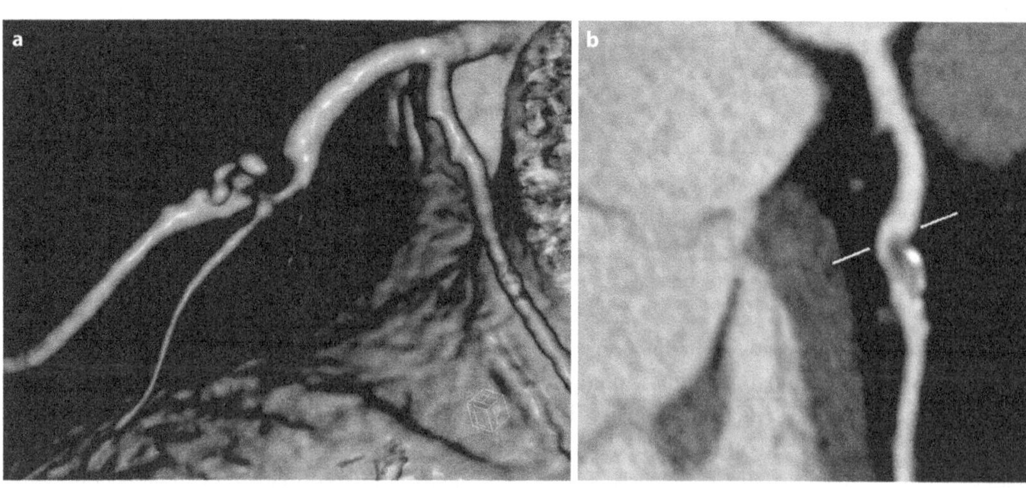

Fig. 5.12 a Ulcerated plaque of the anterior descending artery; b calcific parietal nodules appear as eccentric, often almost extraluminal

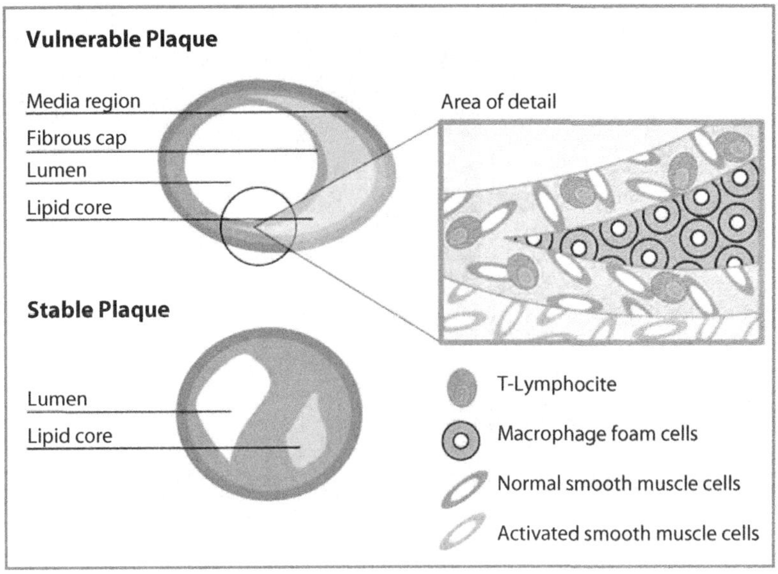

Fig. 5.13 The *stable* plaque and *vulnerable* plaque, with differing cellular compositions

5.4.2 Assessment of Plaque During Medical Therapy

CT can not only identify and characterize coronary atherosclerotic plaques, but also can follow the temporal evolution of the disease. Medical therapy, with antiplatelet drugs and high dose statins, can lead, over time, to a reduction of the volume and the extent of atherosclerotic plaques. We understand, therefore, what might be the importance of this non-invasive technique in the follow-up of patients with non significant coronary plaques or of patients who still underwent to coronary angioplasty or by-pass graft surgery.

5.4.3 Coronary Stenoses and Occlusions

The next step in the identification and characterization of atherosclerotic coronary plaques is the determination of the reduction of the diameter and area of the vessel lumen. This is done initially with three-dimensional technique, which gives an overview, and then with planimetric multiplanar reconstruction technique. The degree of reduction of the calibre of the lumen is generally measured as a percentage compared to the size of the normal vessel (calibre of reference), upstream of the plaque. If the reduction of calibre is above 70% there is a great reduction of flow, such as to determine a reduction in oxygen supply to the myocardium, with possible development of anginal symptoms. The main purpose of coronary CT is, therefore, to select patients to be sent to interventional and invasive cardiologists. The high sensitivity of the method for the diagnosis of significant coronary stenosis should ensure that a high percentage of patients, who previously underwent CT, are appropriately sent to perform a coronary angiography or can be directly treated with percutaneous angioplasty with or without stent implantation. In these patients, the coronary CT provides a preview to the interventional cardiologist, who will schedule possible interventional procedures with savings in execution time of the examination (for example, a stenosis involving the bifurcation between anterior descending artery and the first diagonal branch which provides a special procedure, more complex, aiming not at sacrificing the diagonal branch). In other words, invasive coronary angiography seems to have become increasingly more therapeutic and less diagnostic. In conclusion, we can imagine a new scenario in the diagnostic iter of patients with suspected coronary artery disease: after a non diagnostic functional test (for example, the presence of chest pain in the absence of changes in the electrocardiogram

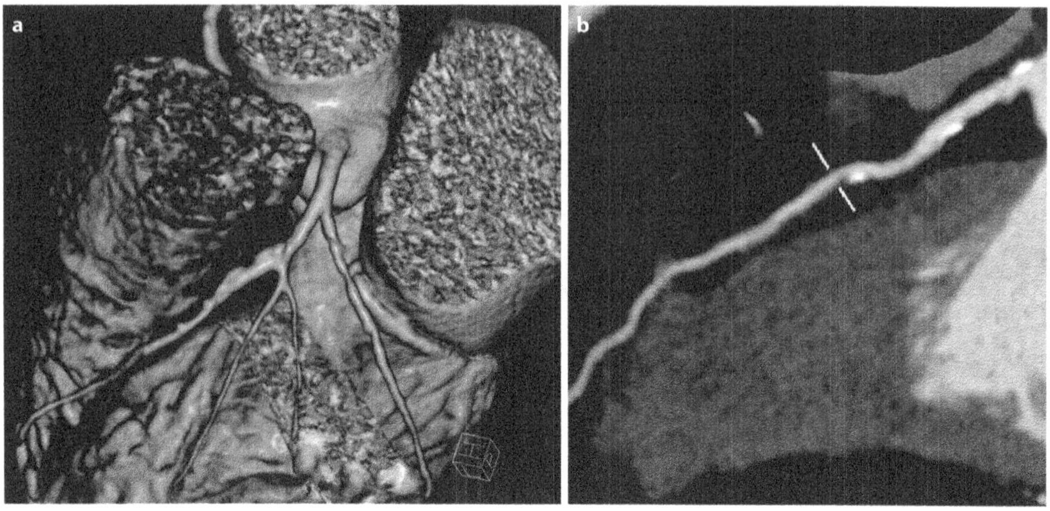

Fig. 5.14 a Extensive atherosclerotic disease with intensely calcific plaques; blooming effect

or non-diagnostic EKG changes at exercise test in the absence of chest pain) a coronary CT could be scheduled. If this examination reveals the presence of normal coronary arteries (negative predictive value close to 100%), we can rule out coronary artery disease and the patient can be followed simply to correct any risk factors. If the CT shows the presence of significant stenosis (reduction of the lumen >50%) the patient will be sent directly to the cathlab to undergo percutaneous angioplasty with or without stenting. Finally, if the CT scan revealed no significant stenosis, which obstructs the vessel lumen <50%, a rigorous preventive programme to reduce risk factors will be established and it will represent a preventive preclinical phase, before the acute event.

5.4.4 Calcified Plaques: Problems in the Definition of Stenosis

Calcium is pathognomonic of coronary atherosclerosis: its presence is common in patients with coronary artery lesions. An important problem is to quantify the degree of stenosis of these plaques. The calcification of the atherosclerotic plaque determines an effect, defined *blooming*, in which the volume of the plaque displayed in the image reconstructed with bi-or three-dimensional techniques is amplified with respect to what it is in the reality. This type of artefact occurs also with metal objects, for example with the wires of the pacemaker, which appear as bright streaks with exceeded real size. Calcifications, which have very high density, create artefacts that make the plaque more voluminous, with possible overestimation of the stenosis (Fig. 5.14 a,b).

5.4.5 Significant Stenosis

Atherosclerotic plaques that cause significant stenosis grade may be concentric or eccentric. For the exact analysis of these plaques is necessary to make the three-dimensional analysis on the three planes of the space, which allows to better evaluate the degree of reduction of the lumen. Another important aspect in the definition of atherosclerotic disease is to define the extent of the plaques on the three major epicardial vessels. The extension of the atherosclerotic disease in more coronary vessels is an important element of the clinical relevance of the disease and its possible treatment.

5.4.6 Remodeling

The presence of an atherosclerotic plaque does not necessarily mean that it should be a consensual

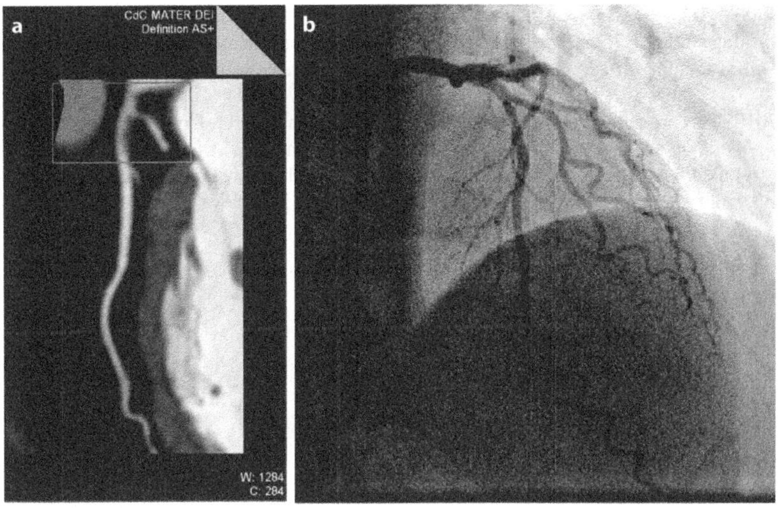

Fig. 5.15 Vascular remodeling. **a** CT imaging shows the presence of an eccentric marginal lipidic plaque (*arrows*); **b** coronagraphy shows a normal vessel without appreciable stenosis (*arrow*)

stenosis of vessel lumen. In fact, the coronary arteries are able to remodel themselves: we can have a plaque with large volume, without reducing significantly the vascular lumen (Fig. 5.15 a,b). In these cases the atherosclerotic plaque is increased within the vessel wall (positive remodeling), maintaining the normal size of vessel lumen. Thus, during the CT evaluation it is necessary to accurately measure the vessel upstream of the plaque, where the vessel is free from disease, to determine whether there is a remodeling which could make the plaque stenosis of a significant or non-significant grade.

5.4.7 Coronary Occlusion and Collateral Circulation

Failure of the display of a section of artery downstream of an atherosclerotic plaque, often with characteristics of calcification, is diagnostic of coronary occlusion. Coronary heart disease is, as already mentioned, a slowly progressive disease, so if a coronary artery is totally occluded, over time it creates collateral, albeit partially compared with normal vessels that allow it to bring the blood to the surrounding myocardial tissue. Generally they are very thin vessels that are created at the level of myocardial peripheral branches, whose cells undergo hypertrophy and hyperplasia and create a flow of blood with reverse flow in the direction of the not perfused area. Being very thin vessels, they often do not appear at least during invasive coronary angiography. With CT, the diagnosis of collateral circulation is often done in an indirect way: if we see an occluded vessel that re-inhabits further downstream, we can assume that there is developed enough collateral circulation, that allows the opacification of the occluded vessel downstream. Sometimes, the collateral circulation is highly developed and winding and it appears as a *corkscrew*. In conclusion, the collateral circulation may also develop from the same occluded coronary artery (omocoronaric circle) with thin peripheral vessels that provide blood flow immediately downstream of the occlusion of the vessel itself.

Suggested Reading

Brenner DJ, Hall EJ (2007) Computed tomography. An increase source of radiation exposure. N Engl J Med 357:2277-2284

Budoff MJ, Shinbane JS (2006) Cardiac CT imaging: diagnosis of cardiovascular disease. Springer, Berlin Heidelberg New York

Cademartiri F, Mollet N, Midiri M (2007) La TC del cuore nella pratica clinica. Springer, Milano

Chiurlia E, Menozzi M, Ratti C (2005) Follow-up of coronary artery bypass graft patency by multi-slice computed tomography. Am J Cardiol 95:1094-1097

Feuchtner GM, Cury RC, Jodocy D (2011) Differences in coronary plaque composition by noninvasive computed tomography angiography in individuals with and without obstructive coronary artery disease. Atherosclerosis 215(1):90-95

Gauss S, Achenbach S, Pflederer T (2011) Assessment of coronary artery remodeling by dual-source CT: a head-to-head comparison with intravascular ultrasound. Heart 97(12): 991-997

Maffei E, Seitun S, Martini C (2010) CT coronary angiography and exercise ECG in a population with chest pain and low-to-intermediate pre-test likelihood of coronary artery disease. Heart 96(24):1973-1979

Sun J, Zhang Z, Lu B (2008) Identification and quantification of coronary atherosclerotic plaques: a comparison of 64-MDCT and intravascular ultrasound. AJR Am Roentgenol 190(3):748-754

Voros S, Rinehart S, Qian Z (2011) Coronary Atherosclerosis Imaging by Coronary CT Angiography Current Status, Correlation With Intravascular Interrogation and Meta-Analysis. JACC Cardiovasc Imaging 4(5):537-48

Cardiac MR

6

Leda Galiuto, Gabriella Locorotondo and Elisa Fedele

6.1 Introduction

Magnetic Resonance (MR) is a multi-planar imaging technique, which exploits magnetic fields and radio-frequency (RF) pulses in order to perform anatomic and tissue assessment of body structures. Cardiac Magnetic Resonance (cMR) has gained a prominent role in the diagnosis and management of cardiovascular system diseases, due to the possibility of combining detailed anatomical images, obtained by scanning different planes of space, with the functional evaluation of the heart. Despite high costs and time-consuming scanning processes, cMR is now of great importance in sports cardiology, because of the pressing need not only to confirm cardiovascular disease assessed by echocardiography but mainly in order to identify apparently healthy subjects, in whom severe cardiomyopathy is latent, which carries the risk of death during physical effort. The clinical indications for cMR have recently been defined by Consensus Panel Report [1].

6.2 Basic Principles of Cardiac Magnetic Resonance

Image processing is based on the *magnetic resonance* phenomenon: each atomic nucleus generates an intrinsic magnetic field that can interact with an applied external magnetic field [2]. Many atomic nuclei exhibit the phenomenon of magnetic resonance, such as hydrogen (^{1}H), carbon (^{13}C), sodium (^{23}Na), phosphorus (^{31}P) and fluorine (^{19}F). However, despite the availability of a large number of chemical elements, the ^{1}H nucleus is preferred in clinical practice owing to its simple chemical structure (comprising one proton) and its widespread availability in water, fat and other biochemical compounds in the human body. The ^{1}H nucleus is able to rotate on itself at high speed, generating an intrinsic magnetic field with its own direction and orientation (*spin*). When placed in a magnetic field (M_z), spins rotate on their own axis, aligning themselves to Mz and behaving like small spinning magnets. In such way, they perform a rotational movement called *precession* (Fig. 6.1). The number of rotational movements around the axis of the magnetic field per unit of time is defined as *precessional frequency*, or *Larmor frequency*, which is correlated with the kind of atomic nuclei and the intensity of applied magnetic field. In the setting of cardiovascular medicine, the intensity of the main magnetic field is 1.5 Tesla (1 Tesla = 10,000 Gauss), which corresponds to an intensity 30,000-60,000 times greater than the magnetic field of the earth. Moreover, despite the availability of higher-intensity magnetic fields (3 Tesla), which can improve signal-to-noise ratio, these systems are not actually used due to the significant risk of radiation absorption.

When all spins precess along the direction of the main magnetic field (*longitudinal magnetization*), the whole system enjoys a state of equilibrium and net MR signal is thus nil. Conversely, when a (RF) pulse with the same frequency as the Larmor frequency is applied perpendicularly to the main magnetic field, the protons flip into the transverse plane

L. Galiuto (✉)
Medicine and Surgery
Università Cattolica del Sacro Cuore
Rome, Italy

M. Fioranelli and G. Frajese (eds.), *Sports Cardiology*,
DOI: 10.1007/978-88-470-2775-6_6, © Springer-Verlag Italia 2012

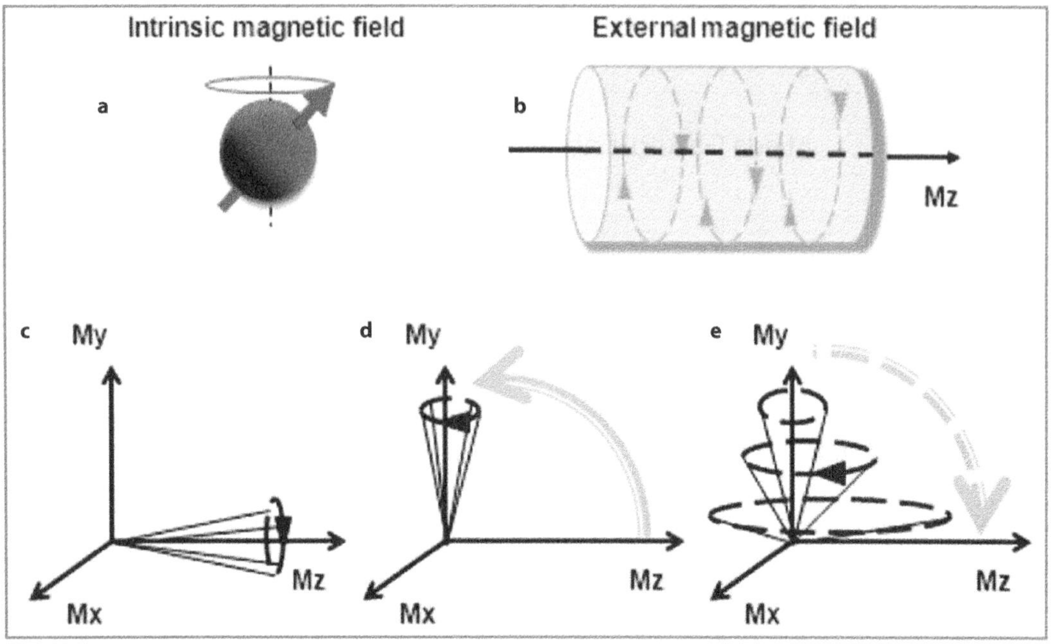

Fig. 6.1 The *Magnetic Resonance phenomenon*: panel a shows the atomic hydrogenous nucleus (^1H), which rotates on its own axis, generating an intrinsic magnetic field; panel b shows how electricity, flowing through coils of a superconductive magnet, provides the main magnetic field. If protons are positioned within the main magnetic field, they rotate in the direction of the magnetic field (*Mz*) (c); the application of a radiofrequency (*RF*) pulse at 90° to the main magnetic field results in a shift of the main magnetization vector towards a plane perpendicular to Mz (d); when the 90° pulse is turned off, protons lose the transversal component of their magnetization and begin a precession movement toward the balanced position

(M_{xy}) (*transversal magnetization*) (Fig. 6.1). The higher the intensity and duration of this RF pulse, the further the magnetization vector moves towards the transversal plane. If the RF pulse is stopped, the excited protons return to their original state of equilibrium within the main magnetic field by releasing gained energy through free precession. This phenomenon, called *free induction decay* (*FID*), occurs in a period of time defined as *relaxation time* (T). There are two different types of T: *T1*, which represents the longitudinal relaxation time and depends on interaction between protons and surrounding environment; and *T2*, which represents the transversal relaxation time, resulting from the interactions between close protons, and is usually $<$T1.

MR signal intensity depends on 3 different parameters:

- proton density, which is indicative of ^1H content (i.e. water content, H_2O) per unit of tissue volume;
- T1 and T2, which are related to the tissue type and its molecular composition: fat is characterized by a short T1 and T2, while free water causes long T1 and T2. Moreover, higher the content of bound water in tissues (i.e. muscle tissue), the shorter T2 is compared to T1, so that T2/T1 < 1;
- T2/T1 ratio.

Spin signals are located within a three-dimensional space, thanks to the introduction of field gradients along three different spatial directions (i.e. z, y and x axes): each point along these axes has a specific degree of magnetization [3]. Therefore, the signal detected by each point is analysed and mathematically revized using *Fourier Transform*.

6.3 Technical Instruments

CMR imaging scans require complex technical instruments, particularly MR tomography equipment, which consists of the following components:

- a magnet, which creates the main magnetic field. It is usually made from superconductive materials: this means that, when electricity flows within coils, it generates a very strong magnetic field without resistance;
- a RF pulse transmitter;
- a receiver coil, capable of detecting the MR signal;
- three external coils, which generate field gradients;
- a computer system, capable of amplifying, elaborating and digitising the MR signal.

Moreover, high quality images are derived from different correction systems (*shim*) applied during both the construction and the utilization phases of the magnet, in order to ensure homogeneity of the magnetic field and correct potential heterogeneities. Cardiac movements greatly affect image quality, producing a large number of artefacts. Thus, an *electrocardiographic gating* system has been introduced, which aims to reduce these errors. It works by synchronising MR pulses to cardiac cycle phases.

6.4 Principal Imaging Sequences Used in cMR

A complete cMR scan is mainly based on the following imaging sequences:

- *spin echo* (SE) sequences, also called *black-blood* or static sequences;
- *gradient echo* (GRE) sequences, also called *white-blood* or dynamic sequences.

SE images are derived from the application of an initial 90° RF pulse that shifts the main magnetization vector into the transversal plane. However, after the interruption of this RF pulse, MR signals are rapidly weakened because spins tend to dephase. Then a second 180° RF pulse refocuses signals, producing detectable echoes. In SE sequences the blood typically appears as hypointense compared to adjacent tissues, because it can be reached only by the initial RF pulse during its movement across the exited region, and flows out of the selected slice at the time of second RF pulse (Fig. 6.2).

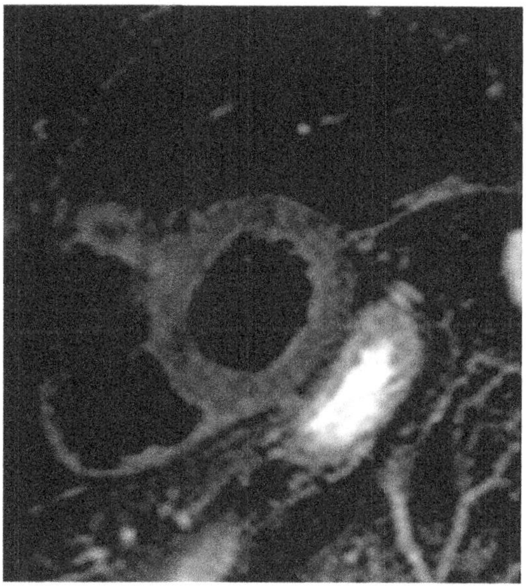

Fig. 6.2 Short-axis view image acquired during a *spin echo* sequence: the blood signal is completely null (*black-blood* sequence), while the cardiac muscle shows moderate intensity signal

The time interval between two subsequent pulsing sequences (*repetition time*) corresponds to a single cardiac cycle (1 R-R interval) in T1-weighted images: fat appears hyperintense, while cardiac muscle tissue is of intermediate intensity. However, the *repetition time* in T2-weighted images involves two or more cardiac cycles (2 R-R intervals), resulting in the visualization of moderately intense fatty tissue and hypo-intense cardiac muscle tissue.

The GRE sequences enable dynamic evaluation of the beating heart, thanks to the possibility of recording both the systolic and diastolic frames (*cine* sequences) throughout an entire cardiac cycle. In particular, the excitation process relies on the delivery of multiple RF pulses with a very short repetition time: the blood, receiving a series of subsequent pulses, typically appears hyper-intense.

In order to optimise blood-tissue contrast, some *inversion recovery* (IR) pulses can be delivered prior to performing standard sequences. During the SE sequence, until three IR pulses (*triple IR*) can be released, it results in complete saturation of the fat signal in T1-weighted images and visualization of hyperintense tissue edema in T2-weighted acquisitions. Moreover, IR pulse application to GRE sequences is powerful to detect necrotic and fibrotic tissue that can be visualized as hyperintense areas compared with adjacent tissue, after the administration of a contrast agent.

The main contrast agent used in cMR is gadolinium: it can be injected into peripheral veins and enables a reduction of T1 blood from 1,200 ms to 100 ms.

6.5 Scan Planes and Views in cMR

Cardiac evaluation by cMR consists of scanning different planes along the three axes of the space and the two main axes of the heart. Because of patient-to-patient anatomic variation (with the heart lying at an arbitrary angle compared to scanner coordinates), the early images, called *scouts*, are acquired along standard orthogonal planes (axial, coronal and sagittal) in order to assess the orientation of the heart axes. By using these orthogonal planes as locators, double oblique views are acquired along the long and short axes of the heart: horizontal long-axis, vertical long-axis and short-axis views. The acquisition planes are placed at about 90° to each other. Moreover, several short-axis slices can be scanned at the basal, medium and apical level. In addition to the standard protocol, assessment of the right ventricular outflow tract (RVOT) and the morphological evaluation of intra- or para-cardiac masses, the pericardium, mediastinum, superior and inferior vena cava, pulmonary veins and coronary arteries (coronary MR imaging) are made possible by acquiring other cardiac planes.

6.6 Study of Morphology, Function, Perfusion and Viability of the Heart

The morphologic evaluation of the heart is performed by *black-blood SE* sequences. In fact, their high spatial resolution (1-1.5 mm) makes the prompt assessment of cardiac and vascular structural abnormalities, as well as congenital heart diseases or cardiac wall abnormalities, reliable. Instead, studies of cardiac function are achieved by using *white-blood GRE* sequences, which show a clear definition of the endocardial border. Thanks to the possibility of accurately delineating endocardial borders, these sequences are used to estimate the thickness of the interventricular septum and posterior ventricular wall, as well as the end-diastolic diameter of the left ventricle and the diameter of the right ventricular inflow and outflow tracts. During *cine GRE* sequences, the whole cardiac cycle is usually scanned by a series of 15-30 consecutive frames for each slice. The estimation of left ventricular volumes relies on the measurement of the area of each ventricular slice, from the base to the apex, encompassing the entire left ventricle. Each area is assessed by tracing sub-endocardial borders at both end-systole and end-diastole, multiplied by the slice thickness, in order to obtain the slice volume. The sum of all slice volumes enables an estimation of the end-diastolic and end-systolic left ventricular volumes, as well as the ejection fraction, without geometric assumptions. The same algorithm can be used for assessing the right ventricle. Furthermore, in addition to the study of overall left ventricular function, cMR enables analysis of regional contractile function, based on a 17 segment model, in which the last one (apex) is evaluated only in long-axis views.

The evaluation of diastolic function is derived by flow analysis during *Phase Contrast* (PC) sequences: after tracing vessel contours or selecting a region of interest, dedicated software automatically analyses the signals of blood flow crossing this area over time and extrapolates a flow curve. Moreover, the *tagging* modality has been recently introduced, which is able to show movements of the left ventricular wall (i.e. rotation, relaxation, shortening or torsion) during the cardiac cycle, thanks to an analysis of demagnetization lines.

Nowadays, cMR is valid for the detection of myocardial perfusion at rest and during stress. For this purpose, the administration of a venous contrast agent (i.e. gadolinium) has to be matched by the execution of peculiar T1-weighted GRE sequences, preceded by saturation recovery preparation pulses. Stacks of short-axis slices (6-8 mm thickness), show, following a dye injection, the physiological gadolinium route, which first fills the right ventricle and then the left ventricle and coronary circulation. Therefore, myocardial perfusion is evaluated by visualising the initial passage

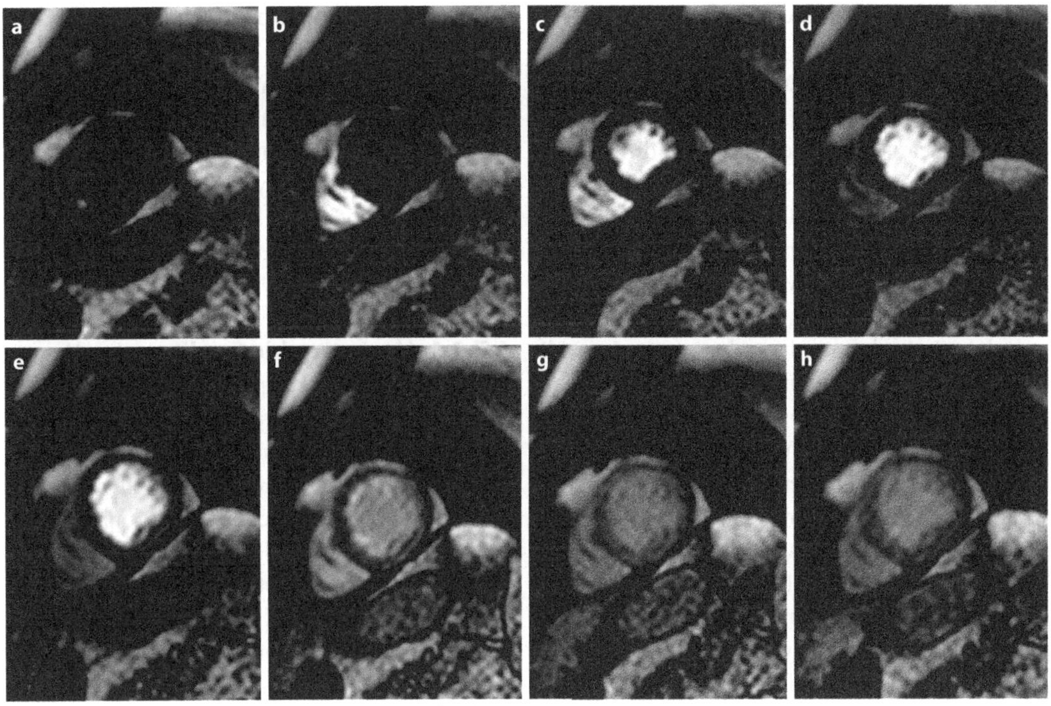

Fig. 6.3 A series of short-axis view images scanned during a *GRE* T1-weighted sequence at the time of the first pass of gadolinium. The images show the same slice, detected consecutively frame by frame, at a brief interval from each other (a-h). Gadolinium flows primarily within the right ventricle (a-b), and then in the left ventricle (c-e) as far as the coronary circulation (f-h)

of gadolinium within the coronary circulation, and, for this reason, such sequences are labelled as *first-pass sequences* (Fig. 6.3). The signal intensity of blood distribution is directly related to myocardial flow: a reduction of blood flow is visualized as a hypointense area, which can extend from endocardial to epicardial layers according to the severity of myocardial ischemia. The stress test is performed using pharmacologic vasodilator stimuli, such as adenosine or dipiridamole. Adenosine is usually preferred due to its short half-life and it is administered according to a standard protocol: the venous infusion of 140 mg/kg/min adenosine for at least 3 minutes is followed by the administration of 0.05-0.1 mmol/kg gadolinium and saline flush (20 ml at a flow rate of 2ml/sec). The evaluation of myocardial perfusion at rest is performed about 15 minutes after the end of the stress phase, in order to allow for complete contrast agent wash-out. Qualitative evaluation of the perfusion defect area implies creation of a regional perfusion map, called the *bulls-eye,* whereas a semi-quantitative method consists of the comparison of curves showing the pattern of signal intensity over time at rest and after stress. Conversely, the quantitative method, based on myocardial flow indexes, is rarely adopted in the assessment of myocardial perfusion.

Injection of gadolinium is followed, after 1-2 minutes, by contrast agent redistribution within the coronary microcirculation (*early enhancement*). Subsequently, gadolinium typically tends to flow out of the vessels and lie in the interstitial space, accumulating at the extravascular level. Necrotic muscle cells, characterized by sarcolemma rupture, capture gadolinium, which fixes within them with a slow *wash-out*. In the late stage (10-12 minutes after dye administration), GRE IR T1-weighted sequences (*delayed enhancement*) can detect necrotic or fibrotic tissue as a hyperintense area (*late enhancement*) compared to normal myocardium, which appears hypointense.

6.7 Clinical Use of cMR

6.7.1 Athlete's Heart

Athletes' hearts have been shown to differ from the hearts of non-athletes, due to the increase in volume and symmetrical thickening of the left ventricular walls: hypertrophy develops eccentrically and is associated with a mass increase [4]. Moreover, remodeling is not confined to the left ventricle. Indeed, both the right ventricular wall thickness and mass [5] and the left atrium, which dilates proportionally to left ventricular expansion and exercise duration, have been shown to increase: the result is an overall and balanced remodeling of the athlete's heart.

In the setting of sports medicine, cMR enables careful estimation of volumes, contractile function, wall thickness and myocardial mass for both ventricles. In particular, *SE T1-weighted* sequences, which are useful for morphological evaluation, are made by selecting short-axis slices at the end of the diastolic phase, while *cine GRE sequences,* acquired in the same view, aim to assess end-diastolic and end-systolic volumes and the myocardial mass of both ventricles.

The presence of *late enhancement* areas in athletes' hearts could adversely affect the long-term prognosis of subjects but its significance is actually under debate. In fact, only a minority of athletes show a sub-endocardial fibrosis pattern indicative of coronary disease. Moreover, the presence and extent of these late enhancement areas seem mainly to be related to exercise and duration, suggesting a probable role of physical activity in determining myocardial fibrosis, with or without obvious myocardial ischemia.

On the other hand, some clinical studies have demonstrated the occurrence of reverse cardiac remodeling in athletes who have stopped physical activity. Particularly, the majority of patients experienced a significant reduction in cavity size, wall thickness and left ventricular mass after long-term de-training. In some cases, however, the resolution of ventricular dilatation was incomplete, and this probably has an important clinical and prognostic significance [6].

6.7.2 Cardiomyopathies

MR plays an important role in diagnostic and long-term prognostic stratification of patients affected by different forms of cardiomyopathy, thanks to the possibility of accurately assessing heart morphology and helpfully identifying patients with a high risk of suffering from major cardiovascular events [7].

6.7.2.1 Hypertrophic Cardiomyopathy

Hypertrophic cardiomyopathy (HCM) is a complex myocardial disease, characterized by abnormal hypertrophy and hyperplasia of cardiac muscle cells, which results in varying degrees of left ventricular wall thickening. In particular, hypertrophy can homogeneously involve all left ventricular walls or can be limited to the septum or apex levels. Moreover, the appearance of intra-myocardial fibrotic tissue, in addition to myocardial hypertrophy, is a distinctive feature of this disease (see Chapter 19).

In the setting of hypertrophic cardiomyopathy, cMR is widely used for assessing heart morphology and function, for identifying typical intra-myocardial fibrotic patterns and apex hypertrophy, and for estimating myocardial mass. Moreover, it is also recommended in the follow-up of patients who have undergone partial myectomy or alcohol ablation of the interventricular septum.

Despite the presence of severe regional hypertrophy, total myocardial mass can be normal.

Black-blood sequences are used to check the distribution of hypertrophy in different planes, while *white-blood* sequences are powerful enough to estimate diastolic wall thickness and systolic thickening (Fig. 6.4), ventricular volumes and ejection fraction. Ventricular volumes may be normalized or reduced. Furthermore, evaluation of diastolic function relies on *PC* sequences or *tagging* methods, which can typically show the presence of reduced posterior rotation and a small radial distension of the inferoseptal wall. Notably, a clear differential diagnosis between pathological hypertrophy of HCM and physiological hypertrophy of an athlete's heart can be achieved by quantitative comparison of cMR data with geometric indexes [8]. Moreover, it has been shown that atrial volume is also correlated to cardiac per-

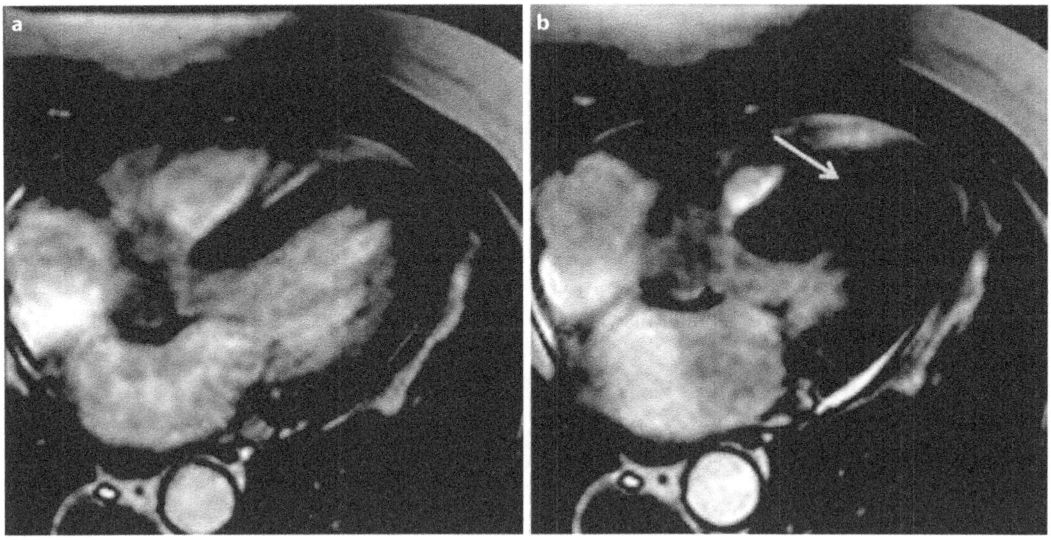

Fig. 6.4 Horizontal long-axis view images obtained during *cine white-blood* sequences in a patient with an apical variant of hypertrophic cardiomyopathy, in the end-diastolic (a) and end-systolic (b) phases: panel b clearly demonstrates the complete obliteration of the ventricular cavity during apical contraction (*arrow*)

formance indexes, suggesting its probable role in long-term prognostic stratification of patients [9].

Additionally, cMR provides a comprehensive assessment of fibrotic tissue distribution by using *delayed enhancement* sequences. Typically, myocardial fibrosis extends, with a focal or diffuse pattern, in the middle third of the left ventricular walls, mainly at the level of the right ventricle, to left ventricle insertion points. The appearance of fibrotic tissue in HCM is certainly not in keeping with the distribution territory of coronary arteries and, consequently, it can easily be distinguished from ischemic coronary disease. In most patients affected by HCM (more than 80%) hyper-enhancement areas, seem to be directly related to wall hypertrophy and inversely related to regional systolic thickening. In particular, they are considered to be the result of multiple factors, such as muscle cell disarray, the fibrotic replacement of the damaged myocardium and the establishment of focal microvascular ischemia. Moreover, several studies have successfully demonstrated that the entity and the extent of these areas are significantly correlated with long-term outcomes for patients, and consequently they can play a decisive role in the identification of patients at high risk of sudden cardiac death. T2-weighted sequences allow for detection of focal edemas in the same areas of fibrotic tissue, mainly in thickened segments.

Obstructive HCM is characterized by the systolic anterior movement (SAM) of the anterior mitral leaflet towards the antero-septal wall. This finding is detectable in horizontal long-axis views, in the left ventricular outflow tract (LVOT) view and in short axis slices through the valvular plane, perpendicularly to LVOT. Moreover, in patients with obstructive HCM, cine GRE sequences can reveal the presence of hypointense turbulent flow in the sub-valvular aortic region during blood ejection. The smallest area between the anterior mitral leaflet and inter-ventricular septum, as visualized in the short-axis view during the systolic phase, can be used as an index of the severity of obstruction, due to its independence from preload.

6.7.2.2 Dilated Cardiomyopathy

Dilated cardiomyopathy (DCM) is a worsening muscle disease characterized by progressive enlargement of cardiac chambers and the deterioration of contractile function, both of which are related to gradual muscle cell replacement by interstitial fibrotic tissue.

MR, by exploiting the properties of *cine white-blood* sequences, allows for careful evaluation of the volumes and function of the left ventricle, in addition to a precise estimation of wall thickness (which can usually be normal or reduced) and regional systolic thickening. *Black-blood* sequences are also able to detect the increase in cavity size and wall thinning, but with contrast levels between myocardium and blood lower than those provided by GRE sequences. Assessment of the morphology and function of the right ventricle, and the size of both atrial and valvular diseases, is also required. In the setting of DCM, the execution of *PC* sequences is helpful to identify diastolic dysfunction of both the right and left ventricles. Additionally, *delayed enhancement* evaluation can show different patterns:

- areas of mid-wall late enhancement, caused by a progressive increase of interstitial fibrotic tissue, particularly in peripheral myocardial cells lying within the interventricular septum (28% of cases);
- completely absent *late enhancement* (59% of cases).

It should be noted that about 13% of patients with a clinical suspicion of DCM have some *late enhancement* areas, which resemble the typical appearance of ischemic heart disease, resulting from coronary artery occlusion. In order to distinguish between DCM and ischemic heart disease, cMR is a useful tool for visualising the distribution pattern of a necrotic myocardium [10]. Instead, in patients with an established diagnosis of DCM, the entity and the extent of mid-wall interstitial fibrotic tissue are predictors of long-term cardiovascular events [11]. Nowadays, cMR is greatly taken into consideration for follow-up evaluation too, because the occurrence of small changes in cardiac volumes and the ejection fraction can be identified with a diagnostic accuracy rate that is higher than that of other imaging methods.

6.7.2.3 Restrictive Cardiomyopathy

Restrictive cardiomyopathy (RCM) is a rare myocardial disease, characterized by considerable impairment of ventricular filling with reduced ventricular volumes. Although systolic function is preserved, the main abnormality is severe diastolic dysfunction, which results in atrial dilatation and venous stasis.

In the setting of RCM, heart chamber morphology is usually evaluated by means of *black-blood* sequences: enlargement of both atria with possible right ventricular dilatation due to severe pulmonary hypertension is a typical finding. In addition, some cases are also characterized by atrial thrombi, and *cine white-blood* sequences are performed to estimate the left ventricular ejection fraction (which sometimes is reduced) and to evaluate the concomitant presence of mitral disease. Moreover, left ventricle size and wall thickness are measured on *GRE* images, by using short- and long-axis views.

Due to the similar clinical presentation, RCM can require differential diagnosis with constrictive pericarditis. Constrictive pericarditis can be clearly distinguished on the basis of pericardial thickening (more than 4 mm), which is assessed using Gradient-echo sequences. However, some clinical cases of constrictive pericarditis can be associated with normal pericardial thickness: in this case, specific *GRE real time* sequences enable abnormal movements of the interventricular septum to be revealed during different phases of breathing, since it typically becomes flat or concave during early breathing in and returns convex during breathing out. Obviously, these abnormal movements are not present in RCM.

6.7.2.4 Arrhythmogenic Right Ventricular Dysplasia

Arrhythmogenic Right Ventricular Dysplasia (ARVD) is a complex disease of unknown origin, characterized by the progressive apoptotic degeneration of cardiac muscle cells, which are gradually replaced by fibrotic and fatty tissue. In particular, this replacement process begins in the sub-epicardial layer and progresses to the sub-endocardial layer, finally becoming transmural. Myocardial atrophy can appear focal or diffuse and is mainly located within the outer two-thirds of the right ventricular wall. Similarly, at times, the left ventricle is also involved in the myocardial degeneration process. Therefore, these tissue alterations can induce the onset of severe arrhythmias that represent one of the most common causes of unexpected sudden cardiac death in young athletes.

There are two different forms of ARVD:

- the fatty variant, which mainly involves the free wall of right ventricle in the absence of wall thickening changes;
- the fibro-fatty variant, which is characterized by the progressive thinning of the free wall that causes the appearance of aneurysm at the infundibulum, apex and basal segment of the inferior wall of the right ventricle, which is known as the *triangle of dysplasia*. This process commonly induces the overall enlargement and segmental dyskinesia of the right ventricular chamber. Moreover, this ARVD variant can also affect the left ventricle, which shows an increase in volume and contractile abnormalities at the apex and posterior wall.

MR allows for the prompt evaluation of the morphology and contractile function of the right ventricle. In particular, *black-blood* sequences are useful when performing an accurate morphological study, using axial and oblique view scans that encompass the entire right ventricle as far as the outflow tract. Instead, the assessment of contractile function requires the execution of *cine white-blood* sequences, oriented along the right ventricular long-axis, horizontal long-axis and short-axis and, additionally, specific scans covering the infundibulum and RVOT. Thus, with these images, it is possible to estimate ventricular volumes, free wall thickness (normal value is about 4-6 mm), the presence of thinning or hypertrophy of the trabeculae and moderator band, in addition to the evaluation of overall and segmental contractile function, which includes the identification of regional dyskinesia, systo-diastolic wall bulging and ventricular aneurysms.

However, the absence of contractile function abnormalities is not an adequate criterion for ruling out ARVD, due to the possibility of late occurrence. Consequently, tissue characterization is a fundamental step and relies on *SE* T1-weighted images, in order to identify the fatty tissue that appears hyperintense compared to the normal adjacent myocardium. Conversely, owing to fat signal saturation, fatty tissue can be seen as hypointense in *triple IR T1-weighted* sequences. Moreover, *delayed enhancement* sequences can reveal fibrotic or fibro-fatty areas that seem to be closely related to the onset of ventricular arrhythmia and contractile dysfunction of the right ventricle. Some cases also display involvement of the left ventricle, which is characterized by the detection of subepicardial or transmural fibro-fatty replacement, at the level of inferoseptal and posterolateral walls.

However, the identification of myocardial fat does not represent a major diagnostic criterion for ARVD because it can derive from different pathophysiological processes, such as aging, increased body surface area or myocardial damage, which results in reparation or healing. In fact, subepicardial fat, which is not matched with degenerated or apoptotic muscle cells, has been widely demonstrated in elderly and obese subjects, as well as alcoholics and diabetics. Therefore, the sensitivity and specificity of fatty tissue as an ARVD marker can vary from 22 to 100%, while the detection of contractile ventricular dysfunction more accurately matches ARVD. However, the diagnosis of ARVD has to fulfil a series of clinic and instrumental findings, known as the McKenna criteria [12]. Finally, the high risk of sudden cardiac death for ARVD patients implies that they are not permitted to practice competitive sport. Thus, it is necessary to carry out a secure diagnosis in order to ensure the best management of patients.

6.7.3 Myocarditis

Myocarditis is a pathological condition characterized by the inflammation of myocardial tissue. Most cases are commonly related to infectious disease, frequently triggered by viruses. However, myocardial inflammation may also be caused by other infective agents, such as bacteria or parasites, or a large number of immune reactions. Inflammation processes can vary in their extent and intensity, and the resulting myocardial injury relates to differing degrees of contractile dysfunction. Moreover, when it evolves rapidly, the resulting prognosis is poor. In the setting of myocarditis, cMR has been revealed to have important advantages, thanks to its ability to reliably evaluate cardiac function and additionally characterize the tissue of a damaged myocardium. Furthermore, it provides an estimation of wall thickness, mass, volumes and hemodynamic indexes (such as ejection fraction, stroke volume and cardiac output) regarding the left ventricle. Despite the presence of myocardial damage, the overall ventricular function can remain within normal limits because it is independent from the extent of necrosis.

Morphological analysis, using *black blood* sequences acquired in the three major cardiac planes, may detect, in such patients, a transient increase in wall thickness corresponding to edematous segments; similarly, a transient increase in left ventricular volumes is a typical finding. *Cine* sequences, performed in the same three main cardiac axes, can additionally identify overall and segmental contractile dysfunction. Moreover, *triple IR* T2-weighted sequences are suitable for checking edema distribution, as these can appear localized within limited regions (mainly within the sub-epicardial layer of the inferolateral wall) or be diffuse, with a typically patchy pattern. In a significant number of patients, accounting for approximately 32-57% of cases of myocarditis, inflammatory processes extend to the pericardium, leading to variable degrees of pericardial effusion (Fig. 6.5).

In *black blood* IR T1-weighted sequences, performed just after injection of the contrast agent,

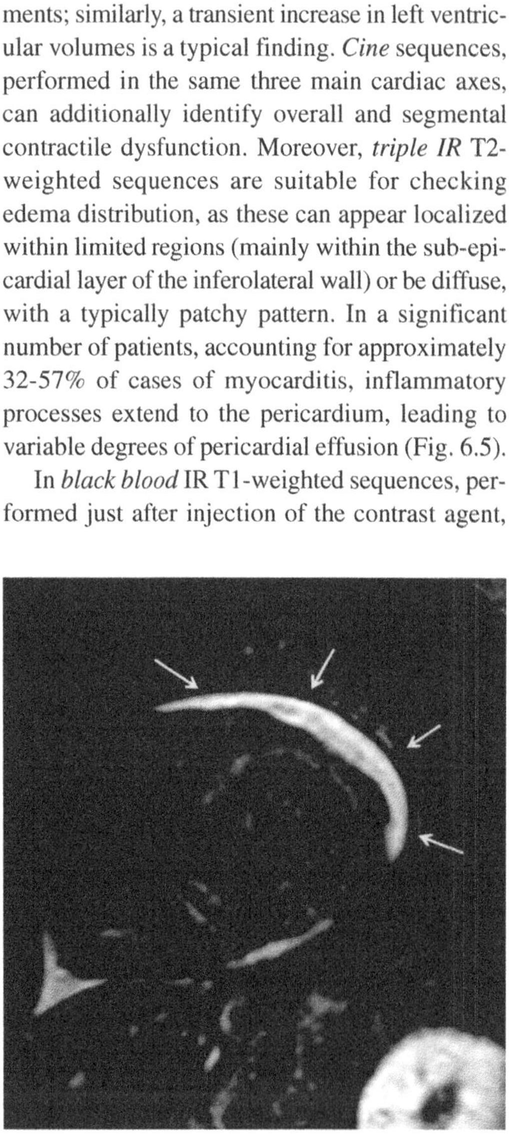

Fig. 6.5 Short-axis view image acquired during GRE T1-weighted sequences in a patient with a recent form of myocardial pericarditis: mild-to-moderate pericardial effusion is seen as a hyperintense signal surrounding the heart (*arrows*)

myocardial regions, which are characterized by intense inflammation, usually show early and significant gadolinium uptake, which is probably partly related to enlargement of the extracellular space due to the presence of edema, inflammatory hyperemia, and the slow gadolinium wash-out from swelling and edematous capillaries, and partly to the entry of gadolinium in injured muscle cells. Such *early enhancement* images reveal tissue inflammation as hyperintense areas compared to the adjacent myocardium. Moreover, *delayed enhancement* sequences are capable of detecting necrosis and irreversible damage to the myocardial tissue. Consistent with edema and inflammation distribution, necrosis is similarly detectable in the sub-epicardial layer and more rarely in the free wall of the right ventricle.

A specific delayed enhancement pattern has been shown in patients with myocarditis caused by human herpes virus 6 (HHV6), which is known for having an important trophism for the myocardial conduction system: late enhancement of the mid-wall interventricular septal is common, which explains the association of this form of myocarditis with different types of arrhythmias and bundle branch block.

The lack of involvement of the sub-endocardial layer makes it possible to clearly and confidently distinguish myocarditis from ischemic damage to the myocardium. Additionally, ischemic necrosis is characterized by a high-intensity and homogenous signal, while myocarditis-related damage is identified as soft and nuanced, due to the presence of diseased myocardium interspersed with normal tissue.

During follow-up, cMR can reveal complete regression of active tissue inflammation in patients with a favourable course. On the other hand, the persistence of hyperintense areas in T1 and T2 images has been correlated to a worse prognosis. Moreover, hyperintense signal areas, which are clearly visible in *delayed enhancement* sequences during follow-up, are suggestive of the deposition of fibrotic tissue as a consequence of myocardial necrosis. The presence and extent of these late enhancement areas are strongly related to dysfunction and late adverse remodeling of the left ventricle, leading to dilated cardiomyopathy.

The diagnosis of myocarditis at cMR is derived from the identification of different features and relies on the combined analysis of all imaging sequences. Nowadays, at least two of the following criteria are required for confirming a clinical suspicion (Lake Louise Consensus Criteria [13]):

- focal or diffuse hyperintense areas (edema) in *triple IR T2 -weighted* sequences;
- hyperintense areas (inflammation) in *early enhancement* sequences;
- sub-epicardial *late enhancement*, which represents necrosis (in acute myocarditis) or fibrosis (in chronic myocarditis).

Moreover, evidence of regional contractile dysfunction and pericardial effusion supports the diagnosis of myocarditis. Sometimes, despite the strong clinical suspicion of myocarditis, cMR findings do not fulfil established criteria. In such cases, the repetition of cMR about two weeks after the first scan is recommended.

6.7.4 Ischemic Heart Disease

Ischemic myocardial damage, triggered by acute occlusion of the coronary artery, results from a series of pathological events that can be easily detected by cMR. The early recanalization of an infarct-related artery allows the viability of a significant portion of the at-risk myocardium to be preserved. However, it has been widely demonstrated that about half of successfully treated patients show impaired reperfusion of the coronary microcirculation and that microvascular damage probably results from ischemia/reperfusion injuries. In addition to *infarct size*, post-infarct microvascular damage is the most important predictor of long-term prognosis.

In the setting of myocardial infarction, cMR enables the accurate evaluation of overall and regional cardiac function, as well as an estimation of reversible (edema) and irreversible (necrosis) myocardial damage. Acute myocardial infarction is characterized by the appearance of a tissue edema in *SE triple IR T2*-weighted sequences: in particular, the edema shows maximum signal intensity during the first week after the acute event and then has a tendency to gradually regress over time and eventually disappears in the chronic phase. Certainly, evidence of persistent inflammatory activity several weeks after an acute myocardial infarction is correlated to negative long-term prognosis.

However, cMR can detect increased diastolic thickness of the infarcted wall. Moreover, in some cases, hyperintense edematous areas show a central core characterized by low signal intensity. Several studies, performed by combining imaging data with histopathological features, have demonstrated that this pattern is due to hemorrhages within the edematous areas (Fig. 6.6). Venous administration

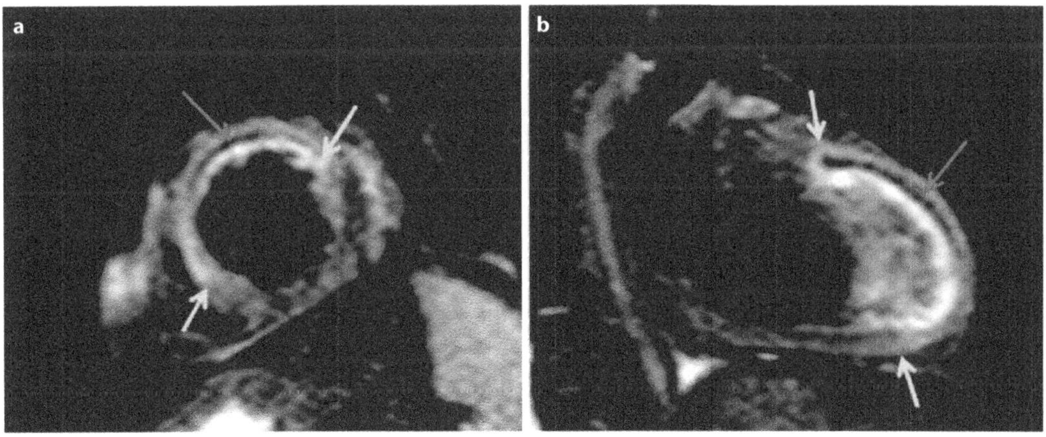

Fig. 6.6 Short-axis (a) and vertical long-axis (b) view images taken during *SE triple IR* T2-weighted sequences in a patient with a recent myocardial infarction of the anteroseptal and lateral walls: the edematous area (*yellow arrows*) is seen as a transmural hyperintense signal, compared to the adjacent myocardium, within the septum, apex and anterior wall of the left ventricle. Moreover, in the centre of the edema, a hypointense area (*red arrows*), suggestive of intraparietal hemorrhage, is evident

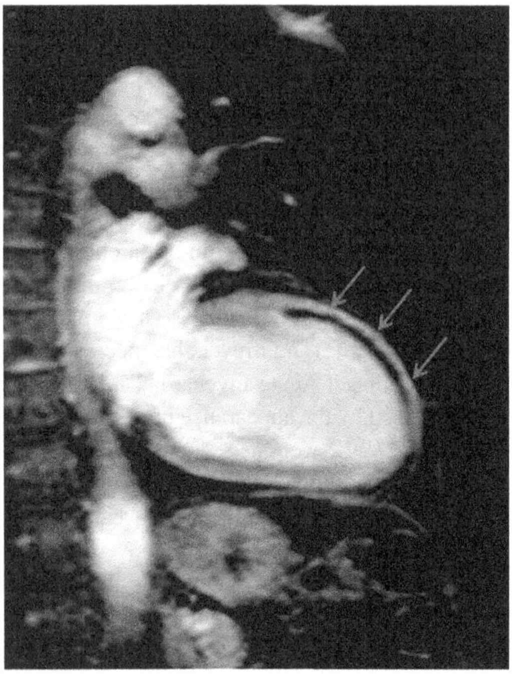

Fig. 6.7 Vertical long-axis view image scanned during *early enhancement* GRE T1-weighted sequences, about 2 minutes after the venous administration of gadolinium: a perfusion defect within the left ventricular anterior wall is detectable, from the mid-cavity to the apex, as a *hypoenhancement area* (*red arrows*) in the context of a hyperenhanced adjacent myocardium showing normal perfusion

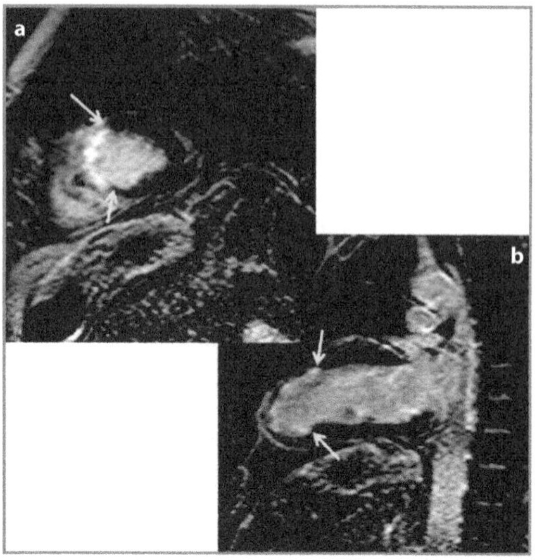

Fig. 6.8 Short-axis (a) and vertical long-axis (b) view images acquired during *delayed-enhancement* GRE IR T1-weighted sequences in a patient with a recent myocardial infarction of the anterior and anteroseptal walls: myocardial necrosis (*arrows*) is identifiable as a hyperintense transmural area within the interventricular septum, apex and anterior wall of the left ventricle

of gadolinium enables myocardial perfusion to be assessed. In the acute phase of myocardial infarction, MR sequences, which are scanned just after dye injection (*first pass*), can reveal the slow and impaired *wash-in* of gadolinium within the infarcted myocardial wall due to the presence of microvascular damage. This perfusion defect can also be seen in *early enhancement* sequences, as *hypoenhancement* areas (Fig. 6.7). Necrotic tissue is clearly identifiable during *delayed enhancement* imaging as a *hyper-enhancement* area, compared to the normally dark adjacent myocardium (Fig. 6.8). A *hypo-enhancement* signal, which may be detected within the late enhancement area, is the usual appearance of post-infarct microvascular obstruction (MVO) (Fig. 6.9). The chronic phase of myocardial infarction is typically characterized by healing, as the replacement of necrosis with fibrotic tissue. A *late enhancement* area leads to significant wall thinning, until reaching measurements less than 5.5 mm. Certainly, cMR plays an important role in the follow-up of patients with acute myocardial infarction, thanks to the ability to reliably estimate ventricular volumes and contractile function, thus allowing an accurate evaluation of cardiac remodeling and, consequently, of the long-term prognosis of patients.

6.7.5 Abnormal Origins and Course of Coronary Arteries

The abnormal origin and course of coronary arteries are congenital abnormalities of the coronary tree. Most cases are merely an anatomic variation that can be identified during a coronary artery scan. However, some cases are so severe that they show a poor prognosis, particularly in young athletes. In fact, coronary arteries, which lie in the space between aorta and main pulmonary artery, may be constricted when the demand for myocardial oxygen increases, as is the case during physical activity. Moreover, coronary arteries can have normal origins from Valsalva sinuses but they can

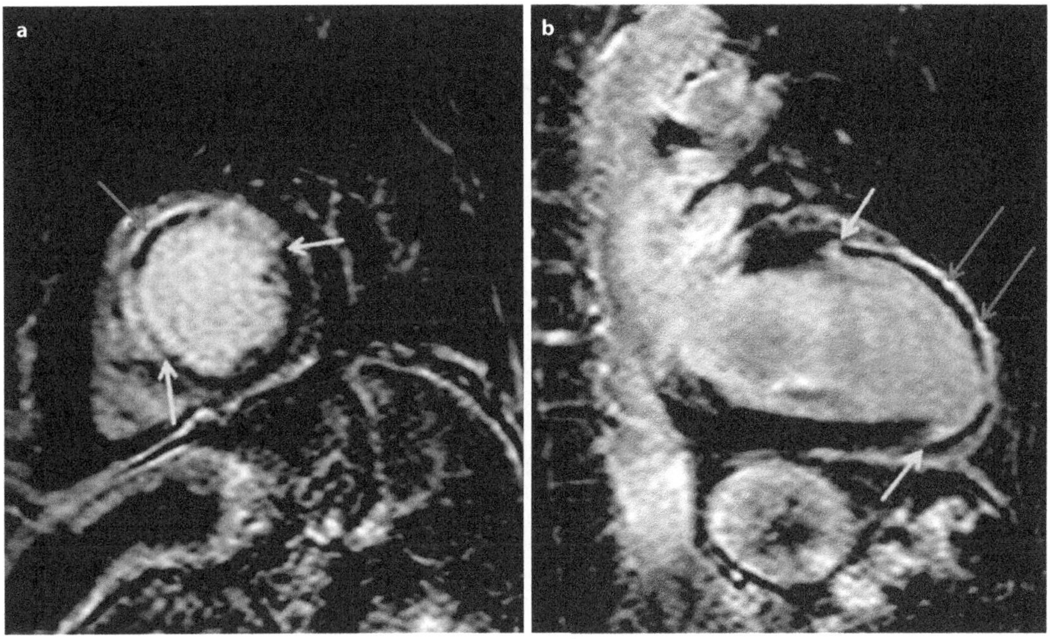

Fig. 6.9 Short-axis (a) and vertical long-axis (b) view images obtained during *delayed-enhancement GRE IR* T1-weighted sequences in a patient with a recent myocardial infarction of the anterior wall: a wide transmural and hyperintense area (*yellow arrows*) representing necrotic tissue is detectable at the level of the interventricular septum, apex and anterior wall of the left ventricle. Moreover, a hypointense area (*red arrows*), which is an expression of microvascular obstruction, is clearly identifiable within the necrosis area

tunnel through the myocardium, rather than rest on the top of it, forming a *myocardial bridge*. In particular, the myocardial bridge consists of a band of heart muscle that overrides and *tightens* the artery and intermittently decreases blood flow during the systolic contraction. Patients with myocardial bridges can experience different clinical patterns, ranging from stable angina to arrhythmias, signs of ventricular dysfunction or sudden cardiac death.

In the setting of sport cardiology, evaluation of the coronary arteries is an essential phase in the adequate diagnostic management of athletes, and their normal appearance is a fundamental requirement for receiving a license to practice sport. Thus, a high number of diagnostic imaging tools have been developed in order to accurately visualise coronary circulation. Actually, despite significant technical progress in the evaluation of coronary circulation through specific planes and sequences, cMR still has a limited application due to the small size of coronary arteries (about 5 mm in diameter, less than the current spatial resolution of cMR), their possibly tortuous course and rotational and translational movements during heart beat and breathing. The assessment of coronary arteries by MR is based on *white-blood* sequences, preceded by saturation recovery preparation pulses, which allow a high contrast to be obtained between blood flow and adjacent fatty tissue, in addition to *SE triple IR* sequences that cause fat signal abolition with a consequent increase in the difference between coronary lumen and epicardial fat. Moreover, using the *whole heart coronary angiography,* which is characterized by free-breathing three-dimensional acquisition of a field of view involving the whole heart and based on GRE method, thin multi-planar slices, scanned during brief phases of the cardiac cycle, are subsequently reassembled in a similar way to computed tomography. During each sequence, the blood signal can be widely enhanced by the administration of a paramagnetic contrast.

The diagnostic accuracy of enhanced magnetic resonance coronary angiography does not change between sequences. Nevertheless, it seems to be higher for the evaluation of the left main and proximal tract of the coronary arteries.

References

1. Pennell DJ, Sechtem UP, Higgins CB et al, Society for Cardiovascular Magnetic Resonance; Working Group on Cardiovascular Magnetic Resonance of the European Society of Cardiology (2004) Clinical indications for cardiovascular magnetic resonance (CMR): Consensus Panel report, Eur Heart J 25:1940–1965
2. Lombardi M, Bartolozzi C (2004) Risonanza magnetica del cuore e dei vasi. Springer, Milano
3. Manning WJ, Pennell DJ (2010) Cardiovascular magnetic resonance. Saunders, Elsevier, Philadelphia
4. La Gerche A, Taylor AJ, Prior DL (2009) Athlete's heart: the potential for multimodality imaging to address the critical remaining questions. JACC Cardiovasc Imaging 2:350–363
5. Scharhag J, Schneider G, Urhausen A et al (2002) Athlete's heart: right and left ventricular mass and function in male endurance athletes and untrained individuals determined by magnetic resonance imaging. J Am Coll Cardiol 40:1856–1863
6. Pelliccia A, Maron BJ, De Luca R et al (2002) Remodeling of left ventricular hypertrophy in elite athletes after longterm deconditioning. Circulation 105:944–949
7. Wu KC, Weiss RG, Thiemann DR et al (2008) Late gadolinium enhancement by cardiovascular magnetic resonance heralds an adverse prognosis in nonischemic cardiomyopathy. J Am Coll Cardiol 51:2414–2421
8. Petersen SE, Selvanayagam JB, Francis JM et al (2005) Differentiation of athlete's heart from pathological forms of cardiac hypertrophy by means of geometric indices derived from cardiovascular magnetic resonance. J Cardiovasc Magn Reson 7:551–558
9. Sachdev V, Shizukuda Y, Brenneman CL et al (2005) Left atrial volumetric remodeling is predictive of functional capacity in nonobstructive hypertrophic cardiomyopathy. Am Heart J 149:730–736
10. Assomull RG, Lyne JC, Keenan N et al (2007) The role of cardiovascular magnetic resonance in patients presenting with chest pain, raized troponin, and unobstructed coronary arteries. Eur Heart J 28:1242–1249
11. Assomull RG, Prasad SK, Lyne J et al (2006) Cardiovascular magnetic resonance, fibrosis, and prognosis in dilated cardiomyopathy. J Am Coll Cardiol 48:1977-1985. Epub 2006 Oct 31
12. McKenna WJ, Thiene G, Nava A et al (1994) Diagnosis of arrhythmogenic right ventricular dysplasia/cardiomyopathy. Task Force of the Working Group Myocardial and Pericardial Disease of the European Society of Cardiology and of the Scientific Council on Cardiomyopathies of the International Society and Federation of Cardiology. Br Heart J 71:215-218
13. Friedrich MG, Sechtem U, Schulz-Menger J et al (2009) International Consensus Group on Cardiovascular Magnetic Resonance in Myocarditis. Cardiovascular magnetic resonance in myocarditis: A JACC White Paper. J Am Coll Cardiol 53:1475-1487

Myocardial Radionuclide Imaging

7

Nishant R. Shah, Eduardo A. Hernandez,
J. Alberto Lopez and Warren H. Moore

7.1 Introduction

Radionuclide imaging of the myocardium is based on the principle that a photon-emitting radiotracer is extracted from the blood by viable cardiomyocytes and retained intracellularly long enough for detection by a sensitive detector (commonly called a scintillation camera or gamma camera). The two most common myocardial radionuclide imaging techniques in modern clinical practice are single-photon emission computed tomography (SPECT) and positron emission tomography (PET). Older myocardial radionuclide imaging techniques, including planar perfusion imaging and radionuclide angiography, have been largely replaced by other cardiac imaging procedures.

7.2 Appropriate Use

According to the 2009 ACCF/ASNC/ACR/AHA/ASE/SCCT/SCMR/SNM Appropriate Use Criteria for Cardiac Radionuclide Imaging, SPECT myocardial perfusion imaging (MPI) and PET MPI to detect coronary artery disease (CAD) are appropriate in the everyday clinical scenarios for sports cardiology listed in Table 7.1. It is important to note that Table 7.1 assumes that, in general, patients participating in sports/exercise regimens: 1) have at least a fair functional capacity, 2) do not have an intermediate/high pretest probability of CAD, and 3) have not had previous ACS or undergone a previous revascularization procedure. The first and third assumptions may not be true for older patients with CAD risk factors who wish to initiate a new sport/exercise regimen. The second assumption is not valid in patients of any age with diabetes, peripheral arterial disease, or a family history of early CAD.

The 2009 Appropriate Use Criteria do not specifically address patients with abnormal coronary artery origin from the opposite sinus of Val-

Table 7.1 Appropriate use criteria for SPECT/ PET MPI in sports cardiology

1. Acute ischemic equivalent* and suspected acute coronary syndrome (ACS).
2. Chronic ischemic equivalent, low pretest probability** of CAD, and either: a) an uninterpretable ECG¥; or b) an inability to exercise.
3. Asymptomatic with new-onset/newly diagnosed heart failure with left ventricular systolic dysfunction and no prior CAD evaluation and no planned coronary angiography.
4. Asymptomatic with ventricular tachycardia.
5. Asymptomatic with elevated troponin and no additional evidence of ACS.
6. Prior abnormal stress test with new/worsening symptoms.

Criteria derived from [4].
* Ischemic equivalent: any combination of clinical findings (including symptoms and/or ECG abnormalities) that the physician feels is consistent with obstructive CAD.
** Low pretest probability: less than 10% pretest probability of CAD.
¥ Uninterpretable ECG: resting ST-segment depression ≥ 0.10 mV, complete left bundle branch block, preexcitation/Wolff-Parkinson-White syndrome, or paced rhythm.

N.R. Shah (✉)
Texas Heart Institute, Baylor College of Medicine
Houston, USA

M. Fioranelli and G. Frajese (eds.), *Sports Cardiology*,
DOI: 10.1007/978-88-470-2775-6_7, © Springer-Verlag Italia 2012

Table 7.2 Appropriate use criteria for SPECT/ PET MPI in sports cardiology

Right ACAOS
Perform SPECT/PET MPI to demonstrate the existence/absence of reversible ischemia or scar. If positive, proceed with an invasive cardiac catheterization study.
Left ACAOS
Patients < 35 years - Proceed with surgical repair. SPECT/PET MPI not necessary.
Patients > 35 years - Symptomatic (chest pain, dyspnea, dizziness, syncope, sudden cardiac arrest) • Proceed with surgical repair. SPECT/PET MPI not necessary. - Asymptomatic • Perform SPECT/PET MPI to demonstrate the existence/absence of reversible ischemia or scar. If positive, proceed with surgical repair.

With permission from [10].

salva with an intramural course (ACAOS). Because of this gap, the algorithm in Table 7.2 has been proposed.

7.3 SPECT Stress Myocardial Perfusion Imaging (MPI)

SPECT stress MPI is by far the most commonly used myocardial radionuclide imaging procedure and is based on the following important concepts:

1) Oxygen extraction by the myocardium is nearly maximal at rest, so any increase in myocardial oxygen demand during stress is normally met by increasing coronary artery blood flow via modulation of downstream resistance in the arteriolar bed;
2) Maximum coronary artery blood flow reserve (the degree of blood flow increase with stress over resting flow) decreases when upstream stenosis is >50%, causing relative perfusion heterogeneity between the coronary arteries;
3) Differential uptake of SPECT radiotracers reliably reflects relative perfusion heterogeneity (i.e., areas of reduced coronary artery blood flow reserve).

7.4 SPECT Perfusion Radiopharmaceuticals

Four FDA-approved SPECT perfusion radiotracers are currently available for clinical use: thallium-201 chloride, technetium-99m sestamibi, and technetium-99m tetrofosmin, and (rarely used) technetium-99m teboroxime. The clinically relevant properties of the commonly used radiopharmaceuticals are summarized in Table 7.3.

7.4.1 Thallium-201

Thallium-201 (^{201}Tl) is a monovalent cation with biological properties similar to potassium. Peak myocardial concentration of thallium occurs within 5 minutes of injection by active transport into myocytes. Less than 5% of radiothallium appears in the heart and concentration also occurs in other tissues (i.e., splanchnic and limited lung uptake). Uptake is followed by concentration gradient-related redistribution back into the bloodstream, beginning almost immediately after injection. Clearance is more rapid from a normal myocardium with good perfusion and high thallium activity than from ischemic myocardium with reduced initial thallium activity, resulting in *differential washout*. This property can

Table 7.3 Properties of SPECT radiotracers

Radiotracer	Primary Energy (keV)	Physical Half-Life (Hr)	Uptake	Redistribution/ Differential Washout	First-Pass Extraction Fraction
Thallium-201	80*	73	Active	Prominent	0.85
Technetium-99m sestamibi/tetrofosmin	140	6	Passive	Minor	0.55-0.65

* Thallium imaging is based primarily on X-ray emissions of the daughter mercury, rather than the limited gamma rays of thallium.

be used to determine myocardial ischemia and viability, which is discussed in further detail below. Two significant disadvantages of ^{201}Tl are the low 80 keV primary energy (producing lower-quality images) and relatively higher radiation exposure (limiting dosages administered to patients to keep patient radiation as low as reasonably achievable).

7.4.2 Technetium-99m

Technetium-99m (^{99m}Tc) sestamibi and tetrofosmin are lipid-soluble cationic compounds. Unlike ^{201}Tl, these ^{99m}Tc agents are retained within myoctes after passive cellular uptake and do not significantly redistribute, even several hours after injection. ^{99m}Tc MPI protocols require separate injections, one at peak stress and one at rest, and may be performed in several different clinical protocols, including:

1) single-day study (rest followed by stress or vice versa);
2) two-day study (commonly used for larger patients);
3) dual-isotope study with thallium injected at rest and ^{99m}Tc at peak stress.

^{99m}Tc imaging often results in better image quality and has potentially improved test specificity in patients with significant breast tissue and in obese patients. Furthermore, ^{99m}Tc test protocols in general result in lower radiation exposure to patients than ^{201}Tl protocols. A notable disadvantage of ^{99m}Tc is prominent hepatic and other gastrointestinal activity that may interfere with cardiac imaging, particularly of the inferior wall of the left ventricle.

7.5 Stress Protocols

7.5.1 Exercise Stress

Adequate treadmill or bicycle exercise stress (i.e., achievement of >85% of maximum predicted heart rate for age) increases coronary flow to 2-3 times resting flow. Exercise stress uniquely provides the opportunity to link exercise-induced symptoms to perfusion abnormalities, and provides important supplementary information on functional capacity and stress-induced ECG-changes or arrhythmias. Additionally, exercise stress allows for calculation of the Duke Treadmill Score, heart rate reserve, and heart rate recovery, all of which are validated measures for assessing CAD probability and/or prognosis. For these reasons, exercise stress is the preferred stress method in nearly all patients. Exercise stress is contraindicated in patients who: 1) cannot be expected to achieve >85% of maximum predicted heart rate for age, or 2) have an uninterpretable baseline ECG abnormality (e.g., resting ST-segment depression ≥ 0.10 mV, complete left bundle branch block, preexcitation/Wolff-Parkinson-White syndrome, or paced rhythm). Additionally, caution is advized in patients with severe baseline hypertension or known arterial aneurysm(s).

7.5.2 Vasodilator Pharmacologic Stress

When exercise stress is not possible, pharmacological stress with a coronary arteriolar vasodilator such as adenosine or dipyridamole should be used. Adenosine results in coronary dilatation by direct stimulation of adenosine A2 receptors on smooth muscle cells. Dipyridamole indirectly results in coronary dilatation by inhibiting adenosine deaminase, an intracellular enzyme responsible for adenosine degradation. Pharmacological stress with these vasodilators increases coronary flow to up to 4-5 times the resting flow. The increase in hyperemia with pharmacological vasodilators compared to exercise should theoretically make pharmacological stress MPI more sensitive than exercise stress MPI for the detection of CAD. This has not been clinically observed, however, because both ^{201}Tl and ^{99m}Tc uptake are diffusion-limited at hyperemic blood flow levels.

It is important to note that myocardial oxygen demand usually does not change significantly with vasodilator stress – peripheral vasodilation mediated via A_{2B} receptors results in an 8-10 mmHg reduction in blood pressure, accompanied by a mild (10-20 bpm) increase in heart rate. Approximately 50% of patients experience side effects from adenosine or dipyridamole infusion. These side effects can include: chest pain (mediated by A_1 receptors in the nociceptive pathway), shortness of breath/bronchial constriction (mediated by A_{2B} receptors in the bronchioles), and AV block (mediated by A_1 receptors in the AV node). In the case of adenosine, which has a very short serum half-life of 20-30 seconds, these symptoms usually resolve quickly after termination of the infusion. For dipyridamole, which has a longer half-life, methylxanthine compounds such as aminophylline or caffeine may be given 1-2 minutes after radiopharmaceutical injection for their adenosine receptor antagonism. Adenosine-mediated bronchospasm, though rare, is a serious side effect and must be carefully managed.

Because of the potential for bronchospasm, patients with a history of significant reactive airways disease should not be subject to pharmacological stress with adenosine or dipyridamole. In these patients, a newer coronary vasodilator agent, regadenoson, can be considered. As a selective adenosine receptor A_{2A} agonist, regadenoson has very little affinity for A_{2B} receptors and thus a significantly lower risk of inducing bronchospasm. Additional advantages of regadenoson include uniform dosing and no requirement for an infusion pump.

Finally, adenosine, dipyridamole, and regadenoson pharmacologic stress is absolutely contraindicated in patients with unprotected (i.e., no artificial pacemaker) baseline sinus node dysfunction, second-degree atrioventricular (AV) block, or third-degree AV block. Additionally, due to the risk of peripheral vasodilation and hypotension, caution is advized when administering these agents in patients with autonomic dysfunction, hypovolemia, left main coronary artery stenosis, stenotic valvular heart disease, pericarditis/pericardial effusion, or stenotic carotid artery disease with cerebrovascular insufficiency.

7.5.3 Dobutamine Pharmacologic Stress

Dobutamine is a broad adrenergic receptor agonist that should be used as a *last resort* in terms of pharmacological stress in patients who cannot exercise and have a contraindication to vasodilator pharmacological stress. Dobutamine increases myocardial oxygen demand by initially increasing contractility at lower doses and then incrementally increasing heart rate at doses above 10 μg/kg/min. Additionally, up to 20 μg/kg/min, there is a modest increase in systolic and diastolic blood pressure. In a typical stress protocol, a continuous intravenous infusion is started at 5 μg/kg/min and is increased in a stepwise fashion until 85% of the maximum predicted heart rate for age is reached, or the maximum dose rate of 40-50 μg/kg/min. Up to 1 mg of intravenous atropine can be additionally administered to achieve the 85% threshold in patients not responding adequately to dobutamine alone. Expected side effects from dobutamine infusion include chest pain, palpitations, and arrhythmias. Due to the short half-life of dobutamine, these symptoms usually rapidly resolve on termination of the infusion. If symptoms persist, intravenous beta-blocker medications can be used.

7.6 ECG-gating

ECG-gating involves simultaneous recording of the patient's ECG with image acquisition. Whenever the peak of an R wave is detected on the ECG, an imaging *gate* opens and stores a certain number of milliseconds worth of data (*frame*). The imaging gate then closes and immediately opens again to store a second frame of imaging data. This process is repeated for a total of eight frames, each of which lasts an eighth of the R-to-R interval of the ECG. This process is then repeated for several hundred R-R intervals over 8-15 minutes. Once this process is complete, the eight frames of data can be displayed sequentially in a cine loop format. The result is the depiction of a single *average* cardiac cycle where normal left ventricular (LV) function is depicted as brightening of the wall during systole. By allowing for simultaneous assessment of LV function and perfusion, ECG-gating increases the specificity of SPECT MPI. An important caveat of ECG-gated image acquisition is its dependence on recording imaging information during cardiac cycles that are relatively homogenous in length. For this reason, beats fluctuating up to 10-15% around the average beat length are accepted, and other beats are rejected (*beat-length windowing*).

7.7 Image interpretation

7.7.1 Analysis of Perfusion Images

After ^{99m}Tc or ^{201}Tl SPECT rest-stress or stress-rest MPI, areas of the myocardium that have normal perfusion at rest and decreased perfusion with stress represent viable regions with blunted coronary flow reserve and the perfusion abnormalities are labelled *reversible*. (Figure 7.1)

Areas of myocardium with decreased perfusion both at rest and with stress either represent an attenuation artefact (see discussion below) or non-viable regions of fibrosis, with the perfusion abnormalities labelled as *fixed*. Finally, areas of the myocardium with decreased perfusion at rest and worse perfusion with stress represent a mix of a viable and fibrotic myocardium, and the perfusion abnormalities are labelled *partially reversible*. The extent of a perfusion abnormality is the total amount of the myocardium that falls below the lower limit of normal, while the severity of a perfusion abnormality is the depth of the abnormality related to the lower limit of normal.

In clinical practice, perfusion images are assessed visually, semi-quantitatively, and/or quantitatively. Visual analysis is operator-dependent and equipment-dependent but well-trained readers can adjust their threshold for interpreting an abnormality based on other factors, including review of the raw data information (e.g., breast attenuation or elevated diaphragm), overall image patterns, and technical- and patient-related artefacts. On the other hand, semi-quantitative and quantitative analyses are highly reproducible and can often account for potential artefacts by the comparison of data to normal, gender-matched subjects. Semi-quantitative analysis involves, for example, assigning a perfusion score of between 0 (normal perfusion) and 4 (severe perfusion defect) to each of the 17 standard myocardial segments on the stress images and then adding the scores to create a summed stress score (SSS), representing the extent and severity of ischemia and infarction. The same process is use with rest images to create a summed rest score (SRS), representing the extent and severity of fixed defects. The SRS is then subtracted from the SSS to determine the summed difference score (SDS), representing the extent and severity of stress-induced ischemia (or flow redistribution in the case of vasodilator stress). Further analysis can be performed by most modern analysis programs and results in a 2-dimensional polar coordinate display representing the entire 3-dimensional myocardium (Figure 7.2).

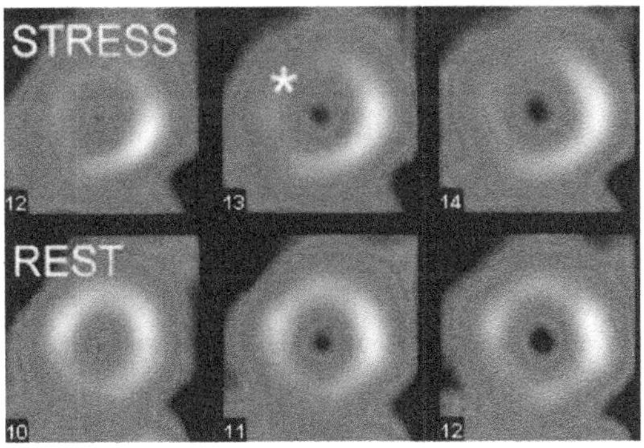

Fig. 7.1 Reversible perfusion defect on SPECT MPI. The bottom row of short-axis tomograms shows normal ^{99m}Tc sestamibi uptake (*orange*) throughout the myocardium at rest. The top row of short-axis tomograms, obtained after stress, shows moderately severe decreased ^{99m}Tc sestamibi uptake in the anterior, anteroseptal, and septal segments (*purple-orange region with asterisk*). These findings suggest that these myocardial territories have reduced coronary artery blood flow reserve

It is important to note that SPECT stress MPI is limited by its dependence on relative perfusion heterogeneity. This is most salient in the case of three-vessel CAD, where the least hypoperfused myocardium will appear *normal* and the extent of CAD can be underestimated. However, taking into account regional functional abnormalities from ECG-gated images decreases this risk.

Regardless of its potential shortcomings, analysis of perfusion data from SPECT stress MPI has important implications for clinical risk and prognosis of CHD. In patients with a normal SPECT stress MPI study, the rate of CHD death and non-fatal MI over the next two years is 0.7%. On the other hand, for patients with an abnormal SPECT stress MPI result, the extent and severity of the perfusion abnormality is significantly correlated with the subsequent likelihood of CHD death and non-fatal MI. It is important to note, however, that only a minority of patients with an abnormal SPECT stress MPI result will suffer such an event during follow-up. If these patients undergo subsequent intervention, it is to prevent events in the minority.

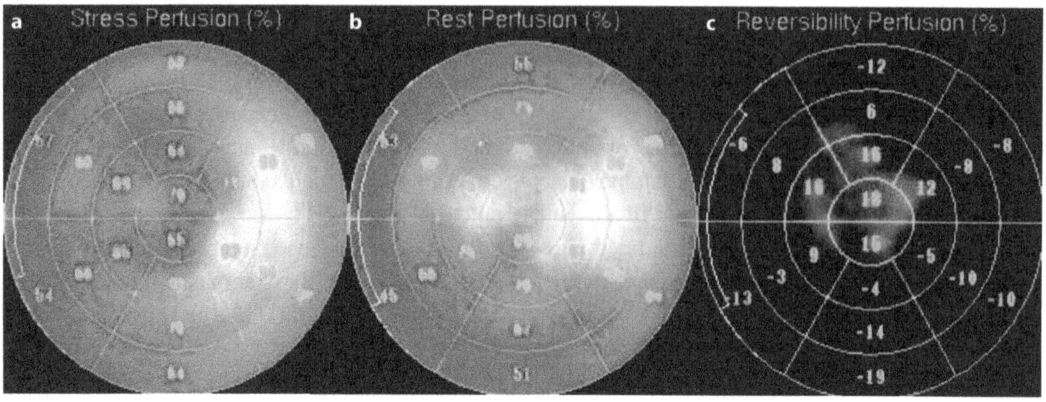

Fig. 7.2 Two-dimensional (2D) polar coordinate display with reversible perfusion defect on SPECT MPI. The rest 2D perfusion polar coordinate display (b) demonstrates essentially normal uptake (*orange*) throughout the myocardium at rest. The stress 2D perfusion polar coordinate display (a) demonstrates decreased perfusion (*purple*) in the anterior, anteroseptal, and septal regions. c is a 2D perfusion polar coordinate display that represents the quantitative difference between the rest and stress displays, highlighting the reversible perfusion defect (*blue*).

7.7.2 High-risk Findings

In addition to a significant perfusion deficit, two additional *high-risk* findings can occur on SPECT stress MPI perfusion images: transient ischemic dilatation (TID) and significant lung uptake. TID refers to one of 2 imaging patterns: 1) the LV cavity appears larger at stress than at rest, signifying extensive ischemia and prolonged post-ischemic systolic dysfunction, or 2) apparent dilatation of the LV cavity with an unchanged epicardial silhouette between rest and stress, signifying diffuse subendocardial ischemia and severe CAD. The presence of either TID pattern raises the possibility of multivessel or left main CAD, especially in the presence of greater than 2 mm of ST depression or hypotension during ECG treadmill testing. Similar to TID, substantial perfusion radiotracer uptake in the lung following stress but not at rest suggests severe multivessel CAD. The mechanism for this finding is thought to be related to the elevation of pulmonary capillary wedge pressure and decreased left ventricular ejection fraction (LVEF) during exercise.

A third finding that could be *high-risk* particularly in athletes is increased tracer uptake in the septum relative to the lateral wall. This creates an apparently mild lateral wall defect, especially on polar maps. This finding suggests the possibility of asymmetric septal hypertrophy or hypertrophic cardiomyopathy.

7.7.3 Analysis of ECG-gated Images

In clinical practice, ECG-gated SPECT MPI images to evaluate LV function are usually evaluated visually and quantitatively. Visually, myocardial segments that brighten normally during systole are labelled as normally contractile. Segments that have diminished brightening during systole are labelled as hypokinetic/severely hypokinetic. Finally, those segments that do not brighten during systole are labelled as akinetic. As with perfusion images, quantitative analysis of ECG-gated SPECT images is automatically performed by most modern analysis programs, which calculate LV volumes and LVEF. These programs can also display the left ventricular function in a three-dimensional surface-rendered or two-dimensional polar map format.

7.7.4 Analysis of ^{201}Tl Redistribution Images

As noted above, the differential washout property of ^{201}Tl can be used to determine myocardial viability in the following manner:

1) reversibility of a ^{201}Tl defect from initial *rest* images to delayed 3-4 hour or 24-hour redistribution images signifies viable myocardium with resting hypoperfusion;
2) reversibility of a ^{201}Tl defect from initial *stress*

images to delayed redistribution images signifies reversibly ischemic, viable myocardium;
3) an irreversible ^{201}Tl defect present on rest, stress, and delayed redistribution images signifies fibrotic myocardium.

7.7.5 Normal Variants and Common Artefacts

Normal variations on perfusion images include *dropout* of the upper septum due to the muscular septum merging with the membranous septum. Additionally, the lateral wall can appear brighter than the contralateral septum; one of the explanations proposed for this phenomenon is that the lateral wall is closer to the gamma camera with less soft tissue attenuation. Finally, in patients with left bundle branch block, an isolated reversible perfusion defect of the septum can be observed, especially with high heart rates. In these patients, apical or anterior involvement of the perfusion defect increases the specificity for CAD.

Common artefacts include:
1) breast attenuation artefact – more common in women and manifests as a mild-moderate fixed defect in the anterior/anterolateral wall with preserved wall motion;
2) inferior attenuation artefact (often misleadingly called diaphragmatic attenuation) – more common in men and manifests as a mild-moderate fixed defect in the inferobasal wall with preserved wall motion;
3) *ramp filter* artefact – occurs when perfusion radiopharmaceutical uptake in an extracardiac structure immediately adjacent to the myocardium either *steals* counts away from the myocardium and makes it appear falsely *cooler*. (The opposite can also occur and radiopharmaceutical uptake in the extracardiac structure can add counts to the adjacent myocardium and makes it appear falsely *hotter*.)

7.8 PET

PET is based on the following important concepts:
1) when PET radiopharmaceuticals undergo decay, a positively-charged beta particle (positron) is released;
2) positrons travel a few millimetres in the tissue and then collide with a negatively-charged beta particle (electron), resulting in complete annihilation of both particles and the release of two 511 keV gamma rays (photons) travelling approximately 180 degrees away from each other;
3) PET gamma cameras attempt to map only those photons that strike with temporal coincidence at directly opposing detectors.

The major advantages of PET over SPECT are:
1) improved spatial resolution;
2) potential for absolute quantitative measurement of myocardial perfusion and metabolism (less susceptibility to false negative results with *balanced* multivessel disease as with SPECT);
3) use of naturally-occurring elements (carbon, oxygen, nitrogen, fluorine) allows *in vivo* interrogation of physiologically relevant processes in normal and diseased states;
4) dynamic mode PET allows interrogation of the rate of change of a physiological process.

Aside from minor differences, PET stress MPI is essentially identical to SPECT stress MPI with regard to stress protocols, ECG-gating and image interpretation. The major difference relates to the perfusion radiotracers used. There are currently two FDA-approved PET perfusion radiopharmaceuticals, ^{82}rubidium and ^{13}N-ammonia.

7.9 PET MPI Radiotracers

7.9.1 ^{82}Rubidium

^{82}Rubidium (^{82}Rb) is a cation with biological properties similar to potassium and thallium. It is actively transported into cardiomyocytes and, like the SPECT perfusion tracers, uptake reflects absolute blood flow up to 2-3 ml/g/min. The advantages of ^{82}Rb are that it has a higher first-pass extraction fraction than thallium and that it is generator-produced, rather than cyclotron-produced. With regard to disadvantages, ^{82}Rb's half-life of 75 seconds restricts its use to pharmacologic stress protocols and there is a high cost associated with monthly generator replacement.

7.9.2 ^{13}N-ammonia

^{13}N-ammonia is similar to ^{82}Rb as a non-diffusible radiotracer whose uptake reflects absolute blood flow up to 2-3 mL/g/min. Unlike ^{82}Rb, uptake is mediated by both passive and active processes, resulting in a higher first-pass extraction fraction (>90%). Although it has a slightly longer physical half-life than ^{82}Rb (10 minutes), it is still restricted for use in pharmacological stress protocols. Another significant disadvantage of ^{13}N-ammonia is the requirement of a nearby cyclotron.

References

1. Cerqueira MD, Weissman NJ, Dilsizian V, et al (2002) Standardized myocardial segmentation and nomenclature for tomographic imaging of the heart: a statement for healthcare professionals from the Cardiac Imaging Committee of the Council on Clinical Cardiology of the American Heart Association. Circulation Jan 29;105(4):539–42
2. Dilsizian V, Narula J, editors (2009) Atlas of Nuclear Cardiology. 3rd ed. Philadelphia: Springer
3. Heller GV, Hendel RC, editors (2011) Nuclear Cardiology: Practical Applications. 2nd ed. China: McGraw Hill
4. Hendel RC, Berman DS, Di Carli MF, et al (2009) ACCF/ASNC/ACR/AHA/ASE/SCCT/SCMR/SNM 2009 Appropriate Use Criteria for Cardiac Radionuclide Imaging: A Report of the American College of Cardiology Foundation Appropriate Use Criteria Task Force, the American Society of Nuclear Cardiology, the American College of Radiology, the American Heart Association, the American Society of Echocardiography, the Society of Cardiovascular Computed Tomography, the Society for Cardiovascular Magnetic Resonance, and the Society of Nuclear Medicine. J Am Coll Cardiol Jun 9;53(23):2201–29
5. McLaughlin MG, Danias PG (2002) Transient ischemic dilation: a powerful diagnostic and prognostic finding of stress myocardial perfusion imaging. J Nucl Cardiol Nov-Dec;9(6):663–7
6. Shaw LJ, Hendel R, Borges-Neto S, et al. Prognostic value of normal exercise and 99mTc-tetrofosmin SPEC imaging: results from the multicenter registry of 4728 patients (2003) J Nucl Med 44:134
7. Udelson JE, Dilsizian V, Bonow RO (2008) Nuclear Cardiology. In: Libby P, Bonow RO, Mann DL, Zipes DP, editors. Braunwald's Heart Disease: A Textbook of Cardiovascular Medicine. 8th ed. Philadelphia: Elsevier p. 345–91
8. McGhie AI, Gould KL, Willerson JT (2007) Nuclear Cardiology. In: Willerson JT, Cohn JN, Wellens HJ, Holmes DR, editors. Cardiovascular Medicine. 3rd ed. London: Springer-Verlag p. 137–160
9. Zaret BL, Beller GA (2010) Clinical Nuclear Cardiology: State of the Art and Future Directions. 4th ed. China: Elsevier
10. Angelini P (2012) Coronary Artery Anomalies. In: Moscucci M (ed) Grossman's Cardiac Catheterization, Angiography, and Intervention. 8th edn. Springer (ahead of print)

Cardiac Catheterization 8

Stefano Tonioni, Carlo Gonnella and Fabrizio D'Errico

8.1 Introduction

Cardiac catheterization [1-3] is an invasive method that makes it possible to evaluate the physiological parameters of the cardiovascular system.

In recent years the use of this method has been considerably reduced due to the more extensive and accurate use of echocardiography. However, this method still plays a vital role especially in clinical conditions in which non-invasive methods are unable to obtain comprehensive information about the status of a specific cardiovascular disease.

Cardiac catheterization can provide information regarding the physiology by evaluating cardiovascular hemodynamic parameters such as: blood pressure values, the calculation of cardiac output and a measurement of vascular resistance.

In the cardiovascular system, pressure varies with cardiac contraction; therefore, when recording blood pressure it must be considered that this is a dynamic measurement. For this reason the morphology of the wave is important rather than its absolute value. Furthermore, each cardiovascular district has a defined type of pressure wave, which takes into account the different anatomical features.

Generally, during an examination of cardiac catheterization the pressures of the right heart (pulmonary capillary wedge, pulmonary artery, right ventricle, right atrium) and the left ventricle and aorta are measured. In addition, blood samples are performed for the determination of any shunt.

S. Tonioni (✉)
Cardiology Department
"San Carlo di Nancy" Hospital, Rome, Italy

8.2 Indications to Cardiac Catheterization

The forms of cardiac catheterization currently indicated are: estimation of pulmonary artery pressure and subsequent changes due to pharmacological tests in patients with pulmonary hypertension, evaluation of pulmonary resistance before and after pharmacological stimulation in patients with valvular heart disease (primarily mitral) or transplant candidates for hearts, lungs or both. Recognizing and analyzing the various components of the different morphologies of the pressure curves is essential to identify any abnormalities associated with various cardiopulmonary diseases. The waveform of central venous pressure is perhaps one of the best known, and the morphology is almost the same for both atria, right and left. In the cath lab, wedge pressure is considered to be the left atrial pressure, because there are no valves between the left atrium and pulmonary veins. Between the right atrium and venae cavae the measured pressure will be almost similar in both districts, because there are no valves to divide these districts. The only real difference between the direct measurement of left atrial pressure, and pressure at the level of the pulmonary capillaries is temporal, as there is a latency time that indicates the transmission time of the pressure wave through the pulmonary vascular district.

The main components of venous pressure are the *a* wave, the *x* collapse, the *v* wave and the *y* collapse. These individual components correspond to contraction, relaxation, atrial filling and emptying. It is possible to detect in correspondence with

M. Fioranelli and G. Frajese (eds.), *Sports Cardiology*,
DOI: 10.1007/978-88-470-2775-6_8, © Springer-Verlag Italia 2012

the *x* collapse a positive wave called the *c* wave, which is the protrusion of the closed atrioventricular valves into the atrium. In normal conditions, the *a* wave has a peak greater than the *v* wave, if the pressure wave is measured in the right atrium, while in the left atrium or in capillary wedge pressure the peak of the *v* wave is greater than the peak of the *a* wave. Many factors can influence the morphology of the atrial curves: the degree of continence of the atrioventricular valves, the contractile state of the atria (in the case of atrial fibrillation the wave is missing) and of the ventricles, atrioventricular synchronism (giant *c* wave, also called cannon wave, in the case of complete atrioventricular dissociation), heart rate and blood volume.

The morphology of the right and left ventricular waves is similar and differs mainly in size. During systole the isovolumic contraction and relaxation phase is longer in the left ventricle, with a lower ejection phase compared to the right ventricle. In the ventricular pressure curve there is an *a* wave, caused by atrial contraction, which occurs immediately after the *P* wave of the electrocardiogram. Ventricular systole, however, begins immediately after the *QRS* complex of the electrocardiogram. The phase of isovolumic relaxation lies between the closure of the semilunar valves and the opening of the atrioventricular valves, corresponding to the fall in pressure values that ends with the protodiastole. Then, the filling phase begins, first quickly and then slowly (telediastole), which leads to a new increase of blood pressure. The values that are generally measured are: the peak value of systolic pressure, protodiastolic pressure and telediastolic pressure (measured after the *a* wave or the peak of the *R* wave on the electrocardiogram). The morphology and values of the ventricular pressure curves are conditioned by hypertension (systemic and pulmonary), acute coronary syndromes, ischemic heart disease, pressure and volume overload, cardiomyopathy, heart valves, ventricular dysfunction and cardiac tamponade.

The pressure curves of the pulmonary artery and aorta are given by waves, coinciding with ventricular systole (immediately after the *QRS* complex of the electrocardiogram), by a dicrotic notch corresponding to the closure of the semilunar valves and a subsequent decrease until the telediastolic phase. The values measured are generally: the peak systolic value, diastolic value and mean value. The measurement and analysis of the aorta and pulmonary artery pressure values are important, for example, in the differential diagnosis of primary pulmonary hypertension and chronic pulmonary microembolism or aortic valvular disease.

The aortic pressure wave morphology is of particular importance during coronary angiography. In fact, in the presence of alterations in the morphology of the pressure curve (damping, ventricularized waveform), it is possible to identify significant ostial stenosis or occlusion by the catheter. Another important piece of information that is obtained during cardiac catheterization is the calculation of the cardiac output. Cardiac output is given as the amount of blood that ejected from the heart, expressed in l/min and directly proportional to body surface area (l/min/m^2).

Cardiac output is measured by thermodilution or by the Fick method. The thermodilution method is based on the principle that the volume of a liquid can be calculated if a known amount of an indicator is added after uniform mixing with the liquid itself. In practical terms, a Swan-Ganz catheter must be inserted into the pulmonary artery and a cold saline solution (5-10 ml) injected, with simultaneous recording of the temperature/time curve, which is inversely proportional to cardiac output. The calculation of cardiac output is made available directly from the equipment by using the Stewart-Hamilton equation.

The Fick method is based on the principle by which the absorption and release of a substance to be part of an organ depends on blood flow and the difference in the arteriovenous concentration of the substance.

To measure the cardiac output, oxygen is used. Normally, in the absence of shunts, systemic blood flow is equal to pulmonary blood flow. Therefore, the cardiac output is calculated using the following formula:

$$Q\ (\text{l/min}) = \frac{\text{Oxygen consumption (ml/min)}}{\text{DA-V } O_2 \text{ (ml/min)}}$$

Oxygen consumption is derived using the tables or normograms. The *DA-V* O_2, in the absence of a shunt, is calculated by performing a blood sample in the pulmonary artery and in the artery to determine peripheral O_2 saturation and hemoglobin and by applying the following formula:

$$\text{Oxygen content} = \text{Hb (g/l)} \times 1.36\ (\text{mlO}_2/\text{g Hb}) \times \text{Oxygen saturation (\%)}.$$

1.36 is the maximum capacity to bind O_2 by 1 g of Hb.

Vascular resistance is calculated by dividing the pressure gradient by the respective cardiac output, using Ohm's law:

$$\text{Systemic vascular resistance (SVR)} = \text{Ao-RA/Qs}$$

$$\text{Total pulmonary resistance (TPR)} = \text{PA / Qp}$$

$$\text{Pulmonary vascular resistance (PVR)} = \text{LA-PA / Qp}$$

Ao: mean aortic pressure; RA: mean right atrial pressure; PA: mean pulmonary artery pressure; LA: mean left atrial pressure and pulmonary capillary wedge pressure (PCW). Vascular resistance is expressed: in Wood's units (resistance units × body surface, m^2), in absolute units (dynes × sec × cm^{-5}) or in resistance units (mmHg/l/min).

Systemic vascular resistance increased in systemic arterial hypertension, in polycythemia in the case of low cardiac output and compensatory arteriolar vasoconstriction. However, there was a decrease in cases of anemia, fever, thyrotoxicosis, sepsis, and arteriovenous fistulae. Pulmonary vascular resistance increases in primitive pulmonary pathologies, in Ebstein's syndrome and in all conditions involving an altered pulmonary vasculature caused by volume overload, in valvular pathologies and in cardiomyopathies.

It is important to consider whether pulmonary resistance is reversible or irreversible, so that the best therapy, pharmacological or surgical, can be chosen, as in the case of valvular disease or cardiomyopathies in transplant patients. In these cases the measurements of vascular resistance are performed in baseline conditions and after pharmacological stimulation (nitric oxide, nitrates).

With cardiac catheterization it is also possible to determine the valve area by measuring the pressure gradients and applying the Gorlin formula:

$$\text{Valve Area} = \frac{\text{Q / (DFP or SEP)} \times \text{HR}}{\text{C} \times \sqrt{\text{D}}}$$

Q: flow rate; DFP: diastolic filling period (used for the atrioventricular valves); SEP: systolic ejection period (used for the semilunar valves), HR: heart rate, C: constant (mitral valve: 37.7; other valves: 44.3); D: average transvalvular gradient.

Currently, cardiac catheterization to determine areas of the tube is a technique used very rarely and is replaced by transthoracic and trans-esophageal echocardiography.

Moreover, cardiac catheterization quantifies the shunts that are generally diagnosed via non-invasive methods.

There are two methods to evaluate shunts: an angiographic method and an oximetry method. The angiographic technique localizes the shunt with the injection of a contrast agent directly into the cardiac chambers and/or great vessels. This method, however, does not make it possible to quantify the shunt. The oximetry method makes it possible to obtain quantitative information and is based on the oxygen concentration or oxygen saturation. Blood samples are taken from the venae cavae (inferior and superior), right atrium (upper, middle and lower), right ventricle (inflow and outflow tracts), pulmonary artery, left ventricle and aorta or peripheral arteries. With this method, however, it is difficult to identify a small shunt, which can be localized by angiography. The formula to quantify left to right shunt is:

$$\text{Qp} = \frac{\text{Oxygen consumption}}{[\text{PV O}_2\ (\text{ml/l}) - \text{PA O}_2\ (\text{ml/l})]}$$

and

$$\text{Qp} = \frac{\text{Oxygen consumption}}{[\text{SA O}_2\ (\text{ml/l}) - \text{MV O}_2\ (\text{ml/l})]}$$

Because QP=QS, the formula is:

$$Qp/Qs = \frac{[AS\ O_2\ (ml/l) - MV\ O_2\ (ml/l)]}{[PV\ O_2\ (ml/l) - PA\ O_2\ (ml/l)]}$$

Qp: Pulmonary blood flow; Qs: Systemic blood flow; PV O_2: Pulmonary venous oxygen content; PA O_2: Pulmonary artery oxygen content; SA O_2: Systemic artery oxygen content; MV O_2: mixed venous oxygen content.

The normal value of Qp / Qs is 1; values between 1 and 1.5 define a shunt of small size, values between 1.5 and 2 define a shunt of medium size to be corrected surgically, and values > 2 indicate a large shunt that if not corrected in a short time will lead to pulmonary hypertension and subsequent dilation of the right ventricle.

References

1. Nishimura RA (2007) Invasive Hemodynamics. In: Murphy JG, Lloyd MA Mayo Clinic Cardiology. Mayo Clinic Scientific Press, Rochester
2. Zanchetta M, Pedon L, Colonna S, Maiolino P (2000) Cateterismo cardiaco e coronarografia. In: AAVV (ed) Trattato di Cardiologia. Excerpta Medica, Milano
3. Baim DS (2006) Grossman's Cardiac Catheterisation, Angiography, and Intervention. Lippincott Williams & Wilkins, Philadelphia

Coronary Angiography

9

Stefano Tonioni, Carlo Gonnella, Fabrizio D'Errico and Maria Antonietta Carbone

9.1 Introduction

Coronary angiography is an invasive radiological diagnostic examination that allows, through the use of radiopaque contrast agents, the visualization of the coronary arteries [1, 2]. It is indicated for the diagnosis and treatment of coronary artery disease (PCI or CABG). It should be performed to rule out the presence of coronary artery disease: in heart valve surgery, before non-cardiac surgery in periprocedural high-risk patients or when the provocative tests are unclear, and in those with a high social risk (airline pilots, bus drivers, police agents, fire-fighters). Coronary angiography is important in congenital anomalies in order to recognize the origin and course of coronary arteries, the presence of fistulas, vasospasm, emboli, arteritis and myocardial bridging [3].

Contraindications can be divided into absolute and relative (Table 9.1). The refusal of the patient to provide informed consent for this examination is the only absolute contraindication to coronary angiography. The relative contraindications, however, include the presence of corrected electrolyte abnormalities or drug toxicity (e.g., hyperkalemia, digitalis toxicity), fever, acute renal failure, heart failure, severe allergy to iodinated radiopaque contrast agents, oral anticoagulants or severe bleeding diathesis, severe uncontrolled hypertension and pregnancy.

S. Tonioni (✉)
Cardiology Department
"San Carlo di Nancy" Hospital, Rome, Italy

Table 9.1 Contraindications to coronary angiography

Absolute
The refusal of the patient
Relative
Electrolyte abnormalities
Drug toxicity
Fever
Acute renal failure
Heart failure
Severe allergy to iodinated radiopaque contrast agents
Oral anticoagulants
Severe bleeding diathesis
Severe uncontrolled hypertension
Pregnancy

Table 9.2 Complications after coronary angiography

Major
Death
Myocardial infarction
Stroke
Minor
Arrhythmia
Contrast-induced nephrotoxicity (CIN)
Allergic reactions
Coronary dissection
Heparin-induced bleeding

9.2 Complications

The possible complications (Table 9.2) can be divided into major and minor.

Major complications are death, myocardial infarction and stroke. The combined frequency of these adverse events is about 0.23%, but it depends on case studies and the standards of each centre. The main risk factors predictive of adverse events

M. Fioranelli and G. Frajese (eds.), *Sports Cardiology*,
DOI: 10.1007/978-88-470-2775-6_9,

are the presence of coronary artery disease and severe aortic valve stenosis. Other important risk factors include advanced age of the patient, angina at rest, left ventricular dysfunction, previous stroke and severe cardiac disease (including renal, cerebrovascular and peripheral vascular diseases, and respiratory failure). Cardiogenic shock increases the risk of coronary angiography approximately six-fold, while acute myocardial infarction raises the risk by about four-fold. Half the complications that occur within 24 hours of the exam were generally considered to be *pseudo-complications*, since they are *complications* that would have occurred equally in the same range even without the execution of coronary angiography.

The minor complications are: local complications in the vascular access, arrhythmia, contrast-induced nephrotoxicity (CIN), allergic reactions, coronary dissection and heparin-induced bleeding. Percutaneous femoral artery access complications include bleeding, distal embolization, pseudoaneurysms, traumatic injury from compression of the femoral nerve, femoral vein thrombosis resulting from venous compression during the removal of the introducer sheath. Complications associated with the use of brachial access are: thrombosis, brachial nerve injury and local hemorrhage/hematoma. The brachial access is most frequently burdened with bleeding and thrombotic events compared to other accesses used (femoral and radial).

Significant vascular complications occur in approximately 1% of patients undergoing diagnostic angiography, and are less likely to occur when the radial approach is preferred. However, this type of access can only be used when there is a palm arch suitable, when the ulnar artery and the radial artery communicate and the ulnar artery supplies adequate blood to the hand. The adequacy of the palm arch can be studied clinically using the Allen test.

Arrhythmic complications, which also include vasovagal reactions, occur in about 1% of patients. They usually resolve spontaneously, but sometimes can be effectively treated with defibrillation or administration of atropine and other antiarrhythmic drugs.

Coronary dissection is fortunately a rare complication. It is due, generally, to the trauma of the catheter on the coronary ostia during diagnostic angiography and can be prevented by observing the morphology of the pressure wave, avoiding injections of contrast agent, pressure and maneuvers for cannulation. Coronary spasm is another possible reaction to cannulation with the diagnostic catheter and is usually sufficient to resolve its retraction, and in cases where such a maneuver is not enough, vasodilators such as nitroglycerin may be administered. Other possible systemic complications, which are fortunately infrequent, are adverse reactions to iodinated contrast agents, which can induce true anaphylactic or anaphylactoid phenomena. Both of these complications should be treated with corticosteroids and antihistamines. Generally, these events occur in patients with a known history of allergy to contrast agents and can be minimized by prior administration of antihistamines and corticosteroids.

An excess of contrast agent can cause acute pulmonary edema, following a volume overload, and, more rarely, cardiogenic shock and acute myocardial infarction.

Acute renal failure from contrast agents, the most feared complication after coronary angiography examination, can be reduced by delaying angiography in patients with known renal failure and avoiding concomitant administration of other nephrotoxic drugs (metformin) and reducing the volume of the contrast medium administered. This can be achieved by minimizing the number of angiographic acquisitions. Adequate hydration and the preventive administration of N-acetylcysteine and bicarbonates can reduce the incidence of nephropathy by the contrast medium.

In case of bleeding during or immediately after coronary angiography, an examination may be useful for the administration of protamine, which antagonizes the effects of heparin.

However, severe reactions can occur with the administration of protamine, such as: wheezing, hypotension, hot flushes.

9.3 Coronary Circulation: Characteristics and Anomalies

Coronary angiography allows both to describe the anatomical course and to identify the type of coronary circulation.

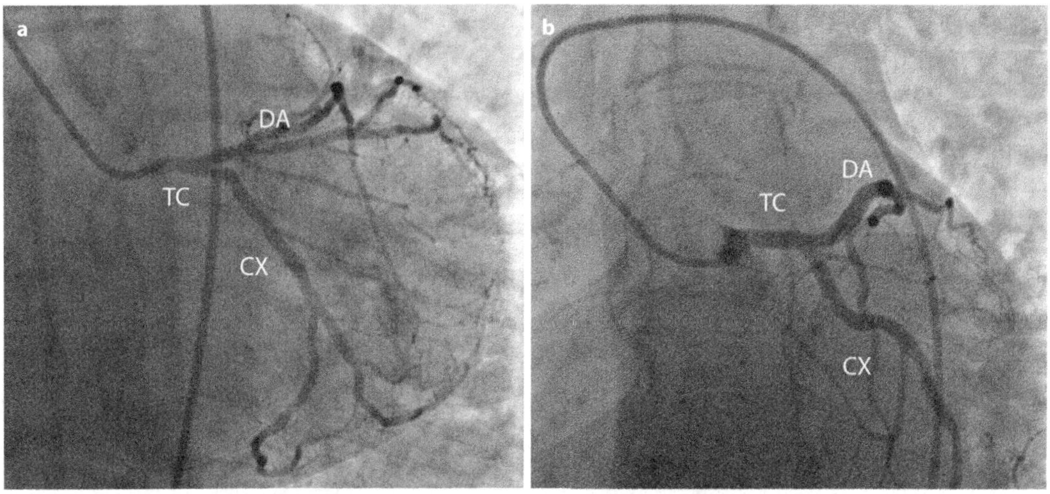

Fig. 9.1 Left coronary artery (a LAO 45°/CAU 25° and b CAU 30°): from the left sinus of Valsalva and the common trunk (*CT*) the origin of the anterior descending (*AD*) artery and the circumflex (*CX*) artery is visualized

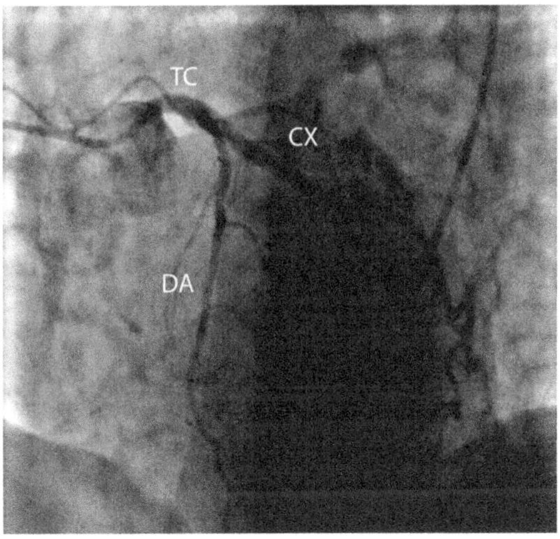

Fig. 9.2 Left coronary artery (LAO 40°/CRA 20°): the common trunk (*CT*), the course of the anterior descending (*AD*) artery as far as the apex, and the circumflex (*CX*) artery are visualized

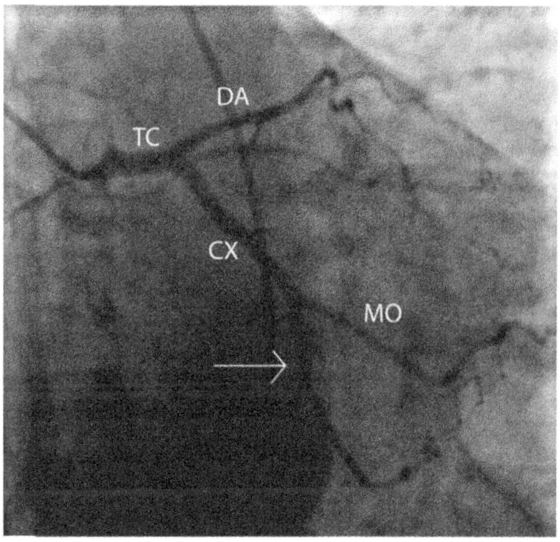

Fig. 9.3 Left coronary artery (RAO 30°/CAU 20°): the common trunk (*CT*), the course of the anterior descending (*AD*), the circumflex (*CX*) artery and an obtuse marginal (*OM*) branch are visualized. The white arrow indicates critical stenosis of the circumflex artery

Coronary circulation is defined by the coronary artery which gives rise to the posterior descending artery (PAD). In about 86% of patients, coronary circulation is dominant on the right; in 7% of patients, it is dominant on the left and the remaining 7% of patients have co-dominant circulation, in which the posterior descending artery arises from the right coronary and the circumflex arteries. The dominance is of no clinical significance.

The left coronary artery (Figs. 9.1-9.4) originates from the first segment of the left sinus of Valsalva, i.e. the left main (LM) coronary artery, and has a variable diameter of generally less than 4 cm. It is divided into the left anterior descending (LAD) and circumflex (CX) arteries, and can sometimes give rise to a third branch called the intermediate branch. The left anterior descending artery runs in the anterior interventricular sulcus, reaching the

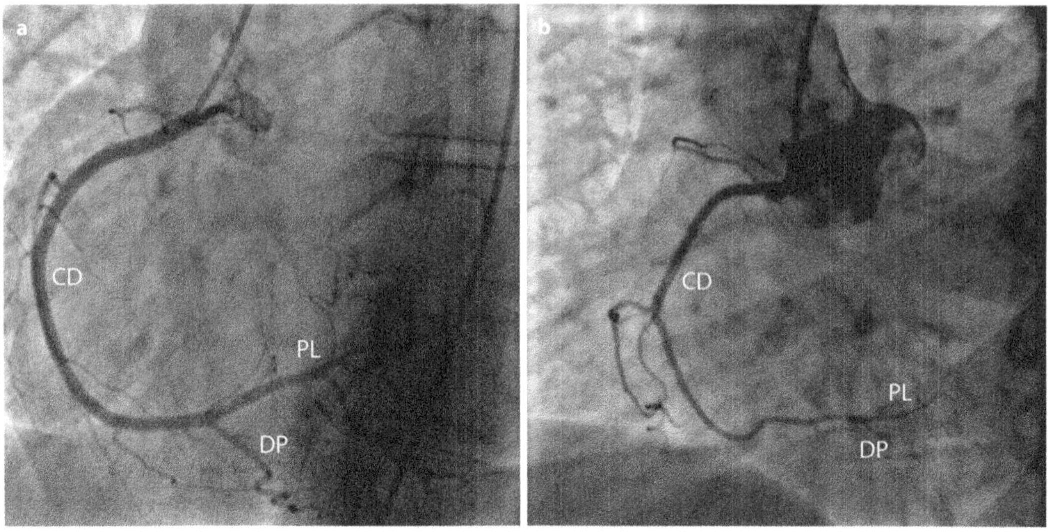

Fig. 9.4 Right coronary artery (CRA 45° and LAO 45°): the right coronary artery (*CRA*) and its dividing branches are visualized: posterior descending (*PD*) artery and posterolateral (*PL*) branch

apex of the left ventricle. Its collateral branches are the diagonal branches that supply the anterolateral wall of the left ventricle and septal branches to the interventricular septum. The circumflex artery runs in the atrioventricular groove and furnishes the left side and back walls. Its collateral branches are obtuse marginal branches.

The right coronary artery (RCA) (Fig. 9.4) runs in the right atrioventricular groove and reaches the posterior interventricular groove back at the crux cordis. Proximally, the artery usually gives rise to the conus branch pulmonary artery (50% of patients), the artery to the sinoatrial node (55% of cases), and acute marginal branches to the right ventricle. At the level of the crux cordis it is divided into the right coronary artery, posterior descending (PDA) and posterolateral branch. In 1.0 to 1.5% of cases it is possible find coronary anomalies during a coronary angiography examination, which are generally benign with no clinical significance. Of these, 90% are abnormalities of the origin or course. Among the most common benign abnormalities are the separated origin of the left anterior descending artery and circumflex artery, in 0.4 to 1% of patients, which is sometimes associated with a bicuspid aortic valve. The circumflex artery may originate from the right sinus of Valsalva or right coronary artery. Its course is generally posterior to the aorta and reaches the left atrioventricular groove. In cases of hypoplastic circumflex artery a superdominant hypertrophic right coronary artery was found running posteriorly in the right and left atrioventricular grooves.

The anomalous origin of the left anterior descending artery from the right sinus of Valsalva and the origin of the right coronary artery from the left coronary sinus have important clinical roles. These abnormalities of origin have a clinical importance because the first stretch runs between the aorta and the pulmonary artery with consequent systolic squeezing and the appearance of symptoms. More rarely, there may be a source of an anomalous coronary vessel, mostly the left coronary artery, directly from the pulmonary artery, with the subsequent onset of left to right shunt, which is responsible for death, myocardial infarction and congestive heart failure.

Other possible anomalies are coronary fistulae, or anomalous connections between one of the coronary arteries and another structure, most commonly a venous structure (i.e., the cardiac vein or coronary sinuses) or a heart chamber. The right coronary artery is responsible for fistulae in 55% of patients. The majority drain directly into the right ventricle, right atrium or coronary sinus. Less common are fistulae that drain into the pul-

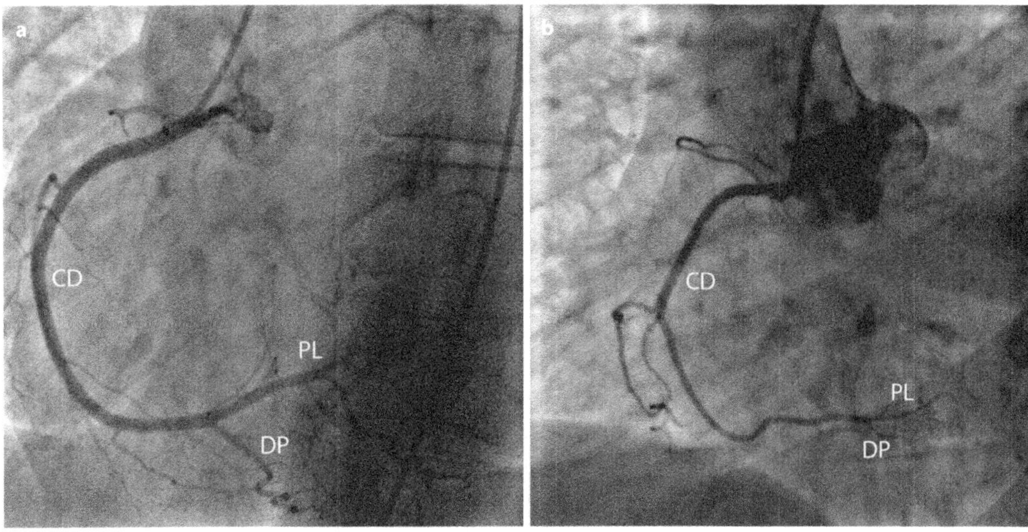

Fig. 9.5 Left ventriculography (RAO 30°): the left ventricle in diastole (*DIA*) and systole (*SIS*) are visualized

monary artery, left atrium or left ventricle. Generally, the shunt is small with no impairment of coronary circulation and for this reason patients are often asymptomatic. However, in cases where there is a large shunt, pulmonary hypertension, congestive heart failure, bacterial endocarditis, rupture and myocardial ischemia may occur. When a coronary angiography is performed, all segments of the coronary arteries should be displayed and any in at least two orthogonal projections should be bypassed. All segments of the coronary arteries must be viewed in their entirety without overlapping, in order to properly evaluate possible abnormalities or stenoses.

The limits of coronary angiography are due to the fact that this diagnostic method consists of a two-dimensional luminogram which therefore provides information of the vessel lumen and not of the vascular walls. To define the degree of stenosis, normal vascular segments are compared with other patients. Therefore, the absence of a normal segment will tend to underestimate the severity and extent of an atherosclerotic plaque. Moreover, the presence of endoluminal thrombi and ulcerated plaques is evaluated indirectly by the type of coronary filling. To do this, other coronary invasive methods such as intravascular ultrasound (IVUS), optical coherence tomography (OCT) or fractional flow reserve (FFR) can be integrated, allowing for a more accurate diagnosis. After coronary angiography ventriculography (Fig. 9.5) can be performed, enabling an assessment of left ventricular function and the presence of mitral valve insufficiency. However, it is possible to obtain the same information on morphology and ventricular function with non-invasive methods, such as echocardiography, with the routine use of angiography considerably reduced, especially in high-risk patients (patients with: severe symptomatic aortic stenosis, moderate to severe congestive heart failure or angina at rest, the presence of thrombotic material in the ventricle, or mitral valve endocarditis involving the aorta, renal failure, and patients with mechanical aortic valve prosthesis).

References

1. Murphy JG, Lloyd MA (2007) Mayo Clinic Cardiology. Mayo Clinic Scientific Press, Rochester
2. Zanchetta M, Pedon L, Colonna S, Maiolino P (2000) Cateterismo cardiaco e coronarografia. In: AAVV (ed) Trattato di cardiologia. Excerpta Medica, Milano
3. Scanlon PJ, Faxon DP, Audet AM et al (1999) ACC/AHA Guidelines for coronary angiography. A report of the American College of Cardiology/American Heart Association Task Force on practice guidelines (Committee on Coronary Angiography). Developed in collaboration with the Society for Cardiac Angiography and Interventions. J Am Coll Cardiol 1756-1824

Endomyocardial Biopsy

10

Stefano Tonioni, Carlo Gonnella and Emiliano Pica

10.1 Introduction

Endomyocardial biopsy (EMB) is an invasive, non-surgical diagnostic technique, which makes it possible to obtain histological samples of myocardial tissue through the use of biopsy forceps. The role of EMB in the diagnosis and treatment of cardiovascular diseases is still controversial. However, EMB is the gold standard for heart disease when the common non-invasive methods (echocardiography, magnetic resonance imaging, computed tomography) do not make precise histopathological diagnosis possible [1-3].

The risks of EMB may be divided into acute and late risks.

The risks include acute perforation with cardiac tamponade, supraventricular and ventricular arrhythmias, cardiac arrest, pneumothorax, perforation of large vessels, thromboembolism, venous hematoma, damage to valves and fistular formation.

The incidence of acute complications is related to the experience of each center and is operator-dependent in relation to the patient's clinical condition. The adoption of particular devices, such as the use of introducers of long dimensions to cross the atrioventricular valves, and appropriate adjuvant drug therapy (antiplatelet and anticoagulant), reduces the possible appearance of intra-procedural complications. Among the most common late complications are: hematoma at the site of vascular access, valvular damage, pericardial effusion, cardiac tamponade, thromboembolism and infections. Biopsy samples, taken percutaneously, transjugularly or transfemorally, by introducing the forceps under fluoroscopic control, must be adequately preserved for histological and isoenzymatic studies using optical microscopy and immunohistochemical, ultastructural and genetic evaluations.

Generally, the samples should be taken from more than one myocardial region, i.e. at least 3-5 samples of an appropriate size. For the analysis using optical microscopy, the biopsy specimens should be stored in paraffin, and a portion subjected to histological staining (hematoxylin-eosin, trichromic stain, Movat pentachromic stain, Congo Red stain and Pearl's iron stain). The samples without prior staining reactions are used for immunohistochemical, ultrastructural and genomic evaluations. The study is useful for histological diagnosis: acute rejection following transplantation, myocarditis (lymphocytic, giant), endocarditis, sarcoidosis, viral infections (cytomegalovirus, Ebstein-Barr virus, Coxackie virus), bacterial and parasitic infections (e.g., *Toxoplasma gondii*), primitive cardiomyopathy (dilated, hypertrophic obstructive pulmonary disease), drug-induced cardiomyopathies (e.g., anthracyclines), accumulation of cardiomyopathy (e.g., amyloidosis, hemochromatosis, glycogen storage, Fabry's disease), secondary cardiomyopathies (e.g., ischemic) and cancer.

10.2 The Role of EMB in the Diagnosis of Cardiovascular Diseases

In 2007 the AHA (American Heart Association), ACC (American College of Cardiology) and ESC

S. Tonioni (✉)
Cardiology Department
"San Carlo di Nancy" Hospital, Rome, Italy

M. Fioranelli and G. Frajese (eds.), *Sports Cardiology*,
DOI: 10.1007/978-88-470-2775-6_10, © Springer-Verlag Italia 2012

(European Society of Cardiology) published a joint paper to define the role of EMB in the management of cardiovascular diseases.

In particular, the joint study group identified 15 conditions (14 clinical scenarios) where, although there is no uniformity of agreement, it is useful to perform EMB.

Clinical Scenario 1

New-onset heart failure of < 2 weeks' duration associated with a normal-sized or dilated left ventricle in addition to hemodynamic compromise [4].

Adult and pediatric patients who present with the sudden onset of severe left ventricular failure within 2 weeks of a distinct viral illness and who have typical lymphocytic myocarditis with EMB have an excellent prognosis. These patients often are in cardiogenic shock and require intravenous inotropic agents or mechanical assistance for circulatory support. The left ventricle is often thick but not dilated, and the ejection fraction (EF) is markedly depressed. However, if other causes of heart failure (such as coronary artery disease) are ruled out, EMB can provide unique prognostic information and rule out clinically more aggressive disorders.

Giant cell myocarditis (GCM) and necrotizing eosinophilic myocarditis may have a fulminant clinical course, but unlike fulminant lymphocytic myocarditis, both disorders have a poor prognosis. This form of eosinophilic heart disease is characterized by the acute onset and rapid progression of hemodynamic compromise. A histological diagnosis on EMB alters the prognosis and would lead to immunosuppressive treatment.

Therapy with combinations of immunosuppressive agents has been associated with improved outcomes in GCM and necrotizing eosinophilic myocarditis.

Thus, EMB may provide unique and clinically meaningful information and should be performed in the setting of unexplained, new-onset heart failure of <2 weeks' duration associated with a normal-sized or dilated left ventricle in addition to hemodynamic compromise.

Clinical Scenario 2

New-onset heart failure of 2 weeks' to 3 months' duration associated with a dilated left ventricle and new ventricular arrhythmias, Mobitz type II second- or third-degree atrioventricular (AV) heart block, or failure to respond to usual care within 1 to 2 weeks [5].

Although most cases of acute dilated cardiomyopathy (DCM) are relatively mild and resolve with few short-term sequelae, certain signs and symptoms predict GCM, a disorder with a mean transplantation-free survival duration of only 5.5 months. GCM is associated with autoimmune disorders, thymoma, and drug hypersensitivity. At presentation, ventricular tachycardia is present in 15% of cases, complete heart block in 5%, and an acute coronary syndrome in 6% – rates higher than are typically seen in non-inflammatory DCM. Thus, clinical clues that suggest GCM and prompt an EMB include association with other autoimmune disorders or thymoma, failure to respond to usual care, and the presence of complete heart block or ventricular tachycardia.

Patients with acute heart failure due to GCM respond well to heart transplantation. Alternatively, treatment with combination immunosuppression may improve transplantation-free survival duration compared with patients with GCM not receiving immunosuppressive treatment. Therefore, a diagnosis of GCM will affect prognosis and treatment.

Clinical Scenario 3

Heart failure of >3 months' duration associated with a dilated left ventricle and new ventricular arrhythmias, Mobitz type II second- or third-degree AV heart block, or failure to respond to usual care within 1 to 2 weeks [6].

Patients who present with heart failure of >3 months' duration associated with a dilated left ventricle and new ventricular arrhythmias, second- or third-degree heart block, or failure to respond to usual care within 1 to 2 weeks are at risk for cardiac sarcoidosis or idiopathic granulomatous myocarditis.

Cardiac sarcoidosis is present in 25% of patients with systemic sarcoidosis, but symptoms referable to cardiac sarcoidosis occur in only 5% of sarcoidosis patients, and up to 50% of patients with granulomatous inflammation in the heart have no evidence of extracardiac disease. Patients with cardiac sarcoidosis may sometimes be distinguished from those with DCM by a high rate of heart block (8% to 67%) and ventricular arrhythmias (29%). The rates of ventricular tachycardia and heart block are therefore similar in cardiac sarcoidosis and GCM, but cardiac sarcoidosis generally has a more chronic course.

Sarcoidosis may respond to treatment with corticosteroids. Corticosteroids may improve clinical status and ventricular function, particularly if used early in the course of disease, but their benefit for ventricular arrhythmias is less certain. Implantable cardiac defibrillators may be effective in treating arrhythmias in patients with ventricular tachycardia related to sarcoidosis. After extensive fibrosis of the left ventricle, steroid use is probably of little benefit.

Clinical Scenario 4

Heart failure associated with a DCM of any duration that is associated with suspected allergic reaction in addition to eosinophilia [7].

Hypersensitivity myocarditis (HSM) is an uncommon disorder with a wide range of presentations, including sudden death, rapidly progressive heart failure, or more chronic DCM. Clinical clues that are reported in a minority of cases include rash, fever, and peripheral eosinophilia. A temporal relation with recently initiated medications or the use of multiple medications is usually present. The ECG is often abnormal, with nonspecific ST-segment changes or infarct patterns similar to other forms of acute myocarditis.

Early suspicion and recognition of HSM may lead to withdrawal of offending medications and administration of high-dose corticosteroids.

The presentation is usually biventricular heart failure, although arrhythmias may lead to sudden death. Usually hypereosinophilia precedes or coincides with the onset of cardiac symptoms, but the eosinophilia may be delayed. Eosinophilic myocarditis may also occur in the setting of malignancy or parasite infection and early in the course of endocardial fibrosis.

Clinical Scenario 5

Heart failure associated with suspected anthracycline cardiomyopathy [8].

Certain chemotherapeutic agents, particularly anthracyclines, are known to be cardiotoxic, particularly at higher cumulative doses. Although cardiotoxicity may be monitored by several methods, including echocardiographic or radionuclide angiography assessment of EF, fractional shortening, or parameters of diastolic dysfunction, these modalities are generally regarded as capable of detecting more advanced stages of cardiotoxicity rather than earlier degrees of cardiotoxicity. Nevertheless, these techniques are non-invasive and thus widely used in routine clinical practice. EMB, though an invasive procedure, is considered to be the most sensitive and specific means of evaluating cardiotoxicity.

Given its invasive nature, EMB in patients treated with chemotherapeutic agents may be best suited for situations in which there is uncertainty about the cause of cardiac dysfunction, as well as in select cases in which ultimate administration of a greater than the usual upper limit of an agent is believed to be desirable, and in clinical studies of chemotherapeutic-related toxicity of newer agents and regimens.

Clinical Scenario 6

Heart failure associated with unexplained restrictive cardiomyopathy [9].

Of the 3 major functional categories of cardiomyopathies (dilated, hypertrophic, and restrictive), restrictive cardiomyopathy is the least common form in adults and in children. Typically, a patient presents with symptoms of heart failure and on echocardiogram is found to have a normal or decreased volume in both ventricles, bi-atrial enlargement, normal or minimally increased wall thickness with no valvular abnormality, or normal or near-normal systolic function with impaired diastolic filling, such as restrictive physiology. This category of cardiomyopathy has been further classified into non-infiltrative processes, infiltrative disorders, and storage diseases that cause characteristic ventricular filling abnormalities. Thus, a variety of pathological processes may result in restrictive cardiomyopathy, although the cause often remains unknown. More importantly, the clinical and hemodynamic features of many types of restrictive cardiomyopathy may mimic those of constrictive pericarditis. EMB, in combination with either CT or MR, can be helpful in differentiating the 2 clinical entities: restrictive cardiomyopathy and constrictive pericarditis. EMB may reveal either a specific infiltrative disorder, such as amyloidosis or hemochromatosis, or myocardial fibrosis and myocyte hypertrophy consistent with idiopathic restrictive cardiomyopathy.

Clinical Scenario 7

Suspected cardiac tumors, with the exception of typical myxomas [10].

EMB is usually performed with the aid of transesophageal echocardiography. Lesions have been biopsied in all 4 cardiac chambers, though most reports are of right-sided tumors. Biopsy has resulted in diagnoses such as primary cardiac lymphoma, non-Hodgkin's lymphoma, cardiac sarcoma, cervical carcinoma, melanoma, hepatocellular carcinoma, and pulmonary microcytoma; lymphoma is the most commonly reported tumor. Most tumors were suspected, although several have been serendipitously discovered during biopsy for other indications. The actual yield of EMB for a suspected cardiac tumor cannot be defined because the number of non-diagnostic and unpublished procedures could never be determined. Therefore, EMB for a suspected cardiac tumor seems a reasonable procedure if (1) the diagnosis cannot be established by non-invasive means; (2) tissue diagnosis can be expected to influence the course of therapy; (3) the chances of successful biopsy are believed to be reasonably high; and (4) the procedure is performed by an experienced operator.

Clinical Scenario 8

Cardiomyopathy in children [11].

As in adults, the major indications for EMB in children include fulminant or acute unexplained heart failure, cardiac transplant surveillance or rejection evaluation, unexplained arrhythmias, and idiopathic forms of DCM. Rarely, patients with other forms of cardiomyopathy, including arrhythmogenic right ventricular dysplasia/cardiomyopathy (ARVD/C), restrictive cardiomyopathy, and hypertrophic cardiomyopathy (HCM), undergo EMB. In nearly all instances, the biopsies are performed in the right ventricle under sedation or anesthesia. Most cases of myocarditis in children are viral induced, have acute onset, and present with heart failure, cardiovascular collapse, or unexplained arrhythmias (usually ventricular tachycardia) or conduction disease (typically AV block). The histopathologic picture is similar to that seen in adults, although it appears to be virus specific.

Clinical Scenario 9

Heart failure of 2 weeks' to 3 months' duration associated with a dilated left ventricle, without *new ventricular arrhythmias or Mobitz type II second- or third-degree AV heart block, that responds to usual care within 1 to 2 weeks [12].*

The utility of EMB in patients with DCM of 2 weeks' to 3 months' duration is less certain than in patients with <2 weeks of symptoms because most patients with uncomplicated acute idiopathic dilated cardiomyopathy improve with standard heart failure care. Lymphocytic myocarditis is the most frequent form of myocarditis seen.

Clinical Scenario 10

Heart failure of >3 months' duration associated with a dilated left ventricle, without *new ventricular arrhythmias or Mobitz type II second- or third-degree AV heart block, that responds to usual care within 1 to 2 weeks [13].*

The role of EMB in chronic, symptomatic DCM has been the focus of recent research articles, particularly in viral-associated cardiomyopathy. EMB may have a greater role to follow the pharmacological therapy in the viral forms or in secondary to hemocromatosis forms.

Clinical Scenario 11

Heart failure associated with unexplained HCM [14].

Hypertrophic cardiomyopathy (HCM) occurs in an autosomal dominant pattern in 1:500 of the general population recognized to have the clinical phenotype, which makes it the most frequently occurring cardiomyopathy. HCM may present as sudden cardiac death in the young and may also cause heart failure at any age. HCM is defined by a hypertrophied, non-dilated left ventricle in the absence of other systemic or cardiac disease that might result in left ventricular wall thickening to the magnitude that is seen in HCM, e.g., systemic hypertension or aortic stenosis.

The diagnosis is made by echocardiography or magnetic resonance imaging, which shows left ventricular wall thickening, small left ventricular cavity, and sometimes a dynamic outflow obstruction. EMB is not usually needed in the evaluation of HCM but may be considered in those cases in which unexplained wall thickening prompts an effort to rule out infiltrative disorders such as Pompe's or Fabry's diseases and non-invasive tests are inconclusive. Senile, transthyretin-associated, and primary (AL) amyloidosis may have cardiac involvement that results in a dilated, restrictive, or hypertrophic pattern of cardiomyopathy.

Clinical Scenario 12

Arrhythmogenic right ventricular dysplasia/cardiomyopathy (ARVD/C) [15].

ARVD/C, an inherited or sporadic form of right and left ventricular cardiomyopathy, is estimated to occur in 1:5000 persons. The disorder involves predominantly the right ventricle, with progressive loss of myocytes that are replaced by fibro-fatty tissue, resulting in ventricular dysfunction and tachyarrhythmias, typically monomorphic ventricular tachycardia. Non-invasive tests, including echocardiography, right ventricular angiography, cardiac CMR, and cardiac CT imaging, often establishes the diagnosis.

The use of EMB for ARVD/C has been controversial because of the perceived risk of perforation of the thin-walled right ventricle with fibro-fatty replacement, but the few reports of EMB for AVRD/C do not report a high rate of complications.

Clinical Scenario 13

Unexplained ventricular arrhythmias [16].

EMB in primary or idiopathic (e.g., without known structural heart disease or predisposing disease) arrhythmias and primary conduction abnormalities had a high incidence of abnormal non-diagnostic findings.

Clinical Scenario 14

Unexplained atrial fibrillation [17].

EMB in unexplained atrial fibrillation do not perform because had non-significant findings.

10.2.1 EMB as a Research Tool

In addition to its clinical roles, EMB may be used to better understand the cellular and molecular pathophysiology of cardiovascular disease.

References

1. Cooper LT, Baughman KL, Feldman AM et al (2007) The role of endomyocardial biopsy in the management of cardiovascular disease. Eur Heart J 28:3076-3093
2. Murphy JG, Frantz RP, Cooper LT Jr (2007) Endomyocardial biopsy. In: Murphy JG, Lloyd MA Mayo Clinic Cardiology. Mayo Clinic Scientific Press, Rochester
3. Arbustini E, Grasso M, Diegoli M, Dal Bello B (2000) Biopsia cardiaca. In: AAVV (ed) Trattato di cardiologia. Excerpta Medica, Milano
4. McCarthy RE III, Boehmer JP, Hruban RH et al. (2000) Long-term outcome of fulminant myocarditis as compared with acute (nonfulminant) myocarditis. N Eng J Med 342:690-695
5. Shields RC, Tazelaar HD, Berry GJ et al. (2002) The role of right ventricular endomyocardial biopsy for idiopathic giant cell myocarditis. J Card Fail 8:74-78
6. Fleming HA, Bailey SM (1981) Sarcoid heart disease. J R Coll Physicians Lond 15:245-253
7. Talierco CP, Olney BA, Lie TJ (1985) Myocarditis related to drug hypersensivity. Mayo Clin Proc 60:463-468
8. Mackay B, Ewer MS, Carrasco CH et al (1994) Assessment of anthracycline cardiomyopathy by endomyocardial biopsy. Ultrastruct Pathol 18:203-211
9. Yazdani K, Maraj S, Amanullah AM (2005) Differentiating constrictive pericarditis from restrictive cardiomyopathy. Rev Cardiovasc Med 6:61-71
10. Alter P, Grimm W, Tontsch D, Maisch B (2001) Diagnosis of primary cardiac lymphoma by endomyocardial biopsy. Am J Med 110:593-594
11. Towbin J (2002) Cardiomyopathy and heart transplantation in childen. Curr Opin Cardiol 17:274-279
12. Grogan M, Redfield MM, Bailey KR et al (1995) Long-term outcome of patients with biopsy-proved myocarditis: comparison with idiopathic dilated cardiomyopathy. J Am Coll Cardiol 26:80-84
13. Parrillo JE (2001) Inflammatory cardiomyopathy (myocarditis): which patients should be treated with anti-inflammatory therapy? Circulation 104:4-6
14. Maron BJ, Towbin JA, Thiene G et al (2006) Contemporary definitions and classification of the cardiomyopathies. Circulation 113:1807-1816

15. Basso C, Ronco F, Abudureheman A, Thiene G (2006) In vitro validation of endomyocardial biopsy for the vivo diagnosis of arrhythmogenic right ventricular cardiomyopathy. Eur Heart J 27:960
16. Sekiguchi M, Nishizawa M, Nunoda S et al (1992) Endomyocardial biopsy approach in cases with ventricular arrhythmias. Postgrad Med J 68:S40-S43
17. Uemura A, Morimoto S, Hiramitsu S et al (2004) Right ventricular endomyocardial biopsy findings in 25 patients with sick sinus syndrome. Jpn Heart J 45:73-80

Integrated Imaging

11

Italo Porto, Rocco Vergallo, Maddalena Piro,
Bruno Pironi and Massimo Fioranelli

11.1 Introduction

In 1957, Sones performed the first human selective coronary arteriography, opening a new era in the assessment of coronary artery disease *in vivo* [1]. More than fifty years since its introduction in the clinical field, coronary angiography remains an irreplaceable diagnostic test in the evaluation of ischemic heart disease. Recently, however, the introduction of other coronary imaging techniques has helped in redefining its limits and usefulness.

The fundamental aim of coronary angiography is to identify and evaluate the basic lesion characterising atherosclerotic disease, the coronary plaque, and its outcome is focused on the quantification of the degree of stenosis determined by such plaque. These data are then used to define the prognosis and to set the therapeutic strategy.

A coronary stenosis can be anatomically defined in two ways: as the reduction of the section of the vessel lumen, according to a purely pathological point of view or to the computed tomography (CT) images, or as the reduction of the diameter in the longitudinal direction, according to a two-dimensional point of view (Fig. 11.1). In particular, quantitative coronary angiography (QCA) evaluates the severity of coronary lesions using the following parameters: stenosis percentage and minimum lumen diameter (MLD).

The assessment of stenosis percentage is obtained by the ratio between MLD, estimated at the narrowest point of the lesion, and the reference diameter of the vessel, which is the average diameter of the lumen in reference segments upstream and downstream the stenosis, judged as apparently healthy. MLD is expressed in millimetres and, compared to the percentage of stenosis, is an absolute variable and it is more easily reproducible [2].

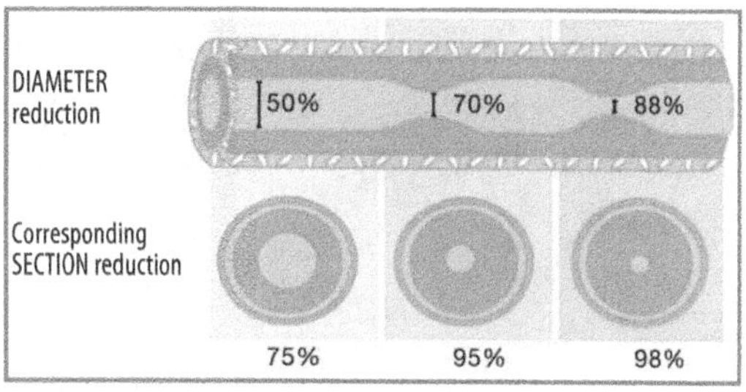

Fig. 11.1 Coronary artery stenosis evaluated as the reduction of the diameter and of the section of the lumen

11.2 The Limitations of Coronary Angiography

Standard coronary angiography has long been shown to suffer from several drawbacks. First of all, stenoses are generally graded on a visual basis (*eyeballing*), which is obviously prone to a high degree of subjectivity. For this reason, several generations of 2D-QCA software have been developed, although all were ultimately shown to have the same limitations of standard angiography. The two principal pitfalls of 2D-QCA are so-called *out-of-plane magnification* and foreshortening. The former is related to the calibration factor measured in a par-

I. Porto (✉)
Cardiovascular and Neurological Department
San Donato Hospital
Arezzo, Italy

M. Fioranelli and G. Frajese (eds.), *Sports Cardiology*,
DOI: 10.1007/978-88-470-2775-6_11, © Springer-Verlag Italia 2012

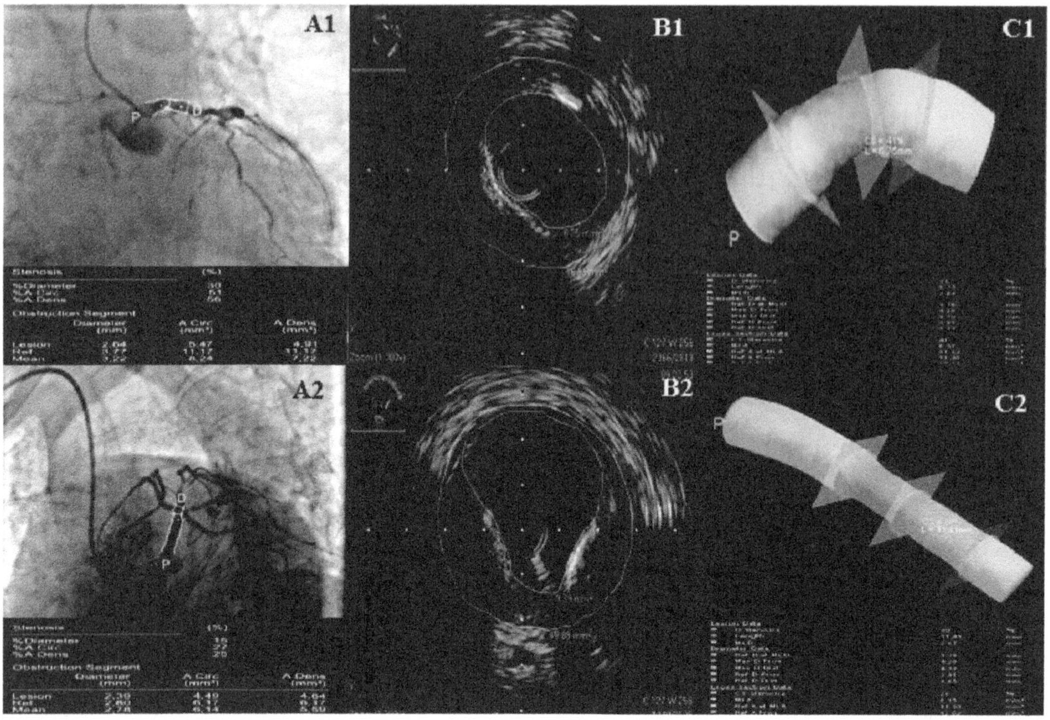

Fig. 11.2 Examples of 2-dimensional and 3-dimensional quantitative coronary angiographic and IVUS analyses of left main coronary artery stenosis. a right anterior oblique caudal view; b anteroposterior cranial view; c showed percent cross-sectional area [CS] stenosis; d 3-dimensional quantitative coronary angiographically measured parameters; e 3-dimensional reconstruction of analyzed left main coronary artery; f IVUS measurement of minimum lumen area (MLA) and external elastic membrane cross-sectional area (EEM CSA) of correspondent left main coronary artery stenosis. D = distal reference segment; P = proximal reference segment. Reproduced with permission from [4]

ticular plane perpendicular to the central projection axis. Foreshortening becomes a significant limitation especially when assessing curved segment length, depending on vessel tortuosity and on the experience of operators [3]. Newer 3D-QCA software, however, may be superior to standard 2D-QCA in specific subsets, such as in the evaluation of the left main segment [4] (Fig. 11.2).

A very important conceptual limit of angiography, moreover, is related to the fact that, while atherosclerotic disease essentially develops within the vessel wall, coronary angiography only detects an image of the vessel lumen, filled with contrast medium. An angiogram thus cannot reliably represent the complex three-dimensional structure of the vessel wall [5]. Indeed, pathology studies and coronary intravascular ultrasound (IVUS) [6] data have consistently shown that segments of the coronary arteries angiographically defined as *normal* often contain a significant atherosclerotic burden, meaning that the degree of angiographic stenosis can be easily underestimated when there is a diffuse atherosclerotic process throughout the examined vessel [7-8]. Finally, it is well known that myocardial infarction generally results from rupture of a *vulnerable* plaque, usually causing only mild to moderate stenosis. Unfortunately, the visualization of these plaques is not possible by coronary angiography [9].

11.2.1 Anatomy vs. Function

In the classical animal model proposed by Gould (Fig. 11.3) [10] the hyperemic flow, and thus the coronary reserve, starts to decrease when an atherosclerotic plaque causes a reduction of at least 50% of the vessel diameter in the case of concentric stenosis, corresponding to a reduction of 75% of the section or the vessel lumen (Fig. 11.1). A

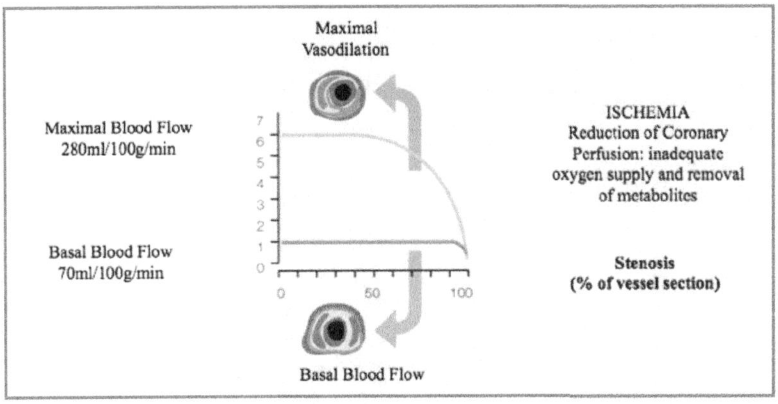

Fig. 11.3 Coronary reserve: stenosis/ischemia relation

stenosis is thus classically defined as hemodynamically *significant* when it reduces the diameter of a coronary vessel by at least 50%. However, this does not mean that this lesion is definitely able to cause ischemia, but only that a given percentage of diameter reduction is the essential and the minimal/least condition in order to have a potential ischemic risk. Indeed, many variables have to be considered in the equation, of which the status of the microcirculation is probably the most important [11]. On the other hand, even in the classical model the baseline flow is not subject to any reduction until the arterial diameter is reduced to about 90%. As a consequence, it is difficult in the single patient to ascribe an ischemic potential to moderately severe stenosis (those with a diameter reduction between 50% and 80%).

Among the various developments that have recently entered the clinical arena, it has to be mentioned that the fractional flow reserve (FFR) is a reliable (and widely validated) functional index in the evaluation of a coronary stenosis. Briefly, FFR identifies the maximal myocardial flow in the distribution area of a coronary artery with a stenosis compared to the theoretical maximum flow. This index represents the fraction of the maximum flow that can be reached in the presence of a coronary stenosis [12]. After administration of intracoronary nitrates and intracoronary or intravenous adenosine, causing maximum epicardial microcirculatory vasodilatation, the trans-stenotic pressure gradient is calculated. The value corresponds to the ratio between the pressure recorded downstream (distal pressure: Pd) and upstream (proximal pressure: Pa) of the stenosis. The normal index is equal to 1 and a value inferior to 0.8 is considered abnormal. For example, if the pressure measured downstream is 52 mmHg, and that measured upstream is 101 mmHg, the FFR value is 0.51, which is clearly abnormal. This index can be easily calculated and it is independent of physiological variations that can affect baseline myocardial blood flow, such as blood pressure or heart rate (Fig. 11.4).

11.3 Intravascular Ultrasound (IVUS)

Coronary Intravascular Ultrasound (IVUS) is an invasive imaging modality performed during coronary angiography, which allows the study of epicardial vessels through intraluminal acoustic assessment. IVUS provides a series of tomographic, cross-sectional images of the vessel of interest, assuring a very accurate and simultaneous assessment of the lumen, vessel wall and atherosclerotic plaque [13]. IVUS has various diagnostic and research applications: its ability to evaluate plaque composition, to objectively measure the degree of stenosis and vessel diameter are useful to guide revascularization procedures, while the identification of lesion vulnerability and the quantification of plaque burden are emerging as risk assessment tools. IVUS imaging requires a specific coronary catheter (2.6 to 3.5 French), with a miniaturized ultrasound transducer mounted at the tip (both mechanical and electronic transducers are available). After vessel engagement with a guide catheter and introduction of a guide-wire (heparinization and nitrates injection are also mandatory steps), IVUS catheter is advanced over a coro-

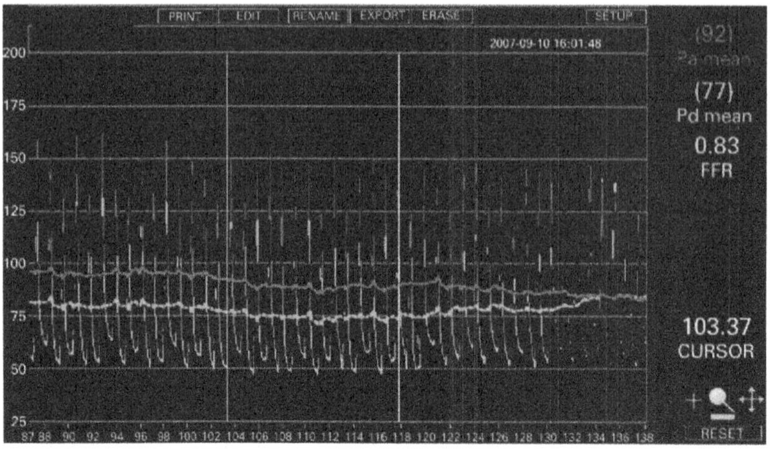

Fig. 11.4 Example of FFR calculation: Pd (distal Pressure)/ Pa (proximal Pressure) = 77/92 = 0.83

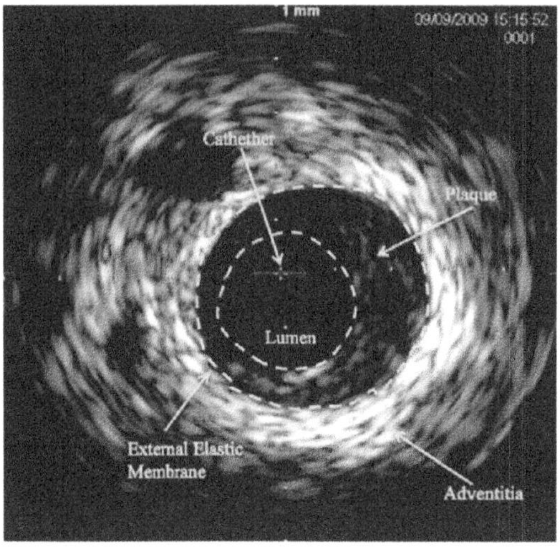

Fig. 11.5 IVUS image. The two borders of the arterial wall are easily recognizable thanks to their different acoustic signal. An echolucent plaque is visible

nary guide-wire and the transducer is placed beyond the target lesion and then pulled back with a distal-proximal direction up to the vessel ostium, in order to obtain a succession of cross-sectional images of the segment of the coronary vessel of interest. The pullback can be performed either manually or using a motorized pullback device, which withdraws the catheter at a constant speed of 0.25-1 mm/s and at a frame-rate of 30 images/s. Motorized transducer pullback and digital storage of IVUS images are necessary to obtain longitudinal imaging (L-mode); this particular computerized technique displays a series of IVUS images along a single cut plane to recreate the longitudinal appearance of the artery. An experienced IVUS operator can also obtain a three-dimensional reconstruction of a vessel segment, which can provide volumetric information.

In the IVUS image (Fig. 11.5), the catheter is at the centre of the vessel, surrounded by the lumen, the vessel wall and adjacent structures. Flowing blood is characterized by a peculiar pattern of echogenicity and it appears as a finely speckled region, allowing the separation of the lumen from the vessel wall. The arterial wall is held between two borders, with the internal one signing the passage between blood and the leading edge of the intima and the second corresponding to the external elastic membrane (EEM), the media-adventitia interface. These two borders can easily be recognized, because ultrasound is strongly reflected at tissue interfaces with different composition and acoustic properties [14]. The leading edge of the media is indeed poorly defined, such as the outer border of the adventitia. Externally to the EEM, some adjacent structures, including arterial side-branches, cardiac veins and the pericardium, can sometimes be recognized.

The strong signal originating at the indicated tissues interfaces allows manual or automated measurements. The most important areas measurements are:

- *Lumen Cross Sectional Area (CSA)*: the area delimited by the lumen border, decreased in presence of a stenosis;
- *EEM Cross Sectional Area (CSA)*: the area de-

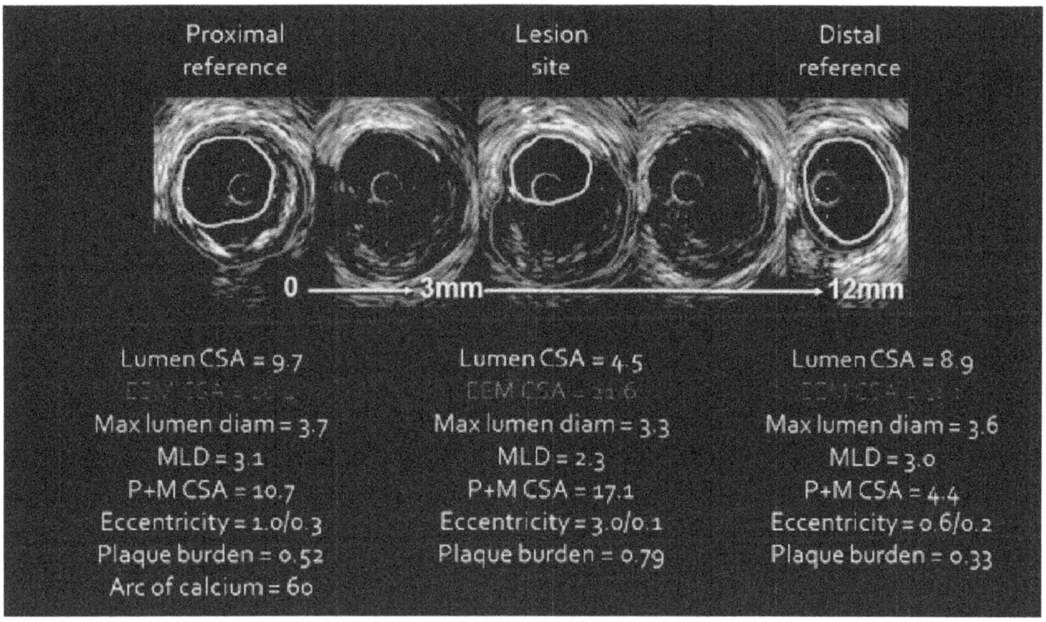

Fig. 11.6 IVUS image depicting successive cross-sectional areas (CSA) acquired with automatic pullback (left to right, proximal to distal). The longitudinal length is indicated at the bottom of the figure. The minimal lumen area is depicted in the middle panel. Yellow circle indicates lumen border, red circle indicates external elastic membrane (EEM). Measured and derived parameters are indicated (in mm^2, see text for details). For the entire lesion, average lumen CSA=9.3 mm^2, average EEM CSA=16.9 mm^2, area stenosis=52%, remodeling index=1.3

limitated by the EEM border; EEM circumference and area cannot be measured reliably at sites where important side-branches depart or in presence of extensive calcification;

- *Plaque Cross Sectional Area (CSA)*: derived by subtracting lumen area from EEM area (EEM CSA – Lumen CSA). Because the leading edge of the media is not well delineated, IVUS cannot determine the true histological plaque area, while it uses the *plaque plus media* area. However, the inclusion of the media into the plaque area does not constitute a major limitation of IVUS because the media represents only a small fraction of the plaque CSA.

The most important linear measurements are:

- *minimum and maximum lumen diameters*;
- *minimum and maximum EEM diameters*;
- *maximum and minimum plaque thicknesses*: the longest and the shortest distances from intimal leading edge to the EEM border.

An example of complete measurements for an entire plaque over its longitudinal length is provided in Fig. 11.6.

Ultrasound provides information about the morphology of atherosclerotic plaques in vivo. It evaluates whether the plaque can be considered as *concentric* (the plaque is present throughout the 360° arterial circumference) or as *eccentric* (the plaque does not cover the whole circumference). Through L-mode, the disease can be considered as *diffuse* (the intimal thickness is abnormal at every site within the studied segment), or as *focal* (sites adjacent to the lesion are normal or have minimal disease). IVUS can also measure the *plaque burden*, that is the area within the EEM occupied by atheroma (the percentage of EEM occupied by atheroma at the lesion site), regardless of the lumen compromise. IVUS studies have shown that the size of the atherosclerotic plaque and the size of the lumen are, in general, weakly related. This is caused by two main elements: the diffuse nature of the atherosclerotic disease, and the so-called positive arterial remodeling. This phenomenon, described at first by Glagov [15], refers to adaptive changes of the arterial wall, which tries to preserve lumen despite plaque development. In case

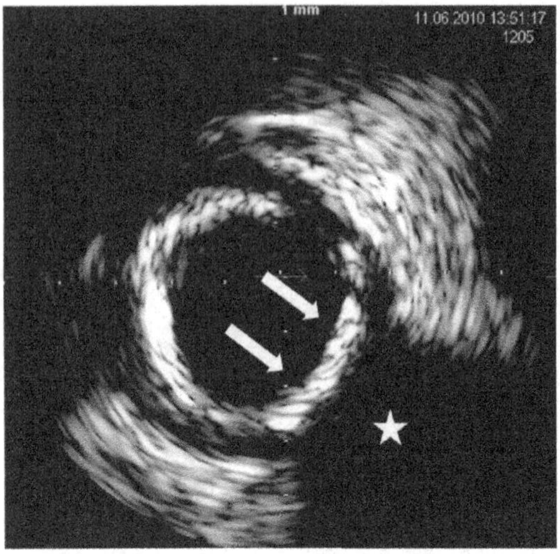

Fig. 11.7 Concentric calcific plaque (*arrows* show leading edge) with signal void and acoustic shadowing (*star*)

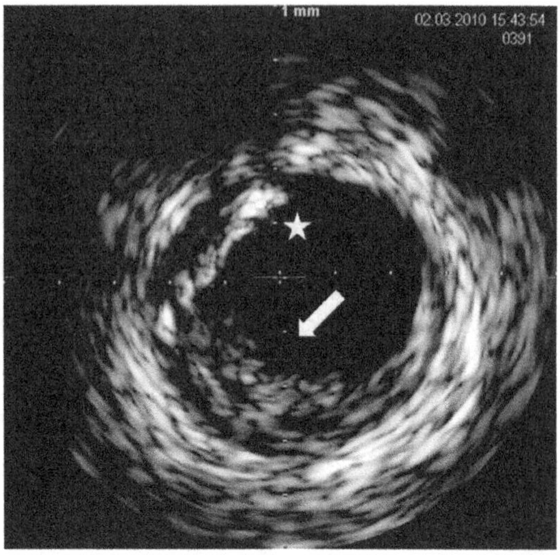

Fig. 11.8 Fibrous plaque (*arrow*) with spotty calcifications (*star*)

of mild or moderate lesions, plaque accumulation is balanced by an increase in arterial size, especially of the EEM area, resulting in a stable lumen area. In more advanced lesions, expansive remodeling is less evident and plaque progression is finally associated with luminal stenosis. Subsequent IVUS studies showed that, at certain diseased sites, the EEM area may actually decrease, contributing to luminal stenosis: this process is called negative remodeling or arterial shrinkage.

IVUS is also able to infer on the tissue components of the atherosclerotic lesions, based on the echogenicity of the structures; this ability is not comparable to histology [16]. In particular, IVUS can identify three different types of plaques:

1) Echolucent (*lipid*) plaque, with low echogenicity (Fig. 11.5); frequently these lesions present an important echogenic border at the lumen/intima interface, which may correspond to the fibrous cap.
2) Echoreflective (*calcified*) plaque, with signal void (acoustic shadowing) (Fig. 11.7).
3) Echodense (*fibrous*) plaque, with an intermediate echogenicity between echolucent lipidic atheromas and highly echoreflective calcific lesions (Fig. 11.8).

Mixed plaques, however, composed by various tissue components and with peculiar acoustic properties, are frequent. IVUS is considered a very sensitive *in vivo* method for the detection of coronary calcium, which is an indicator of atherosclerotic disease. Calcified deposits appear as reflecting and bright echoes that obstacle the penetration of ultrasounds, creating a characteristic phenomenon called *acoustic shadowing*. IVUS can show only the leading edge of the calcified plaque but it cannot determine its thickness and the underlying structures. Although IVUS identifies with high sensitivity and specificity fibrous tissue and calcifications, it is less reliable to detect fatty tissue; lesions with low echogenicity may indeed be attributable to a plaque with high lipidic content, but also to plaque with a necrotic zone within, or to intramural hemorrhage, or to thrombus. More recently, greyscale IVUS has been used to identify a peculiar type of echolucent plaque, the *attenuated* plaque (defined as deep ultrasound attenuation without calcification), associated with periprocedural complications and distal embolization [17].

IVUS has shown to be a safe technique: the rate of complications is indeed very low. Major complications, such as dissection or vessel closure, are uncommon (less than 0.5%); minor complications are more frequent, such as transient coronary spasm, which can be resolved by intracoronary nitroglycerin, and transient ischemia, caused by passage of the catheter in a tight vessel or stenosis [18].

The main clinical and therapeutic indications to perform IVUS are *the assessment of ambiguous (intermediate or indeterminate) angiographic findings* and *the guidance of revascularization procedures* [19-21]. Certain lesion patterns or locations elude accurate angiographic visualization, despite multiple projections. Most of these cases concern lesions of intermediate or subcritical severity, or the localization of the disease at ostial, at bifurcation or at branching sites; other possible angiographic *hazy* results may be caused by aneurysmal lesions, tortuous vessels, sites with plaque rupture, intraluminal filling defect or thrombus. Left main stem lesions are particularly challenging [4]. The precise role for IVUS during percutaneous procedures has not been well defined in large-scale studies, but it has demonstrated to provide important skills in pre-interventional target lesion assessment.

Pre-interventional IVUS is commonly used to select the most appropriate interventional approach and the choice of particular devices. A decision can be taken after the analysis of several plaque characteristics, such as stenosis degree, plaque distribution, depth and extent of calcification, arterial remodeling, and the presence of thrombi or dissections. IVUS can have also a very important role after intervention, allowing monitoring the correct and complete stent symmetry, expansion and apposition. IVUS allows diagnosis and treatment of dissection and other complications.

In general, while latest data have clearly shown that IVUS data should not be used to judge on the severity of a stenosis [22] as it does not reliably predict the degree of reduction of flow reserve as expressed by FFR (see above), important datasets indicate a good negative predictive value in certain specific situations, such as in the left main. Here, an IVUS minimal lumen area of more than 6 mm^2 is associated with a very good long term prognosis [23]. Coupled with the important guidance role of IVUS for left main stenting (which is potentially associated with improved long-term survival), and with the lower reliability of other intravascular imaging techniques (such as OCT, see below) in large-sized vessels, in the authors' opinion IVUS remains a cornerstone for operators willing to evaluate and tackle left main disease.

11.3.1 Limitations of IVUS

IVUS has long evidenced some weaknesses. First of all, the physical size of ultrasound catheter may cause dilatation and distort the measurements in imaging severe stenosis and small vessels. Secondly, IVUS imaging can product some artefacts. The most important one is the characteristic acoustic shadowing caused by calcified lesions, negating the visualization of underlying structures. Another significant problem is the blood *speckle*, more evident with higher-resolution probes and increasing exponentially as blood flow velocity decreases. Therefore flow stagnation, often evident when the catheter is advanced through a tight stenosis, can limit the ability to differentiate lumen from echolucent tissue, such as soft plaque, neointima and thrombus [24].

11.3.2 Radiofrequency Analysis: Virtual Histology, iMAP and Integrated Backscatter

In the last years, information derived from spectral radiofrequency analysis on the reflected acoustic waves (RF-IVUS) has been added to greyscale reconstructions to infer on morphology and composition of the atherosclerotic plaque. With this method, ultrasounds within the RF range are transformed into electrical signals, analysed in the various frequency components and transformed into graphical visualization. Three main post-processing methods for tissue characterization based on RF analysis have been developed [25]: Virtual Histology (VH-IVUS, Volcano Therapeutics, Rancho Cordova, CA, USA), iMap (Boston Scientific, Santa Clara, CA, USA) and Integrated Backscatter (IB-IVUS) (Table 11.1).

VH-IVUS software combines the gross amplitude information of conventional gray-scale IVUS to the underlying frequency content of the tissue assessed by a specific algorithm, in order to obtain a more detailed characterization of plaque morphology [26] (Fig. 11.9). Atherosclerotic plaques are characterized by a classification tree, and different histological components are coded into colors. VH-IVUS is usually performed by a 20 MHz, 2.9 F phased-array catheter (Eagle Eye, Volcano Cor-

Table 11.1 A comparative table showing technical data and strengths/weaknesses for the three types of plaque characterization software based on radiofrequency analysis commercially available at the time of writing. Integrated backscatter (IB) is not available outside Japan

	VH-IVUS	iMAP	IB-IVUS
IVUS	Volcano	Boston Scientific	Terumo
Frequency	20/45 MHz	40 MHz	40 MHz
Parameter	8 data points	13 data points	IB value
Construction	Histology	Histology	Ultrasound
Color Map	Classification tree	Pattern recognition	IB value
Behind Ca	Possible?	Impossible	Impossible
Thrombus	Impossible	Impossible	Possible?
Impression	Different	?	Grayscale-like
Difference	Modified	Modified	Direct analysis

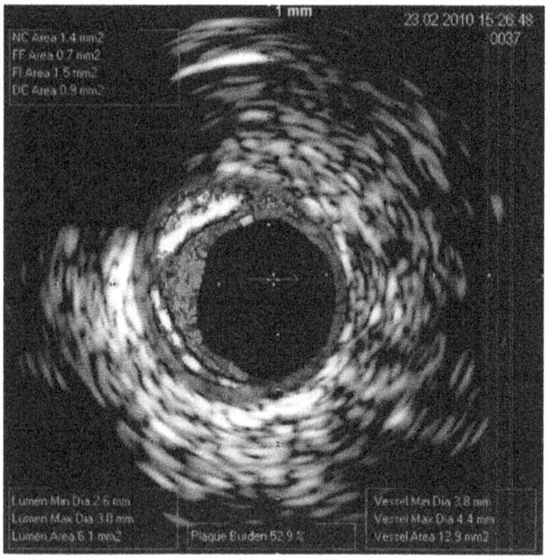

Fig. 11.9 Virtual Histology image: fibrous areas are marked in *green*, fibro-lipid in *yellow* (not visible here), calcium in white and necrotic core in *red*

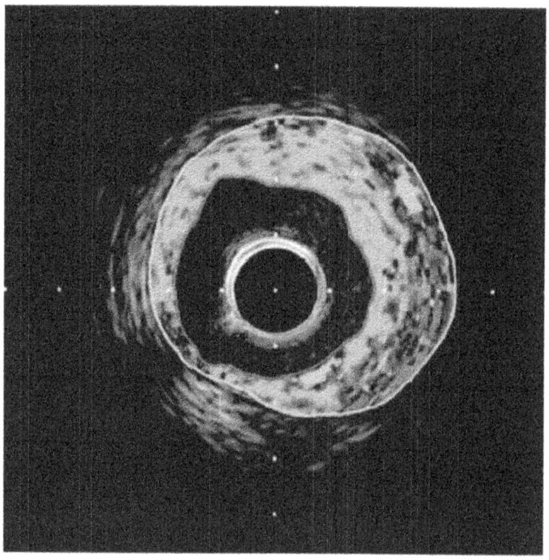

Fig. 11.10 iMAP image: mixed fibrous-calcific plaque. *Green*: fibrous tissue; *blue*: calcium; *pink*: necrotic tissue; *yellow*: lipid tissue. Reproduced with permission from [44]

poration, Rancho Cordova, CA, USA) with an electrocardiogram (ECG)-gated acquisition. Alternatively, a 45 MHz, 3.2 F rotational catheter (Revolution®, Volcano Therapeutics) can be used [27].

iMAP is another novel IVUS-derived technique using spectral analysis for the characterization of plaque morphology. It is performed by a 40 MHz imaging system without ECG-gated acquisition (instead, 2 frames/mm are captured). The color scheme is different from VH-IVUS, marking fibrous tissue in green, lipid area in yellow, calcium in blue and necrotic core in pink. It provides volume, area and percent measurements, by a real-time automatic border tracing and tissue characterization (Fig. 11.10). Thanks to its ability of selecting specific areas in the cross-sectional and longitudinal view, iMAP allows to analyse a particular region of interest rather than just entire atheroma [28].

In vivo plaque characterization can also be obtained by IB-IVUS, performed by a 40 MHz mechanically rotating catheter acquiring ultrasound backscattered signal, which is analyzed by a fast Fourier transform and measured in decibels (dB). At IB-IVUS analysis fibrous areas are marked in green, lipid pool in blue, calcium in red and fibro-fatty tissue in yellow [29] (Fig. 11.11).

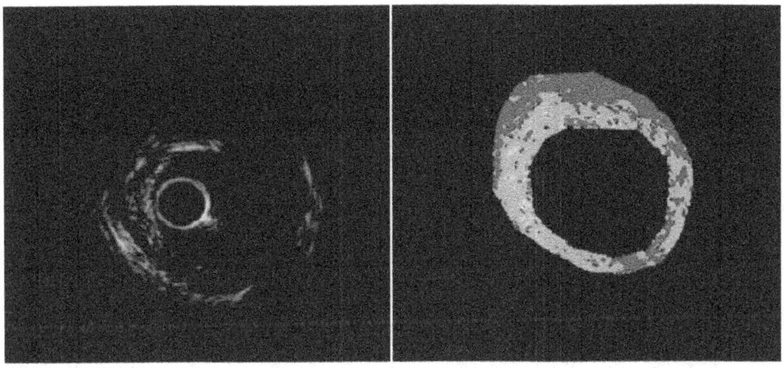

Fig. 11.11 IVUS (*left*) and integrated backscattering (IB) (*right*): fibrous-lipid plaque. *Green*: fibrous tissue; *blue*: lipid pool; *red*: calcium. Reproduced with permission from [44]

11.4 Optical Coherence Tomography (OCT)

Optical coherence tomography (OCT) is a novel high resolution imaging modality that use a light source with a near-infrared spectrum (wavelengths ranging from 1280 to 1350), in order to create cross-sectional images of biological tissues by measuring the *echo time delay* and the intensity of backscattered light [30]. A thin optical fibre (0.019 inches) is introduced into coronary arteries during a traditional coronary angiography and a light source is emitted towards the sample. Because of the high speed of light ($3x10^8$ m/sec), an interferometer is necessary to measure the backscattered signal. The low-coherence light source is split by a fibre optic beam splitter into two separate arms, one directed to the tissue sample and the other to a reference moving mirror. Interference occurs when the light reflected from the tissue and the light returning from the mirror have travelled the same optical distance, arriving to the detector at the same time. In this way, OCT generates images with a spatial resolution (10-15 mm) greatly higher (30 times) than IVUS [31].

There are two main types of OCT:

1) the first-generation, called time domain (TD)-OCT, which requires a cleanness of the images in order to extract information from coronary artery microstructure, due to the blood scattering and attenuation of light. Image acquisition can be performed by two different approaches: the occlusive technique and the non-occlusive technique; the former clears images from blood by inflating a proximal occlusion balloon and flushing a crystalloid solution, such as Ringer's lactate, at a constant rate using a power injector; thanks to the improvement of TD-OCT acquisition speeds, the cleanness of the images from blood can be obtained just by using a transparent media flush (non-occlusive technique), thus reducing the potential risk associated to the procedure (see below).
2) frequency domain (FD)-OCT which provides higher quality images than TD-OCT. Due to a faster pullback rate (10-20 mm/sec), it can be performed by the non-occlusive technique.

OCT can discriminate the three layers of the coronary artery wall (intima, media and adventitia) and structures delimiting the media (internal and external elastic lamina) [31] (Fig. 11.12). The

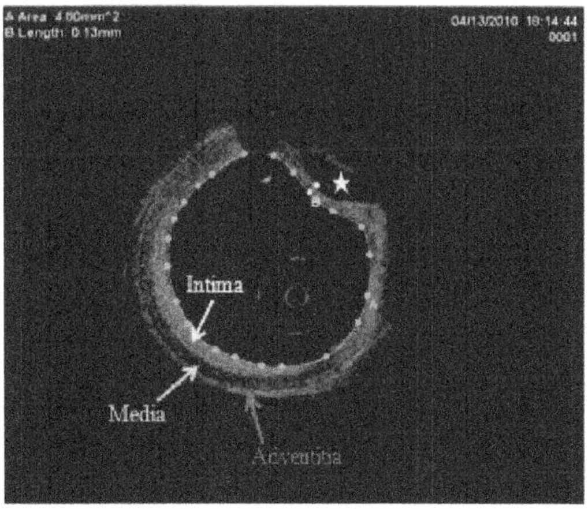

Fig. 11.12 OCT image. The three layers of arterial wall (intima, media, adventitia), luminal area (*green circle*), fibrous cap (*white line*) and calcifications (*star*) can be observed.

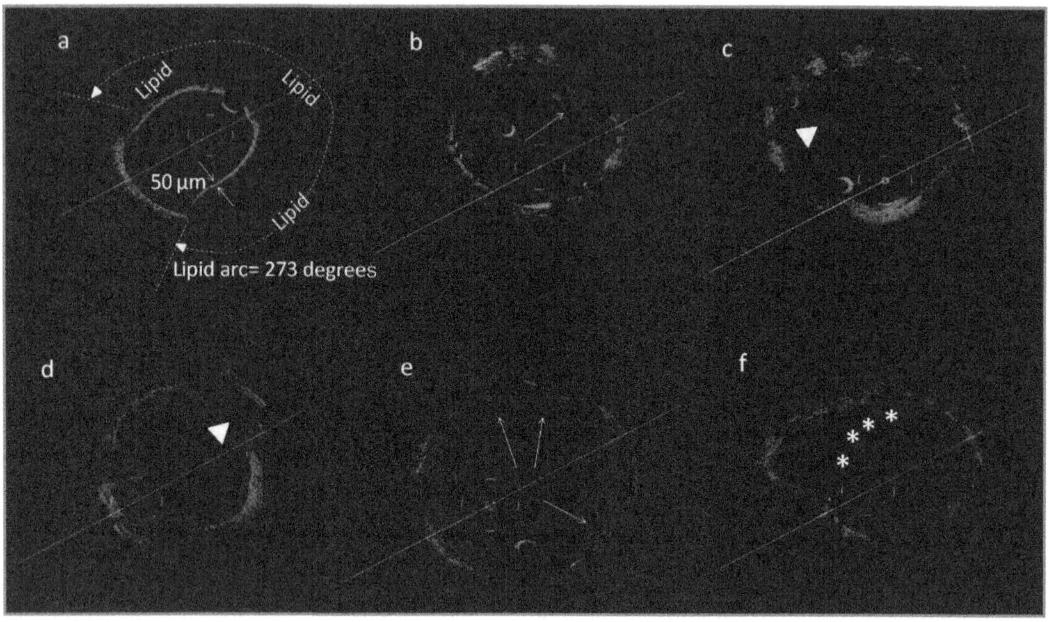

Fig. 11.13 FD-OCT images of main plaque features pre- and post-PCI. a TCFA is imaged. Lipid arc is 273°, and cap thickness at the thinnest portion is 50 µm (*arrows*). b Intrastent thrombus (*arrow*) is imaged as an irregular mass with dorsal shadowing protruding within the lumen. Stent struts can be identified from their bright blooming appearance and characteristic dorsal shadowing. c Dissection (*arrowhead*), located in the body of the stent. d Dissection (*arrowhead*), located at the stent edge. e Tissue prolapse (*arrow*) is imaged as protrusion of tissue between stent struts extending inside a circular arc, connecting adjacent struts. f Malapposed stent struts are shown (asterisks). Reproduced with permission from [42]

intima appears as the signal rich layer nearest the lumen, surrounded by the *media* (signal poor middle layer) and the *adventitia* (external signal rich layer). OCT provides a very detailed characterization of atherosclerosis, making it possible to identify different types of coronary plaque [32-33]:

- *fibrous plaque*, appearing as a signal rich, homogeneous area;
- *fibrocalcific* or *calcific plaque*, identified by a low backscattering, heterogeneous lesion surrounded by sharp borders;
- *lipid rich plaque*, observed as a signal poor, diffuse border area.

Furthermore, OCT is very useful to assess plaque complications, such as plaque ulceration, rupture, dissection or fissure, intracoronary thrombus, thin-cap fibroatheroma (TCFA). *Plaque rupture* is defined as a ruptured fibrous cap connecting the lipid core with the lumen, *plaque ulceration* appears as a recess beginning at the luminal-intimal border, *plaque dissection* or *fissure* can be observed as thin protruding rims of tissue. Sometimes, a thrombotic mass can be appreciated onto these lesions. *Thrombus* appears as a signal rich, low backscattering (white thrombus) or high backscattering, with signal free shadowing (red thrombus) mass protruding into the coronary lumen. Mostly, a mixed thrombus is involved. OCT is able to minutely detect plaque features of vulnerability, such as a *thin fibrous cap* (< 65 mm), a large lipid pool and activated *macrophages* (confluent or punctuate highly backscattering regions which can cause shadowing of underlying tissue) near the fibrous cap. Interestingly, presence of *TCFA* (defined as a lipid-rich plaque with a fibrous cap thickness of ≤65µm) at pre-PCI FD-OCT, and of intra-stent thrombus and intra-stent dissection at post-PCI FD-OCT, have been shown to be independent predictors of periprocedural myocardial infarction (type IVa MI of the Universal Definition) [34] (Fig. 11.13). Additionally, OCT is able to detect *intimal microchannels* as signal-poor, sharply delineated voids, which can play an important role in the pathogenesis of atherosclerotic plaque complica-

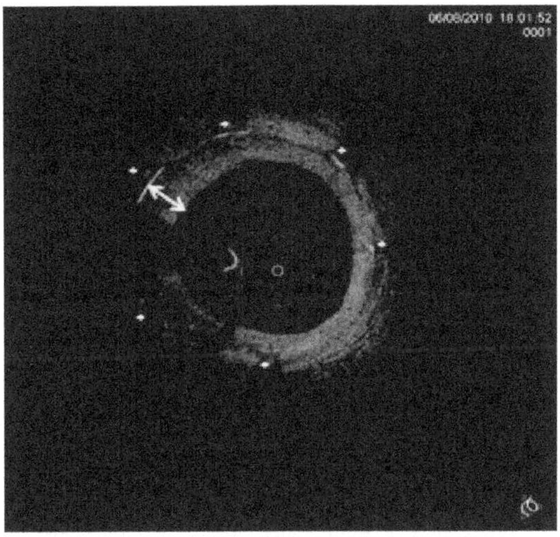

Fig. 11.14 OCT image of neointimal hyperplasia (*double-arrow*), observed 60 days after stent (*asterisks*) deployment

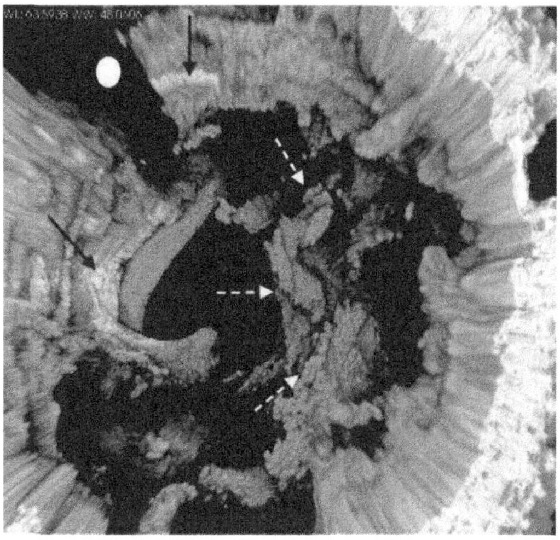

Fig. 11.15 Three-dimensional OCT image showing an intracoronary thrombus (*arrows*). Reproduced with permission from [43]

tions. Besides fibrous cap and lipid pool thickness measurement, OCT allows an accurate assessment of lumen areas and diameters (*luminal area stenosis, minimal lumen area, minimal* and *maximum lumen diameters*). Thanks to its high resolution and contrast, OCT provides valuable information about stent deployment and accurately detects a series of complications, such as *intra-stent thrombus, intra-stent* or *edge dissection, plaque prolapsed* (defined as the projection of tissue into the lumen between stent struts), *incomplete stent apposition* and *malapposition length, strut coverage* [35]. Finally, OCT makes it possible to evaluate *intimal hyperplasia* during the follow-up, providing useful information about the risk of restenosis after percutaneous coronary intervention (Fig. 11.14).

The analysis of atherosclerotic plaque and characterization of components related to instability, such as fibrous cap, lipid necrotic core or plaque angiogenesis, can be improved by three-dimensional reconstructions of OCT segments [36] (Fig. 11.15).

11.4.1 Safety and Feasibility of OCT

The applied energy during an OCT analysis is low (5.0-8.0 mW) and unable to cause a tissue damage, so OCT safety is mainly related to the mechanical features of the catheter and the size of ischemia caused by the occlusion balloon or the amount of contrast injected during the non-occlusive technique [37]. In a study conducted by Prati et al in 64 patients using non-occlusive technique no major complications such as death, myocardial infarction or major arrhythmias were reported, but only transient ECG modifications, angina or ventricular extrasystoles. These data were supported by a multicentre study by Yamaguchi et al, in which no significant adverse events, including vessel dissection or fatal arrhythmia, were observed [38].

11.4.2 Current Clinical Application of OCT

OCT current clinical applications include the analysis of angiographically normal coronary arteries, in order to confirm the absence of significant lesions or assess the degree of subclinical atherosclerosis, and the evaluation of intermediate stenoses and ambiguous lesions, such as disease at branching sites, ostial or left main stem stenoses, sites with focal spasm or angiographically hazy lesions [39]. However, the most interesting emerging OCT field of application is the study of plaque vulnerability and its progression [40].

11.4.3 Limitations of OCT

OCT generates far higher resolution images, allowing an optimal characterization of plaque morphology and accurately detecting some important complications such as fissures, intracoronary thrombus, intra-stent or edge dissection, tissue prolapse, whilst on the other hand it penetrates the arterial wall less deeply than IVUS. In fact, the main limitation of OCT resides in low penetration of near infrared light, which precludes the analysis of plaques whose thickness exceeds 1-1.5 mm. Furthermore, it scarcely distinguishes calcific from lipidic lesions [41].

References

1. Sones FM, Shirey EK (1962) Cine coronary arteriography. Mod Concepts Cardiovasc Dis 31:735-8
2. Garrone P, et al (2009) Quantitative coronary angiography in the current era: principles and applications. J Interv Cardiol 22(6):527-36
3. Agostoni P, et al (2008) Comparison of assessment of native coronary arteries by standard versus three-dimensional coronary angiography. Am J Cardiol 102(3):272-9
4. Porto I, et al (2012) Comparison of Two- and Three-Dimensional Quantitative Coronary Angiography to Intravascular Ultrasound in the Assessment of Intermediate Left Main Stenosis. Am J Cardiol
5. Topol EJ, SE Nissen (1989) Our preoccupation with coronary luminology. The dissociation between clinical and angiographic findings in ischemic heart disease. Circulation, 1995. 92(8): p. 2333-42.
6. Gussenhoven, E.J., et al., Intravascular ultrasonic imaging: histologic and echographic correlation. Eur J Vasc Surg 3(6):571-6
7. Patel MR, et al (2010) Low diagnostic yield of elective coronary angiography. N Engl J Med 362(10):886-95
8. Schmermund A, Erbel R (2001) Unstable coronary plaque and its relation to coronary calcium. Circulation 104(14):1682-7
9. Alfonso F, et al (1994) Intravascular ultrasound imaging of angiographically normal coronary segments in patients with coronary artery disease. Am Heart J 127(3):536-44
10. Gould KL, Kirkeeide RL, Buchi M (1990) Coronary flow reserve as a physiologic measure of stenosis severity. J Am Coll Cardiol 15(2):459-74
11. Camici PG, Crea F (2007), Coronary microvascular dysfunction. N Engl J Med 356(8):830-40
12. Tonino PA et al (2010) Angiographic versus functional severity of coronary artery stenoses in the FAME study fractional flow reserve versus angiography in multivessel evaluation. J Am Coll Cardiol 55(25):2816-21
13. Potkin BN et al (1990) Coronary artery imaging with intravascular high-frequency ultrasound. Circulation 81(5):1575-85
14. Gussenhoven EJ et al (1989) Arterial wall characteristics determined by intravascular ultrasound imaging: an in vitro study. J Am Coll Cardiol 14(4):947-52
15. Glagov S et al (1987) Compensatory enlargement of human atherosclerotic coronary arteries. N Engl J Med 316(22):1371-5
16. Nissen SE et al (1991) Intravascular ultrasound assessment of lumen size and wall morphology in normal subjects and patients with coronary artery disease. Circulation 84(3):1087-99
17. Okura H et al (2007) Atherosclerotic plaque with ultrasonic attenuation affects coronary reflow and infarct size in patients with acute coronary syndrome: an intravascular ultrasound study. Circ J 71(5):648-53
18. Hausmann D et al (1995) The safety of intracoronary ultrasound. A multicenter survey of 2207 examinations. Circulation 91(3):623-30
19. Mintz GS et al (2001) American College of Cardiology Clinical Expert Consensus Document on Standards for Acquisition, Measurement and Reporting of Intravascular Ultrasound Studies (IVUS). A report of the American College of Cardiology Task Force on Clinical Expert Consensus Documents. J Am Coll Cardiol 37(5):1478-92
20. Di Mario C et al (1998) Clinical application and image interpretation in intracoronary ultrasound. Study Group on Intracoronary Imaging of the Working Group of Coronary Circulation and of the Subgroup on Intravascular Ultrasound of the Working Group of Echocardiography of the European Society of Cardiology. Eur Heart J 19(2):207-29
21. Nissen SE, Yock P (2001) Intravascular ultrasound: novel pathophysiological insights and current clinical applications. Circulation 103(4):604-16
22. Kang SJ et al (2011) Validation of intravascular ultrasound-derived parameters with fractional flow reserve for assessment of coronary stenosis severity. Circ Cardiovasc Interv 4(1):65-71
23. De la Torre Hernandez JM et al (2011) Prospective application of pre-defined intravascular ultrasound criteria for assessment of intermediate left main coronary artery lesions results from the multicenter LITRO study. J Am Coll Cardiol 58(4):351-8
24. Kimura BJ, Bhargava V, DeMaria AN (1995) Value and limitations of intravascular ultrasound imaging in characterizing coronary atherosclerotic plaque. Am Heart J 130(2):386-96
25. Garcia-Garcia HM et al (2011) IVUS-based imaging modalities for tissue characterization: similarities and differences. Int J Cardiovasc Imaging 27(2):215-24
26. Tuzcu EM, Weissman NJ (2010) Imaging coronary artery histology: a virtual pursuit? Circ Cardiovasc Imaging 3(4):348-50
27. Nasu K et al (2006) Accuracy of in vivo coronary plaque morphology assessment: a validation study of in vivo virtual histology compared with in vitro histopathology. J Am Coll Cardiol 47(12):2405-12

28. Heo JH et al (2011) Reproducibility of intravascular ultrasound iMAP for radiofrequency data analysis: Implications for design of longitudinal studies. Catheter Cardiovasc Interv
29. Kawasaki M et al (2002) In vivo quantitative tissue characterization of human coronary arterial plaques by use of integrated backscatter intravascular ultrasound and comparison with angioscopic findings. Circulation 105(21):2487-92
30. Tearney GJ et al (2012) Consensus standards for acquisition, measurement, and reporting of intravascular optical coherence tomography studies: a report from the international working group for intravascular optical coherence tomography standardization and validation. J Am Coll Cardiol 59(12):1058-72
31. Bezerra HG et al (2009) Intracoronary optical coherence tomography: a comprehensive review clinical and research applications. JACC Cardiovasc Interv 2(11):1035-46
32. Yabushita H et al (2002) Characterization of human atherosclerosis by optical coherence tomography. Circulation 106(13):1640-5
33. Jang IK et al (2002) Visualization of coronary atherosclerotic plaques in patients using optical coherence tomography: comparison with intravascular ultrasound. J Am Coll Cardiol 39(4):604-9
34. Porto I et al (2012) Predictors of Periprocedural (Type IVa) Myocardial Infarction, as Assessed by Frequency-Domain Optical Coherence Tomography. Circ Cardiovasc Interv
35. Bouma BE et al (2003) Evaluation of intracoronary stenting by intravascular optical coherence tomography. Heart 89(3):317-20
36. Tearney GJ et al (2008) Three-dimensional coronary artery microscopy by intracoronary optical frequency domain imaging. JACC Cardiovasc Imaging 1(6):752-61
37. Yamaguchi T et al (2008) Safety and feasibility of an intravascular optical coherence tomography image wire system in the clinical setting. Am J Cardiol 101(5):562-7
38. Prati F et al (2007) Safety and feasibility of a new nonocclusive technique for facilitated intracoronary optical coherence tomography (OCT) acquisition in various clinical and anatomical scenarios. EuroIntervention 3(3):365-70
39. Prati F et al (2010) Expert review document on methodology, terminology, and clinical applications of optical coherence tomography: physical principles, methodology of image acquisition, and clinical application for assessment of coronary arteries and atherosclerosis. Eur Heart J 31(4):401-15
40. Radu MD, Falk E (2012) In search of vulnerable features of coronary plaques with optical coherence tomography: is it time to rethink the current methodological concepts? Eur Heart J 33(1):9-12
41. Capodanno D et al (2009) Comparison of optical coherence tomography and intravascular ultrasound for the assessment of in-stent tissue coverage after stent implantation. EuroIntervention 5(5):538-43
42. Porto I, Di Vito L, Burzotta F, Niccoli G et al (2012) Predictors of periprocedural (type IVa) myocardial infarction, as assessed by frequency-domain optical coherence tomography. Circ Cardiovasc Interv 5:89-96, S1-6. Epub 2012 Jan 31. PubMed PMID:22298799
43. Porto I, Cautilli G, Di Vito L, Bolognese L (2012) Late stent thrombosis visualized with three-dimensional optical coherence tomography image reconstruction. G Ital Cardiol 13:169-170
44. Amano T, Matsubara T, Uetani T et al (2007) Impact of Metabolic Syndrome on Tissue Characteristics of Angiographically Mild to Moderate Coronary Lesions: Integrated Backscatter Intravascular Ultrasound Study. J Am Coll Card 49:1149-1156

The Intracardiac Electrophysiological Study 12

Caterina Bisceglia and Valentina Boccadamo

The electrophysiological study (EPS) is a diagnostic procedure to study characteristics of heart excitability and conduction properties. It is essential to understand the origin and mechanism of arrhythmias; sometimes it is performed before the catheter ablation, enabling the understanding of critical elements that sustained the arrhythmia itself and that will be the target of radiofrequency lesions.

12.1 Electrophysiological Non-Invasive Transesophageal Studies

Since 1970 electrophysiological non-invasive transesophageal testing has been performed as a diagnostic tool for the diagnosis of supraventricular arrhythmias; a probe is advanced into the esophagus because of its proximity to the left atrium. Both the mouth and the nostril are used for the insertion. Electrical impulses are delivered to the heart, following standard protocols. It is reliable in the diagnosis of supraventricular tachycardia but cannot be helpful for ventricular arrhythmias. Moreover, it cannot offer information about conduction properties behind the His bundle, which are crucial for advanced AV block.

Evaluation during transesophageal testing:

- Sinus node: Recovery time of sino-atrial node;
- Atrial vulnerability, tendency to develop atrial fibrillation (AF) and evaluation of the shortest RR interval with preexcited ventricular activation during AF;
- Atrio-ventricular node properties: coupling interval of the Wenckebach phenomenon; relative and effective refractory periods of AV node;
- Antegrade conduction capability of the accessory pathway: refractory period of the pathway; shortest preexcited RR interval and shortest coupling interval exhibiting pre-excited QRS;
- Supraventricular arrhythmias inducibility.

Maneuvers can be performed in baseline conditions or during drug administration (propanonol or atropine) to eliminate the autonomic nervous system effects. Finally, evaluation can be performed at rest or during exercise.

12.2 Invasive Electrophysiological Studies

In the last years, invasive electrophysiological studies have gained widespread acceptance in the assessment of electrical system properties that may serve as a prologue for catheter ablation procedures.

After local anesthesia, a venous route (mostly the right femoral vein) is gained by the modified Seldinger technique. A variable number of catheters is introduced and they are positioned along critical parts of the electrical system. In athletes, some issues may occur with muscle hypertrophy of the leg, so the course of the femoral vein may be raised. During standard EPS, three standard (fixed curve) catheters are positioned under fluoroscopic view; they are connected to a dedicated system for the analysis of signals, which can also be displayed and

C. Bisceglia (✉)
Electrophysiology Department
"San Raffaele" University Hospital, Milan, Italy

M. Fioranelli and G. Frajese (eds.), *Sports Cardiology*,
DOI: 10.1007/978-88-470-2775-6_12, © Springer-Verlag Italia 2012

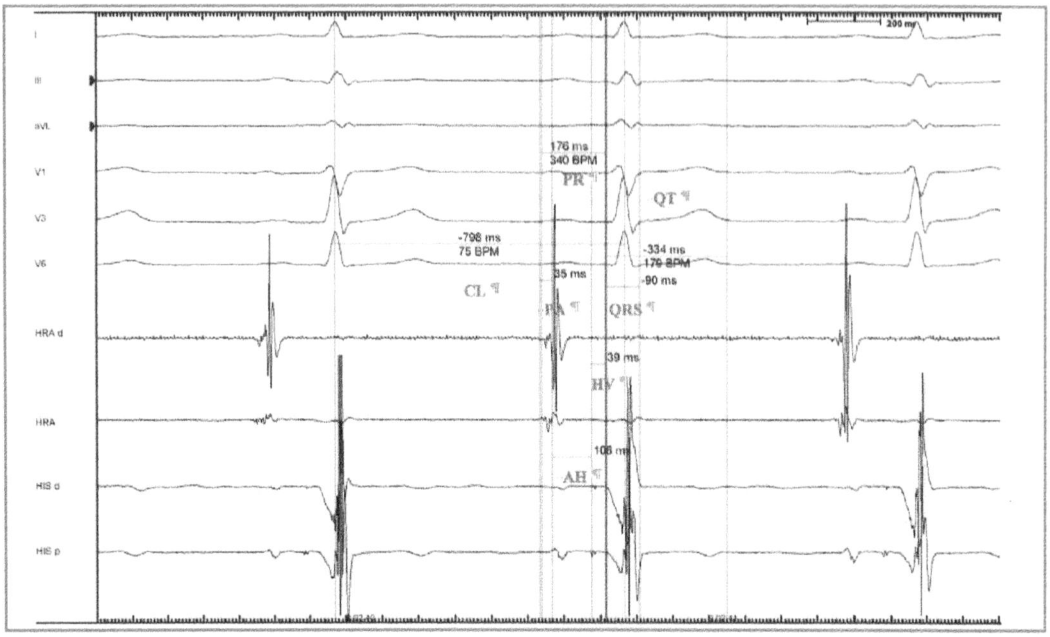

Fig. 12.1 Baseline parameters during EPS. From the top to the bottom: EKG leads DI, DII, aVL, V1, V3, V6; electrograms recorded by quadripolar catheters in right atrium (HRA) and His bundle (HIS p = proximal; HIS d = distal). CL (cycle length) is related to the heart rate. PR interval, QRS duration, QT interval duration. PA: interval between the beginning of the P wave on 12 lead EKG and A electrogram (recorded on HIS d), that is the conduction time between SA node and AV node; AH: from the beginning of the A electrogram to the His potential, which is the time of intranodal conduction (range 50-120 ms); HV: interval between His potential and QRS beginning on the surface EKG, which is the time of conduction behind the His bundle (range 35-55 ms)

recorded on a screen. Catheters are generally advanced toward the:

- Right atrium (or right appendage) close to the SA node;
- His bundle (apex of the Koch triangle), just beneath the septal leaflet of the tricuspid valve;
- Right ventricle: apex and outflow tract.

The approach to the left heart is not generally required, so arterial cannulation is not necessary. When a detailed mapping of the mitral annulus is required, a multipolar catheter is advanced into the coronary sinus; very small catheters can be also advanced into distal portions of the coronary venous tree, to record potentials along the epicardial surface. The access to the left heart, when needed, is obtained through the femoral artery or by transeptal puncture. This kind of maneuver can easily and safely be performed by skilled operators, because it requires the puncture of the fossa ovalis with preformed needle that are also inserted into the femoral vein. The electrodes (poles) are located on the tip of the catheter; their number and distance are variable to enable different anatomical structures to be mapped; they can record the local potential (electrogram), in a bipolar or unipolar modality (connection with a neutral reference) and can serve to stimulate the heart in a wide range of modalities, frequency and amplitude, thanks to the connection with an impulse generator. Signals are detected, amplified and filtered (using high-pass and low-pass filters) to avoid noise interferences; they can be shown in a real-time on a monitor or recorded for off-line analysis.

During baseline rhythm it is possible to evaluate: cycle length (CL, 60,000/heart rate); conduction time along the AV node is recorded (AH interval; range 50-120 ms), as well as the conduction time of the His-Purkinje system (HV, range 35-55 ms); other parameters are shown in Fig. 12.1. In some settings retrograde conduction times are calculated, even during arrhythmias and during ventricular pacing.

Sinus bradycardia is almost the rule in athletes, with heart rate at rest approaching 40 bpm, and first or second degree AV block are also common, but they are generally limited to the AV node. These are generally related to an *autonomic imbalance* of the athlete, with a higher vagal tone that results in modified electrophysiological parameters. These conditions are not harmless in the absence of symptoms and can rapidly be overcome by adrenergic stimulation.

Pacing maneuvers can be performed from each bipole; a series of stimulation with a fixed coupling interval can be delivered (drive) or a programmed stimulation (drive + one or more extrastimuli with different coupling intervals) can be performed. Other protocols are generally performed with incremental stimulation (progressive heart rate increase). It is possible to check:

1. Sino-atrial node recovery time: this refers to the time taken for the SA node to recover its firing after a transient inhibition by stimulation at a fixed drive (for 30-60 sec). It can be corrected for the baseline CL (cSNRT<550 msec).
2. Refractory periods: atrial, AV node and ventricle refractoriness can be determined. When a pre-excitation syndrome is present, the refractory period of the accessory pathway can be evaluated to rule out the risk of atrial fibrillation degenerating into ventricular fibrillation in patients with WPW syndrome.
3. Wenckebach periodism: by incremental pacing, this is the interval with which a stable conduction to ventricular second-degree AV block and Wenckebach phenomenon is calculated. It is normal for heart rate to be >120 bpm. In competitive athletes this parameter is visible for lower rates.
4. Arrhythmic induction (both supraventricular and ventricular): especially when reentry is the leading mechanism of the arrhythmia, the extrastimulus is capable of evoking the functional and unidirectional block responsible for the arrhythmia to start and sustain.
5. Atrial vulnerability: short stimulation sequences at very high rates can be used to test the susceptibility of the atrium to developing atrial fibrillation. Even if there is no strict correlation between this parameter and the clinical risk in the development of arrhythmia, it can be used to induce AF for the risk of sudden death to be assessed in patients with accessory pathways.

Table 12.1 Baseline parameters during EPS: normal values are reported

Conduction intervals	PA	25-55 ms
	AH	55-125 ms
	HV	35-55 ms
	QRS	≤ 100 ms
	QTc	M:≤ 440 ms
		F:≤460 ms
Sino-atrial node function	TRNSA	1500 ms
	TRNSAc	550 ms
	SACT	50-115 ms
	TRT	≤ 5 s
Refractory periods	Atrium	180-330 ms
	AV Node	250-400 ms
	Ventricle	180-290

SACT sino-atrial conduction time, *cSANRT* correct sino-atrial recovery time, *SANRT* sino-atrial recovery time, *TRT* sino-atrial total recovery time (time to baseline heart rate after pacing).

During arrhythmias, the sequence and characteristics of the activation wavefront are evaluated; once the mechanism of the arrhythmia is understood, sites exhibiting the best prematurity in activation are identified and they are generally the target of ablation. Additional clues can be obtained by pacing maneuvers or drug administration (for example adenosine or isoprenaline), or the same mechanism of induction and interruption of the arrhythmia. For ablation, a catheter with a thermocouple is advanced to the target area to enable precise identification of the substrate. Radiofrequency, a kind of alternate current, is applied through the tip of the catheter and the lesion created interrupts the arrhythmia and prevents recurrence (Fig. 12.2).

12.3 Complications

The EPS is a safe procedure, with a complication rate less than 1%, which could be higher if ablation is performed (about 2.5%). The higher risks are in older patients and in those who have under-

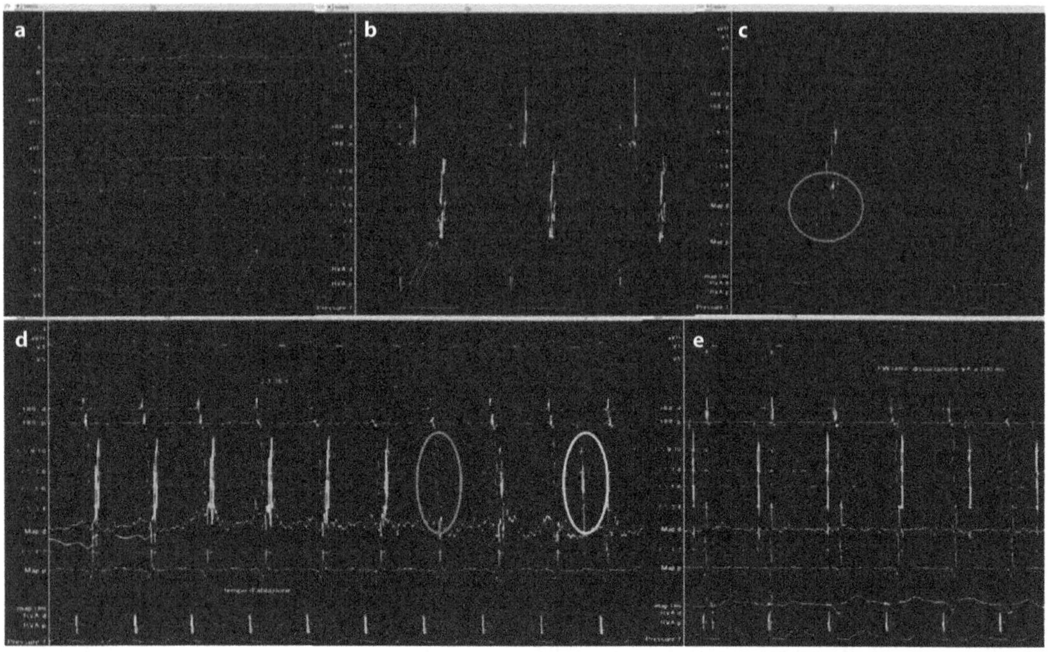

Fig. 12.2 EPS in 22-year-old tennis player with Wolff-Parkinson-White syndrome for left lateral AP. (a) Baseline 12 lead EKG: delta wave, short PR interval and large QRS (arrows). (b) During ventricular pacing an eccentric conduction to the atria is documented (double arrows), with the earliest atrial activation on a distal pair of coronary sinus catheters, corresponding to the antero-lateral wall of the left atrium. (c) During right ventricular pacing a fusion between ventricular and atrial electrograms (map D, circle) is recorded while the ablation straddles the AP. (d) During RF delivery, sudden ventriculo-atrial dissociation (RV pacing) occurred, meaning that the accessory pathway is effectively treated. Results are evident (e) 30 minutes after application

gone ablation in the left chambers. The complications are:

- Hematoma from the vascular access (mostly from the arterial access);
- Thromboembolism: particularly when left heart access is gained;
- Phlebitis: rare;
- Arrhythmia induction, which is generally the purpose but may also require external cardioversion. Ventricular fibrillation can also be induced so an external defibrillator is mandatory;
- Cardiac tamponade: cardiac perforation, with or without tamponade, is generally related to ablation.

Indications of EPS in the athletes are discussed in chapter 16.

An appropriate diagnostic work-up for ventricular arrhythmias in athletes may raise several issues. Even when performed by experienced physicians, it is not free of risk, although the risk is rare. Indications and results have to be evaluated carefully in relation to the presence of structural cardiomyopathy. Sometimes difficulties can be opposed by an asymptomatic patient; on the contrary the indiscriminate application of tests for athletes may provoke stress and fear into these particular populations and their family and friends. On the other hand, the identification of markers of a very high clinical risk, such as sudden death, is crucial in saving these patients, paying dues of exclusion from competitions.

12.4 Unconventional Mapping

Technological evolution has recently led to the development of non-fluoroscopic mapping systems for the heart. They enable the 3D anatomical reconstruction of cardiac chambers, with electrical parameters recorded simultaneously. In fact, they are

Table 12.2 Sensibility and specificity of EPS for detection of arrhythmias in different conditions. It is highly sensitive in patients with coronary artery disease, but rarely useful in long QT syndrome

Condition	Sensibility	Specificity
Normal heart	1	3
Hypertrophic cardiomyopathy	1	1
Ischemic cardiomyopathy	4	4
Abnormal coronary	0	0
ARVDx	3	3
LQTS	0	0
Idiopathic dilated cardiomyopathy	1	1
Idiopathic VT	3	3

ARVDx arrhythmogenic right ventricle dysplasia, *LQTS* long QT syndrome, *VT* ventricular tachycardia.

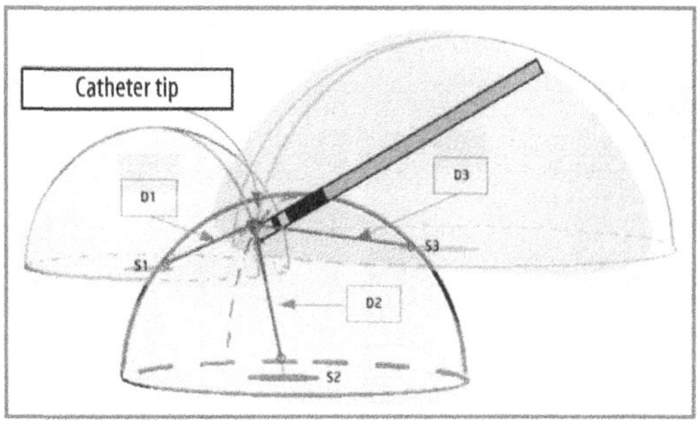

Fig. 12.3 Magnetic field generated by the CARTO system to allow the catheter position to be defined. Three distances enable the acquisition of the position, rotation and direction of the tip of the catheter (D1, D2 and D3)

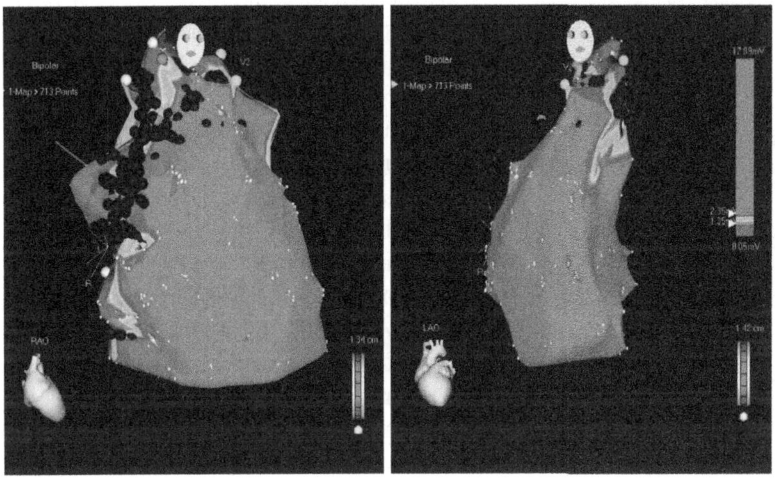

Fig. 12.4 26-year-old competitive athlete. After weakness and syncope, ventricular tachycardia was documented. An electroanatomical voltage map of the right ventricle in RAO (on the left) and LAO view (on the right) by CARTO system. A low-amplitude zone along the tricuspid valve (red band) is shown crossing the free-wall toward RVOT.
Red spots tagged RF applications. Cardiac MRI diagnosed arrhythmogenic right ventricle dysplasia

largely employed to support ablation in very complex settings and to define pathological substrates earlier than standard imaging technique or as a complementary measure. The possibility of performing an endomyocardial biopsy guided by pathological findings on electroanatomical mapping systems holds the promise of enhancing our diagnostic power for the early detection of cardiomyopathies. Finally, the possibility of reaching the epicardial space with subxiphoid percutaneous peri cardial access has opened a new frontier in diagnostic comprehension and therapeutic procedures.

Contact systems are best represented by NaVX and CARTO systems, while the non-contact system employs a balloon catheter (Array). In some centers data can also support navigation with robotic systems, where the catheters are safely maneuvered by a distant operator. The CARTO system allows precise introduction into the cardiac chambers of the tip of a dedicated catheter equipped with a magnet, the chest of the patient being included in a non-homogenous, low-density magnetic field (5×10-6 and 5×10-5 T). Maps are created by systematic acquisition of the spatial coordinate of the catheter and recording of local electrical activity. (Figs. 12.3 and 12.4). Differcnt data can be integrated into maps, to create:

1. voltage map: unipolar or bipolar voltage amplitude is recorded in each part of the chamber, to discriminate a normal myocardium (bipolar voltage amplitude >1.5 mV) from low-voltage areas (amplitude <1.5 mV);

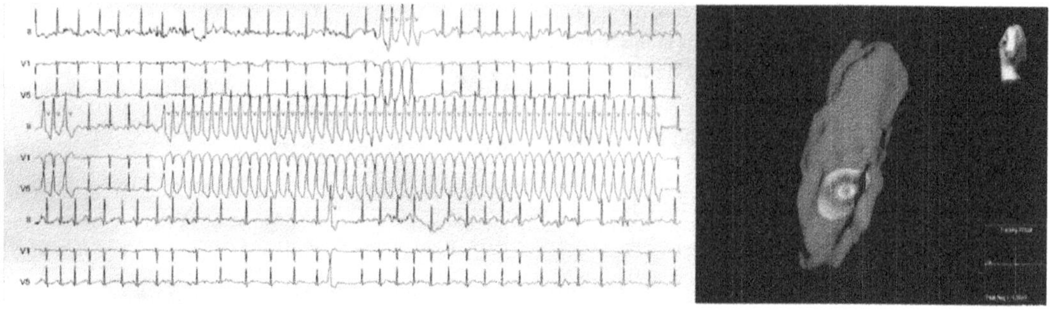

Fig. 12.5 On the left: frequent ventricular premature beats and ventricular tachycardia in a young athlete (basketball player).Twelve-lead morphology suggests the origin to be in the right ventricle outflow tract (RVOT). On the right: multipolar Array catheter delivered into RVOT (in transparency). Map shows the postero-septal portion of the RVOT. On the geometry the color-coded isopotential lines distinguish the earlier activation (*white circle*) during the premature beat. Radiofrequency applications along this area resulted in complete abolition of arrhythmias; VT was no more inducible.

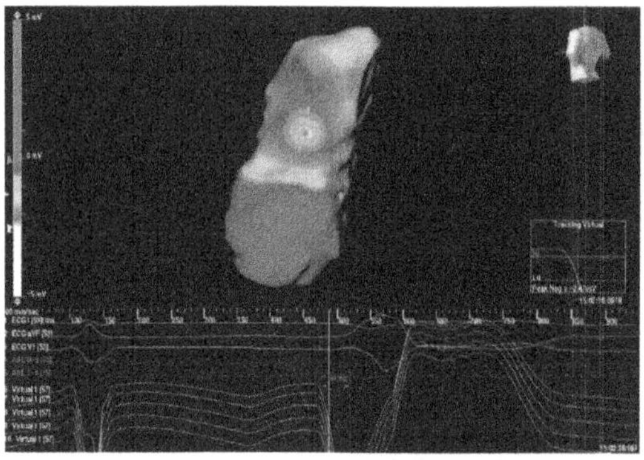

Fig. 12.6 Competitive football player affected by frequent PVCs. Off-line analysis of unipolar signals (*yellow*) and an isopotential map showed the PVCs coming from the postero-septal right ventricular outflow tract (*white circle*). It is possible to see endocardial surface reconstruction and the multi-electrode Array balloon catheter

2. activation map: local activation time (from a reference point) is recorded during arrhythmias to show areas with the earliest activation;
3. isochronal map: narrow lines identify fast conduction areas and large linear areas with slow conduction;
4. propagation map: film displaying the wavefront circuit.

In a similar way, the NaVx system allows visualization of different catheters in the heart chamber by using an electric field created by adhesive patches along the chest. Maps than can be generated can describe the same characteristics as the CARTO system.

Dedicated software (CARTOMERGE and NaVx-Fusion) are employed to merge the 3D reconstruction with imaging techniques like MRI or CT scan. Physicians can operate using a reliable geometry, with time-saving during fluoroscopy. A critical step is the fixed position of the patient: if the initial position is lost, maps can no longer serve as a guide. The Ensite-Array system is conceptually different, because it *feels* the distant-field endocardial potential thanks to the multipolar catheter (Array system, 64 unipolar poles) that has to be placed near the target zone and can record more than 3,000 electrograms/sec (Fig. 12.5). After Array delivery, an ablation catheter is rotated to create a *virtual* chamber; and the process employs the Array catheter as a reference point. The target arrhythmia is analyzed off-line because the system creates high-density color-coded maps to project onto the surface of the wavefront propagation even for a single heart beat (Fig. 12.6).

The role of EPS for the clinical evaluation of athletes is limited by a low negative predictive value and specificity when performed for bradyarrhythmias, because of the specific characteristics of this population. It represents a diagnostic process before the ablation of supraventricular arrhythmias (mostly, AV re-entrant tachycardia or AV node re-entrant tachycardia) and for ventricular idiopathic arrhythmias (like ventricular tachycardia or premature ventricular beats) (Fig. 12.7). Technological support has been implemented to provide additional information about cardiac substrates and the arrhythmia mechanism and to support ablation even in pericardial spaces, which was previously accessible only by surgical techniques.

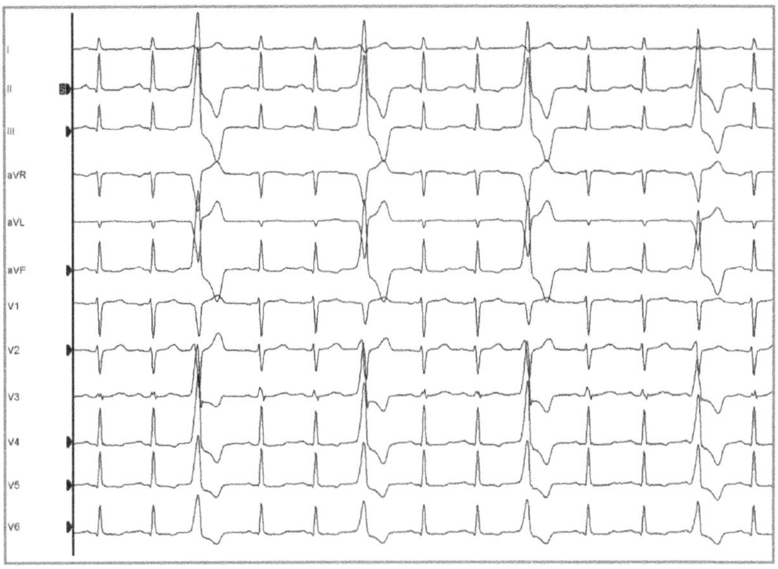

Fig. 12.7 Non-competitive athlete. Twelve-lead EKG showing frequent PVCs from the left aortic cups. Ablation will be performed near the origin of the left main trunk with complete abolition of the phenomenon

Suggested Reading

Avella A, d'Amati G et al (2008) Diagnostic value of endomyocardial biopsy guided by electroanatomic voltage mapping in arrhythmogenic right ventricular cardiomyopathy/dysplasia. J Cardiovasc Electrophysiol 19:1127-1134

Biffi A, Ansalone G, Verdile L et al (1996) Ventricular arrhythmias and athlete's heart. Role of signal-averaged electrocardiography, Eur Heart J 17:557-563

Biffi A, Pelliccia A, Verdile L et al (2002) Long-term clinical significance of frequent and complex ventricular tachyarrhythmias in trained athletes. J Am Coll Cardiol 40:446-452

Bonso A, Corò L, Delise P et al (1996) Bradicardia sinusale e turbe della conduzione. Atti del Convegno Nazionale di Cardiologia della Sport

Delise P (2004) Aritmie: diagnosi, prognosi e terapia. Casa Editrice Scientifica Internazionale, Roma

Delise P, Bonso A, Corò L et al (1991) The endocavitary and transesophageal electrophysiological findings in idiopathic atrial fibrillation. G Ital Cardiol 21:1093-1099

Estes III NA, Link MS, Cannom D et al (2001) Report of the NASPE policy conference on arrhythmias and the athlete. J Cardiovasc Electrophysiol 12:1208-1219

Furlanello F, Galanti G, Manetti P et al (2004) Microvolt T wave alternans as a predictor of electrophysiological testing results in professional competitive athletes. Ann Noninvasive Electrocardiol 9:201-206

Giada F, Barold SS, Biffi A, De Piccoli B et al (2007) Sport and arrhythmias: summary of an international symposium. Eur J Cardiovasc Prev Rehabil 14:707-714

Giustetto C, Gaita F (2008) Sudden cardiac death in athletes with an apparently normal heart: the channelopathies. G Ital Cardiol 9:78S-82S

Heidbüchel H, Corrado D, Biffi A et al (2006) Study Group on Sports Cardiology of the European Association for Cardiovascular Prevention and Rehabilitation. Recommendations for participation in leisure-time physical activity and competitive sports of patients with arrhyttmias and potentially arrhythmogenic conditions. Part II: ventricular arrhrythimas, channelopathies and iplantable defibrillators. Eur J Cardiovasc Prev Rehabil 13:676-86

Heidbüchel H, Hoogsteen J, Fagard R et al (2003) High prevalence of right ventricular involvement in endurance athletes with ventricular arrhythimias. Role of an electrophiologic study in risk stratification. Eur Heart J 24:1473-1480

Inama G, Pedrinazzi C, Durin O et al (2008). Microvolt T wavealternans for risk stratification in athletes with ventricular arrhythmias:correlation with programmed ventricular stimulation Ann Noninvasive Electrocardiol 13:14-21

Josephson ME (2002) Clinical cardiac electrophysiology, techiques and interpretations. Lippincott Williams & Wilkins, Philadelphia

Langdeau JB, Blier L, Turcotte H et al (2001) Electrocardiographic findings in athletes: the prevalence of left ventricular hypertrophy and conduction defects. Can J Cardiol. 17:655-659

Link MS, Wang PJ, Estes III NA (2001) Ventricular arrhythmias in the athlete. Curr Opin Cardiol 16:30-39

Madias JE (2008) Athletes, ventricular arrhythmias, electrophysiologica testing, microvolt T-wave alternans, and a follow-up of 30+/-21 months: a need for follow-up updates. Ann Noninvasive Electrocardiol 13:319-20

Paterick TE, Petrick TJ, Fletcher GF et al (2005) Medical and legal issues in the cardiovascular evaluation of competitive athletes. JAMA 294:3011-3018

Sarubbi B (2006) The Wolff-Parkinson-White electrocardiogram pattern in athletes: how and when to evaluate

the risk for dangerous arrhythmias. The opinion of the pediatric cardiologist. J Cardiovasc Med 7:271-278
Stein R, Moraes RS, Cavalcanti AV et al (2000) Atrial automaticity and atrioventricular conduction in athletes: contribution of autonomic regulation. Eur J Appl Physiol 82:155
Thiene G, Carturan E, Corrado D, Basso C (2010) Prevention of sudden cardiac death in the young and in athletes: dream or reality? Cardiovasc Pathol 19:210-217
Zeppilli P (2004) Cardiologia dello sport. Casa Editrice Scientifica Internazionale, Roma
Zeppilli P, Fenici R, Sassara M et al (1980) Wenckebach second-degree A-V block in top ranking athletes: an old problem revisited. Am Heart J 100:281-294

Part II

Clinical Cardiology in the Athlete

Syncope

13

Caterina Bisceglia and Maddalena Piro

Syncope is properly defined as a transient loss of consciousness and postural tone due to global cerebral hypoperfusion; the onset is sudden, the duration is short, and recovery is generally spontaneous [1].

Syncope is a very common symptom in the general population, accounting for about 1% of emergency department admissions in Italy and a very high number of hospitalizations. It is therefore a major issue for healthcare and the economy, because employment is a great economic source.

Loss of consciousness is estimated to occur in 19% of the population aged over 45 years, but distribution according to age shows an incidence of 5% in children (age < 5 years); there is a higher prevalence in younger patients aged between 10 and 30 years, with peak incidence occurring at the age of about 15 years in both males and females (47% and 31%, respectively). It is very difficult to obtain data in the specific population of athletes; even if the incidence in highly trained competitors may be as high as 10%, and the incidence of syncope is thought to be the same in the general population.

In the pre-participation Italian screening program, the authors found a prevalence of 6.2% (474 athletes) during 5 years of follow-up in a study sample of more than 7,500 athletes. Syncope was independent of exercise in the vast majority of cases (86.7%), occurring during exercise in 1.3% and immediately in the recovery phase in 12%. Vaso-vagal syncope was the most common cause [6]

Generally syncope is a benign condition, even

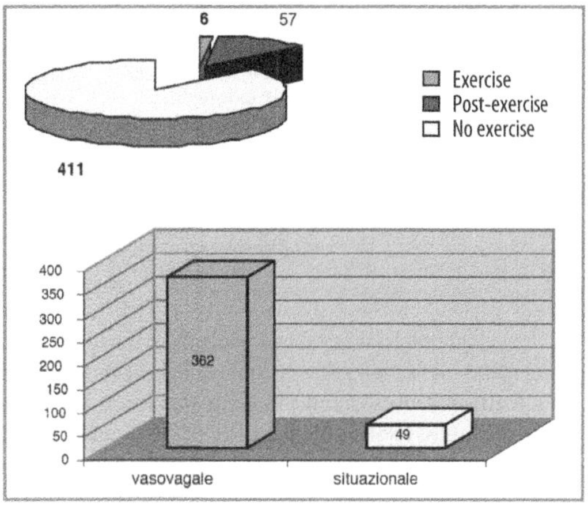

Fig. 13.1 Epidemiology of syncope in athletes

if frequent, and does not require specific medical care [27,28]; when heart disease is responsible for syncope, it is associated with a worse outcome, with a mortality rate of 18-33% after 1 year of follow-up. A cardiac disorder is the best predictor of overall mortality and sudden death in patients with syncope. In athletes it can be a diagnostic dilemma [32,34]. Most episodes are not relevant [35-37], but syncope can be the first clinical manifestation of cardiac conditions associated with a high risk of sudden death, such as HCM, ARVD/C and long-QT syndrome [8,9]. Syncope following effort is defined as a loss of consciousness during exercise or in the early recovery phase. Most episodes due to orthostatic hypotension or extreme exercise occurred in the early recovery phase. The sudden lack of muscle pumping cannot overcome vessel dilation, especially in endurance sports, and postural tone is therefore lost. This is the mechanism

C. Bisceglia (✉)
Electrophysiology Department
"San Raffaele" University Hospital, Milan, Italy

M. Fioranelli and G. Frajese (eds.), *Sports Cardiology*,
DOI: 10.1007/978-88-470-2775-6_13, © Springer-Verlag Italia 2012

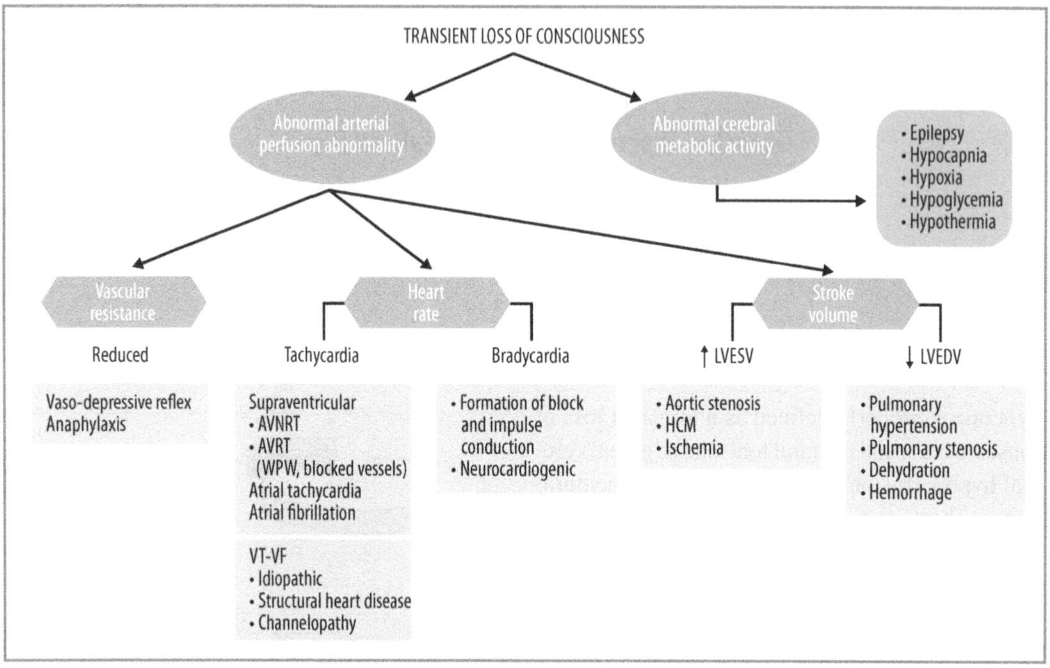

Fig. 13.2 Pathophysiological mechanisms of the loss of consciousness during exercise. Note that episodes of abnormal cerebral metabolic activity do not come under the definition of syncope [10]. *AVNRT,* AV nodal re-entrant tachycardia, *AVRT,* AV re-entrant tachycardia, *WPW* Wolff-Parkinson-White, *VT-VF* ventricular tachycardia, ventricular fibrillation, *LVESV* left ventricular end-systolic volume, *LVEDV* left ventricular end diastolic volume, *HCM* hypertrophic cardiomyopathy

of so-called *exercise faintness*, which is typical of exercise relapse.

A significant reduction in cardiac stroke volume is the leading mechanism of malignant cardiac syncope, due to arrhythmias or structural cardiac abnormalities (Fig. 3.2) [10]. Syncope during exercise is less common, but requires careful evaluation and a proper diagnostic work-up.

Pathophysiology of sudden death during exercise includes:

1. coronary plaque disruption, due to sheer stress and thrombus formation;
2. ventricular arrhythmias due to enhanced catecholaminergic status;
3. great vessel rupture.

In the previously reported Italian series, athletes who experience faintness during the early recovery phase had no adverse events during long-term follow-up; in 2 of the 6 patients with exercise-related syncope, structural cardiomyopathy was diagnosed and patients were therefore categorically excluded from competitions.

13.1 Diagnostic Work-up in Athletes with Syncope

Athletes who experience faintness would have been excluded from competitions until diagnosis had been made. Exhaustive clinical history and physical examination have to be performed, ensuring that the following are covered:

1. circumstances (exercise, recovery...), prodromes (arrhythmic syncope is not generally preceded by symptoms), allergic history, drug assumption, etc.;
2. symptoms suggesting cardiovascular pathology (chest pain, dyspnea, palpitations) or factors that may evoke syncope (in some cases of long-QT syndrome, arrhythmias are triggered by typical sounds, such as alarm clocks);
3. family medical history, in order to understand sudden death in relatives, especially young relatives.

Physical examination has to include:

Table 13.1 Criteria suggestive of benign syncope

Single episode
Negative familial hystory
Normal physical examination
Normal ECG
During recovery
Orthostatic symptoms
Simptoms preceding

1. General appearance;
2. Systemic pressure determination (both arms and legs, in clino-static and orthostatic positions);
3. Cardiac auscultation: heart sounds and murmurs have to be evaluated, even during squatting or Valsalva maneuvers (dynamic auscultation);
4. Arterial pulses (especially the carotid pulse);
5. Overall neurological evaluation.

Further evaluation, when needed, includes 12-lead ECG and laboratory tests. If syncope clearly appears to be a benign condition, no other exams are requested (Table 13.1).

The European Society of Cardiology addressed features that were suggestive of malignant syncope; if present, clinical suspicion of a cardiogenic cause has to remain high (Table 13.2).

Analysis of 12-lead ECG is valuable, because most conditions can be suspected by careful ECG evaluation (Table 13.3).

Further investigations include 2D echocardiogram, Holter ECG monitoring, stress test and Head-Up Tilt Test. Cardiac MRI and CT scan are required only in selected cases, when a high-detailed definition of the cardiac structure and performance is required (especially MRI) or when a non-invasive study of coronary artery patency has to be combined.

If arrhythmias are thought to be the cause of syncope, an electrophysiological study can be performed to confirm the diagnosis and guide catheter ablation if treatment is necessary or desirable. After definitive treatment of the arrhythmia, compe titions can be resumed.

A dedicated team of cardiologists has to be consulted if arrhythmias are responsible for episodes, if cardiomyopathy has been diagnosed, if the cause of syncope remains unclear, or if treatment or specific follow-up has to be provided.

Table 13.2 Cardiogenic syncope

Family hystory of sudden death
Syncope during exercise
Associated symptoms
Symptoms after recovery
No prodromes
Traumatic syncope
Estabilished cardiomyopathy
Previous episodes
12 lead ECG abnormalities
Antiarrhythmic drug assumption

Table 13.3 ECG criteria suggestive of cardiac disorders.

ARVDx	RBB (complete or not), Negative anterior T-wave, ε wave
HCM	Hypertrophy criteria, anterior or lateral Q wave
DCM	LBB, repolarization abnormalities
IHD	Normal or segmental abnormalities of ST-T, presence of Q wave
Abnormal coronary origin	Segmental repolarization abnormalities
Long QT syndrome	long QT, ST-T wave abnormalities
Short QT syndrome	QT interval<320 msec, absent ST tract
Brugada syndrome	RBB (complete or not) ST V1-V2 "coved" o "saddle-back", dynamic pattern
WPW syndrome	δ wave, short PR, slurred QRS

ARVD arrhythmogenic right ventricular dysplasia, *RBB* right branch block, *LBB* left branch block, *CI* cardiac ischemia, *LVH* left ventricular hypertrophy, *DCM* dilated cardiomyopathy, *HCM* hypertrophic cardiomyopathy, *WPW* Wolff-Parkinson White

13.3 Neurally Mediated Syncope

Vasovagal or neurocardiogenic syncope is the most common neutrally-mediated syncope (others are situational syncope and carotid sinus hypersensitivity syndrome). The first occurs when the autonomic response fails to control systemic pressure and sometimes heart rate to support cerebral perfusion and consciousness. Prodromes are generally weakness, confusion, diaphoresis, palpitations,

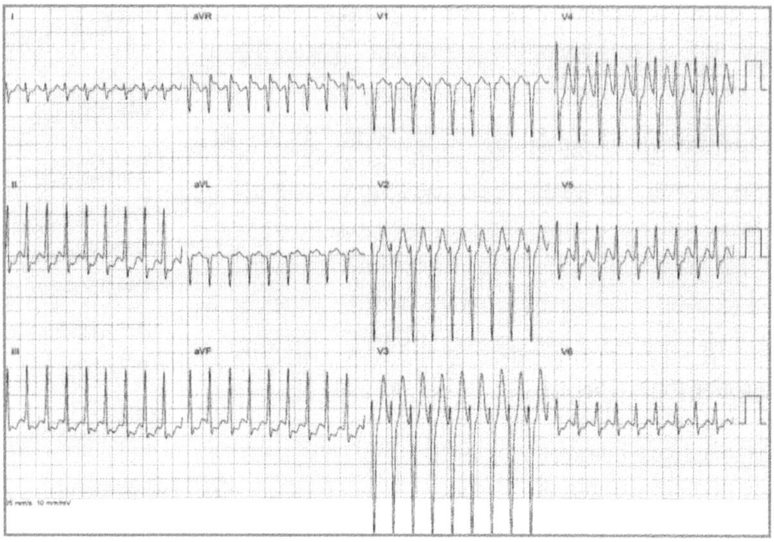

Fig. 13.3 12-lead ECG of orthodromic AV re-entrant tachycardia

sickness and incorrect awareness of body temperature. Subjects showed paleness and sometimes they were nervous, with dilated pupils and yawns. Prodromes can precede the events for a few minutes; recovery of consciousness generally happened within 30 seconds, but faintness may remain for a few hours

When the trigger is unknown, a detailed clinical history may be sufficient to diagnose neurocardiogenic syncope, and in uncertain cases a tilt test can be performed. There is no general agreement about the effectiveness of the tilt test to support diagnosis in athletes, and because of its high sensibility but low specificity; false positive tests in athletes are probably related to enhanced neurovegetative tone. Results of this test require careful evaluation to avoid dangerous misdiagnosis. When frequent unexplained episodes occur, a subcutaneous device may be implanted (loop-recorder) to rule out an arrhythmic etiology; these devices are capable of recording a single-lead trace in an automatic or activated way, for a total of about 45 minutes. Therapy is limited to lifestyle changes, possibly with psychological support. High-sodium intake is recommended, whereas standing up for a long time and dehydration must be avoided.

Tilt training (30-40 min/day until pre-syncope occurs) has been demonstrated to be effective in the prevention of episodes in some reports. If patients need pharmacological therapy, bear in mind that beta-blockers are banned as doping drugs, so elective treatment involves selective serotonin reuptake inhibitors and midodrine.

A history of neurally mediated syncope generally does not prevent participation in competitive sports.

13.4 Cardiac Causes of Syncope

The presence of structural heart disease and/or channelopathies seems to contradict the perception of athletes as a *healthy subjects* by definition. These conditions are frequently related to cardiac and sudden death, as in the general population. Bradyarrhythmias are common in athletes (sinus bradycardia, first-degree AV block or second-degree Mobitz type AV block), but they are rarely symptomatic. Non-invasive assessment of cronotropic response can be a reliable criterion for selecting those who can perform competitions. If high-degree AV block is documented and pacemaker implantation is required, contact sports needs to be avoided (the same is true for congenital AV block if a pacemaker is implanted).

The most common supraventricular arrhythmias (AV node re-entrant tachycardia and AV re-entrant tachycardia) are rarely associated with syncope, but if so, they can be effectively treated by catheter ablation (Fig. 13.3). Radiofrequency

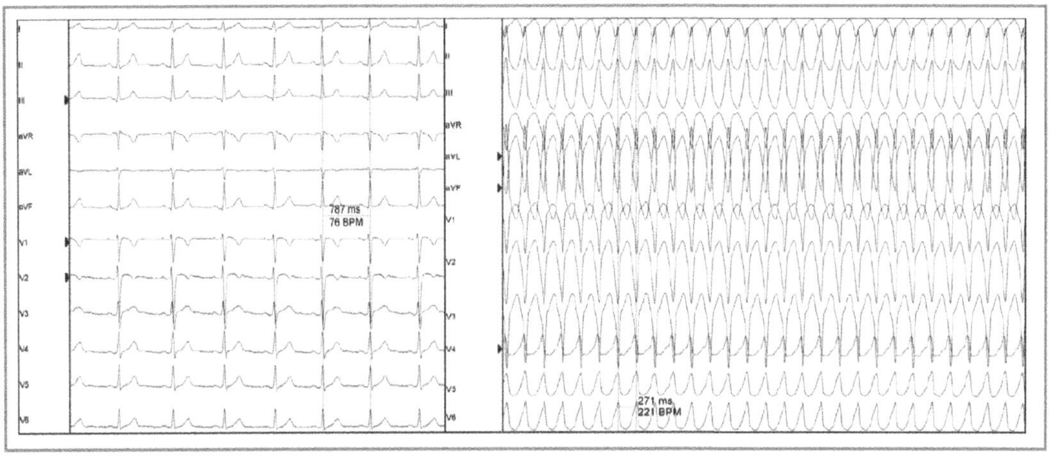

Fig. 13.4 23-year-old football player with pre-syncope, even during exercise. No structural heart disease can be detected. During EP study, induction of monomorphic ventricular tachycardia HR=220 bpm, originating from right ventricular outflow tract. Arrhythmia will be successfully ablated

ablation is the treatment of choice in these patients, because of its high efficacy in the prevention of recurrence. In the absence of structural heart disease, effective ablation therapy enables a return to competitions.

Ventricular arrhythmias associated with syncope are one of the most complex situations in sports medicine. In the absence of structural heart disease, ablation of such idiopathic arrhythmias may enable sports eligibility after a period of at least 3 months (Fig. 13.4).

In the presence of heart disease, the substrate responsible for the arrhythmias is generally progressive; anti-arrhythmic drugs do not offer complete protection against recurrence, and ablation therapy itself does not prevent the pathological evolution of the condition. Only moderate physical effort is allowed for these athletes, because frequently the high physical strength is responsible for the induction of arrhythmias.

13.5 Conclusions

Syncope in athletes leads to specific diagnostic and therapeutic issues for cardiologists and sports physicians. Athletes are often on-stage, and media attention towards their performance is sometimes very high. Those who are at risk of fatal complications are to be carefully screened, and withdrawal from competitions needs to be advised. On the other hand, benign conditions may guarantee normal daily life and safe sports training. Specific therapy is available, when needed. A critical approach to this symptom is mandatory, because the scientific commettees are in agreement about the malignant nature of syncope in patients with underlying heart disorders.

References

1. Guidelines for the diagnosis and management of syncope (2009). The Task Force for the Diagnosis and Management of Syncope of the European Society of Cardiology (ESC). Eur H Journal (Epub ahead of print)
2. Brignole M, Menozzi C, Bartoletti A et al (2006) A new management of syncope: prospective systematic guideline-based evaluation of patients referred urgently to general hospitals. Studio EGSYS-2 (Evaluation of Guidelines in Syncope Study) Studio di popolazione svolto nei Dipartimenti di Emergenza-Accettazione in Italia sull'impatto di una valutazione diagnostica del paziente strettamente aderente alle linee guida della Società Europea di Cardiologia. Eur Heart J 27:76-82
3. Chen LY, Shen WK et al (2006) Prevalence of syncope in a population aged more than 45 years. Am J Med 119:1088
4. Lombroso CT, Lerman P (1967) Breathholding spells (cyanotic and pallid infantile syncope). Pediatrics 39:563-581
5. Ganzeboom KS, Colman N et al (2003) Prevalence and triggers of syncope in medical students. Am J Cardiol 91:1006-1008

6. Colivicchi F, Ammirati F, Santini M (2004) Epidemiology and prognostic implications of syncope in young competing athletes. Eur H Journal 25:1749-1753
7. Soteriades ES, Evans JC et al (2002) Incidence and prognosis of syncope. N Engl J Med 347:878-85.
8. Maron BJ, Roberts WC, McAllister HA et al (1980) Sudden death in young athletes. Circulation 62:218-229
9. Corrado D, Thiene G, Nava A et al (1990) Sudden death in young competitive athletes: clinicopathologic correlations in 22 cases. Am J Med 89:588-596
10. Levine BD, Buckley JC et al (1991) Physical fitness and cardiovascular regulation: mechanism of orthostatic intolerance. J Appl Physiol 70:112-122
11. Kramer MR, Drori Y, Lev B (1988) Sudden death in young soldiers: high incidence of syncope prior to death. Chest 93:345-347
12. Maron BJ, Roberts WC, McAllister HA et al (1980) Sudden death in young athletes. Circulation 62:218-229
13. Corrado D, Migliore F, Basso C et al (2006) Exercise and the risk of sudden cardiac death. Herz 31:553-558
14. Tofler GH (1998) Triggers of sudden cardiac death in the athlete. In: Estes NAM, Salem DN, Wang PJ (eds). Sudden cardiac death in the athlete, pp 221-234. Futura, New York
15. O'Connor F, Levine BD et al (2009) Practical management: a systematic approach to the evaluation of the exercise-related syncope in athletes. Clin J Sport Med 19:429-434
16. Link MS, Eates NA (2007) How to manage athletes with syncope. Cardol Clin 25:457-466
17. Pelliccia A, Di Paolo FM, Corrado D et al (2006) Evidence for efficacy of the Italian national pre-participation screening programme for identification of hypertrophic cardiomyopathy in competitive athletes. Eur Heart J 27:2196-2000
18. Maron BJ, Estes NA III, Link MS (2005) 36th Bethesda Conference: Eligibility recommendations for competitive athletes with cardiovascular abnormalities. J Am Coll Cardiol 45:1371-1373
19. Hosey RG, Carek PJ, Goo A (2001) Exercise-induced anaphylaxis and urticaria. Am Fam Physician 64:1367-1372
20. Sauer AJ, Moss AJ, McNitt S et al (2007) Long QT syndrome in adults. J Am Coll Cardiol 49:329-337
21. Kapoor WN (2002) Current evaluation of and management of syncope. Circulation 1606-1609
22. Link MS, Wang PJ, Estes NA III. (2001) Ventricular arrhythmias in the athlete. Curr Opin Cardiol 16:35
23. Marcus FI (2000) Electrocardiographic features of inherited diseases that predispose to the development of cardiac arrhythmias, long QT syndrome, arrhythmogenic right ventricular cardiomyopathy/dysplasia, and Brugada syndrome. J Electrocardiol 33(Suppl):1-10
24. Grubb BP (2005) Neurocardiogenic Syncope. N Engl J Med 352:1004-1010
25. Benditt DG, Ferguson DW, Grubb BP et al (1996) ACC Expert Consensus Document: Tilt table testing for assessing syncope. J Am Coll Cardiol 28:263-275
26. Grubb BP, Temesy-Armos PN, Samoil D et al (1993) Tilt table testing in the evaluation and management of athletes with recurrent exercise-induced syncope. Med Sci Sports Exerc 25:24-28
27. Driscoll DJ, Jacobsen SJ, Porter CJ, Wollan PC (1997) Syncope in children and adolescents. J Am Coll Cardiol 29:1039-1045
28. Maron BJ, Shirani, Poliac LC et al (1996) Sudden death in young competitive athletes. Clinical, demographic, and pathological profiles. JAMA 276:199-204
29. Maron BJ, Zipes DP (2005) 36th Bethesda Conference: eligibility recommendations for competitive athletes with cardiovascular abnormalities. J Am Coll Card 45:1312-1375
30. Brignole M, Menozzi C et al for the Evaluation of Guidelines in Syncope Study 2 (EGSYS-2) group (2006) A new management of syncope: prospective systematic guideline-based evaluation of patients referred urgently to general hospitals. Eur H Journal 27:76-82
31. Di Girolamo E, Di Iorio C, Leonzio L et al (1999) Usefulness of a tilt training program for the prevention of refractory neurocardiogenic syncope in adolescents: a controlled study. Circulation 100:1798-1801
32. Driscoll DJ, Jacobsen SJ, Porter CJ, Wollan PC (1997) Syncope in children and adolescents. J Am Coll Cardiol 29:1039-1045
33. Maron BJ, Shirani J, Poliac LCet al (1996) Sudden death in young competitive athletes. Clinical, demographic, and pathological profiles. JAMA 276:199-204
34. Kapoor WN (1998) Approach to the patient with syncope. In: Goldman L, Braunwald E (eds). Primary cardiology, pp 144-153. Saunders, Philadelphia
35. Corrado D, Basso C, Schiavon M, Thiene G (1998) Screening for hypertrophic cardiomyopathy in young athletes. N Engl J Med 339:364-369
36. Corrado D, Basso C, Thiene G. (1998) Sudden arrhythmic death in young people: warning symptoms and pathologic substrates. Presented at the 19th Annual Scientific Sessions of NASPE. San Diego, May 6-9, 1998
37. AAVV (1997) When does fainting represent a deadly condition? Exertional syncope: benign hypotension or life-threatening abnormality? Part 1. Sports Med Dig 19:118-120
38. Kapoor WN (1990) Evaluation and outcome of patients with syncope. Medicine 69:160-175
39. Alboni P, Brignole M, Menozzi C et al (2001) The diagnostic value of history in patients with syncope with or without heart disease. J Am Coll Cardiol 37:1921-1928
40. Manari A, Menozzi C, Roti S et al (1996) Syncope in trained athletes: occurrence and clinical significance. New Trends in Arrhythmias 11:13-15
41. Colivicchi F, Ammirati F, Biffi A et al (2002) Exercise-related syncope in young competitive athletes without evidence of structural heart disease: clinical presentation and long-term outcome. Eur Heart J 23:1127-1132
42. Biffi A, Verdile L, Ammirati F et al (2000) Syncope in athletes: how much is neuromodulation involved? In: Santini M (ed). Progress in clinical pacing, pp 84-86. Futura, New York

Epidemiology, Classification and Description of Cardiac Arrhythmias 14

Francesco Perna and Milena Leo

14.1 Introduction

The term *arrhythmia* is used to indicate an alteration of the normal rate or regularity of the heartbeat, as well as an alteration of the physiological conduction sequence of electrical impulse from the sinus node to the His-Purkinje system and the ventricles. The term bradycardia refers to a heart rate (HR) of less than 60 beats per minute (bpm), while the term tachycardia identifies a sequence of 3 or more beats with HR above 100 bpm.

According to the HR, arrhythmias can be classified into two large groups:

- *bradyarrhythmias*, characterized by a reduction in the HR;
- *tachyarrhythmias*, characterized by an increase in the HR.

Further sub-classifications are possible, in both groups, based on the site of onset of the arrhythmia (various levels of the conduction system, atria, ventricles). Table 14.1 shows a classification for arrhythmias.

14.2 Bradyarrhythmias

14.2.1 Sinus Bradycardia and Sinus Arrhythmia

Sinus bradycardia is caused by a reduced automatism of the sinus node. It is a condition characterized by a HR below 60 bpm with normal P wave morphology at ECG (Fig. 14.1). This phenomenon is often physiological. In young athletes, for example, a good level of aerobic exercise may cause a significant slowdown in the HR, due to an increase of vagal tone and a reduction of sympathetic tone. Its prevalence decreases, however, in older subjects. Other causes of sinus bradycardia are drugs (beta-blockers, calcium channel blockers, anti-arrhythmic agents, lithium and others), several clinical conditions (depression, hypothyroidism, inferior myocardial infarction, hypothermia, etc.) or primary sinus node dysfunctions. During sleep, the HR can slow to 35-40 bpm; moreover, this type of bradycardia is often associated, particularly in young people, with sinus arrhythmia, with pauses even longer than 3 seconds. Since this is usually a benign phenomenon, treatment of asymptomatic individuals is not necessary. In rare cases of symptomatic sinus bradycardia (asthenia, dizziness, syncope), treatment with a permanent pacemaker is required, since no drugs are effective for a reliable long-term therapy.

Sinus arrhythmia (Fig. 14.2) is a condition characterized by sinus cycle oscillation of more than 160 ms or 10% (difference or ratio between longest and shortest cycle). It is usually a physiological phenomenon, common in younger individuals, especially when related to the breathing phases (respiratory sinus arrhythmia, characterized by HR increase during the inspiration and HR decrease during expiration), and is less frequent in the elderly.

Non-respiratory sinus arrhythmia is sometimes an indicator of sinus node dysfunction. Symptoms are very rare, except for some cases in which pauses

F. Perna (✉)
Heart Center
Casa di Cura Mater Dei, Rome, Italy

M. Fioranelli and G. Frajese (eds.), *Sports Cardiology*,
DOI: 10.1007/978-88-470-2775-6_14, © Springer-Verlag Italia 2012

Table 14.1 Classification of arrhythmias

Bradyarrhytmias	Tachyarrhytmias
Sinus bradycardia	Sinus tachycardia
Sinus arrhythmia	Sinoatrial re-entrant tachycardia
Sinus pause and sinus arrest	Parasystole
Bradycardia-tachycardia syndrome	- Atrial
Wandering pacemaker	- Junctional
Sinoatrial block	- Ventricular
- First degree	Supraventricular premature beats
- Second degree, type 1 (Mobitz 1)	Atrial tachycardia
- Second degree, type 2 (Mobitz 2)	Atrial flutter
- Second degree, 2:1	- Typical (counter-clockwise and clockwise)
- Third degree	- Atypical
Atrioventricular block	Atrial fibrillation
- First degree	Junctional automatic tachycardia
- Second degree, type 1 (Mobitz 1)	Atrioventricular nodal re-entrant tachycardia
- Second degree, type 2 (Mobitz 2)	Atrioventricular reciprocating tachycardia
- Second degree, 2:1	Accelerated junctional rhythm
- Third degree	Ventricular premature beats
	Accelerated idioventricular rhythm
	Ventricular tachycardia
	Ventricular fibrillation

are long enough to cause syncope. Treatment is rarely required; sedatives, anxiolytics, atropine, ephedrine or isoproterenol are often sufficient for the management of associated palpitations.

14.2.2 Sinus Pause and Sinus Arrest

Sinus pause and *sinus arrest* are disorders of sinus node automatism consisting in a transient or persistent failure of impulse generation. PP interval during sinus pauses is not a multiple of the baseline PP. The absence of atrial depolarization may result in asystole if escape beats/rhythms do not emerge.

Sinus arrest may be caused by acute myocardial infarction, fibrotic degeneration of the sinus node, digitalis toxicity, stroke, or vagal hypertonia; it is very frequent in patients with sleep apnoea syndrome. As for sinus bradycardia, treatment is necessary in rare cases (in general, symptomatic patients and/or pauses longer than 3 seconds), and it is represented by pacemaker implantation.

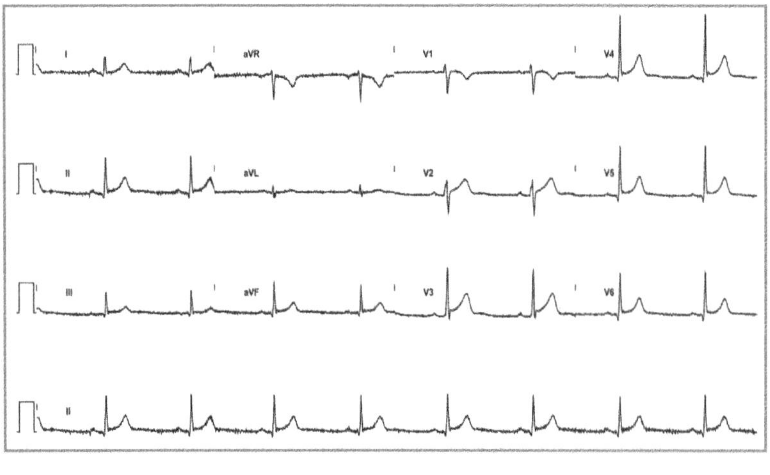

Fig. 14.1 Sinus bradycardia (50 bpm) in a 25-year-old athlete

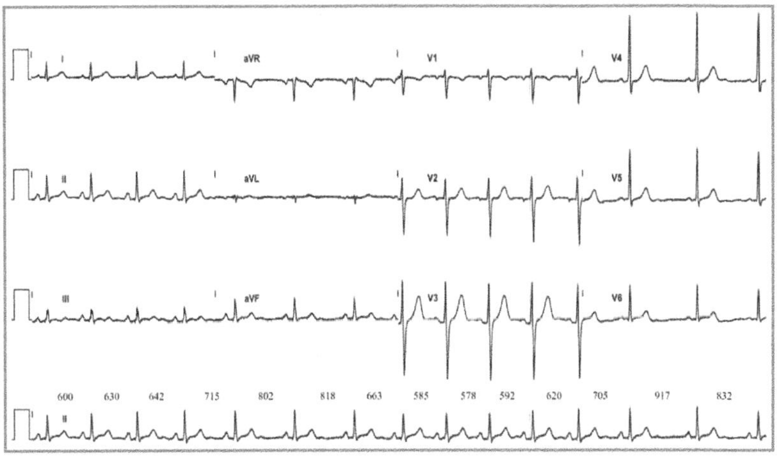

Fig. 14.2 Sinus arrhythmia in a 21-year-old athlete. Numbers indicate the duration of the RR intervals in milliseconds

14.2.3 Sinoatrial Exit Block

Sinoatrial (SA) *exit block* is a condition caused by a disturbance of impulse conduction from the sinus node to the surrounding atria. It can be intermittent or persistent. Furthermore, according to the disease severity, three degrees of block can be distinguished.

First-degree SA block consists of a slow impulse conduction between the sinus node and the surrounding atrium; it is not recognisable on the surface ECG and it has no clinical significance. *Second degree SA block* is characterized by the intermittent absence of a sinus beat. It can be further classified as Mobitz 1 (or Wenckebach SA block), in which the pause caused by the impulse blockade is shorter than double the PP sinus cycle (which tends to be irregular and to progressively shorten before the pause), or as Mobitz 2 and 2:1 types (Fig. 14.3), in which the sinus pause is exactly twice the baseline PP cycle. Mobitz 1 SA exit block is due to diminishing impulse conduction (progressive elongation of the conduction time), while Mobitz 2 and 2:1 types are due to *all or nothing* impulse conduction.

Third degree SA block, in which no sinus impulse reaches the atria, is characterized by the total absence of sinus P waves (although ectopic atrial activity may be present). It cannot be distinguished from sinus arrest at surface ECG.

The principal causes of SA block are vagal hypertonia, myocarditis, myocardial infarction, atrial fibrotic degeneration, drug toxicity. Furthermore, it can frequently occur in trained athletes: it is usually transient and asymptomatic, syncope may rarely occur due to the absence of an effective escape rhythm. The management of this type of arrhythmia is the same as for sinus bradycardia.

14.2.4 Bradycardia-Tachycardia Syndrome

This syndrome is characterized by frequent bradyarrhythmic episodes and pauses due to significant sinus bradycardia, sinus arrest or sinoatrial exit block, alternating with paroxysmal, rapid, regular or irregular atrial tachyarrhythmias, such as atrial tachycardia, atrial flutter and atrial fibrillation. It is likely due to a diffuse alteration of the atrial myocardium, constituting the electrophysiological substrate for both tachyarrhythmias and sinus dysfunction. The management of this condition is complex: it requires pacemaker implantation for bradyarrhythmia treatment and anti-arrhythmic drug therapy for tachyarrhythmia treatment.

14.2.5 Sick Sinus Syndrome

The term *sick sinus syndrome* is used to indicate a series of pathological conditions due to sinus node dysfunction:

- persistent sinus bradycardia, non-appropriate to the circumstances;
- sinus arrest or sinoatrial exit block;
- chronotropic incompetence;
- bradycardia-tachycardia syndrome.

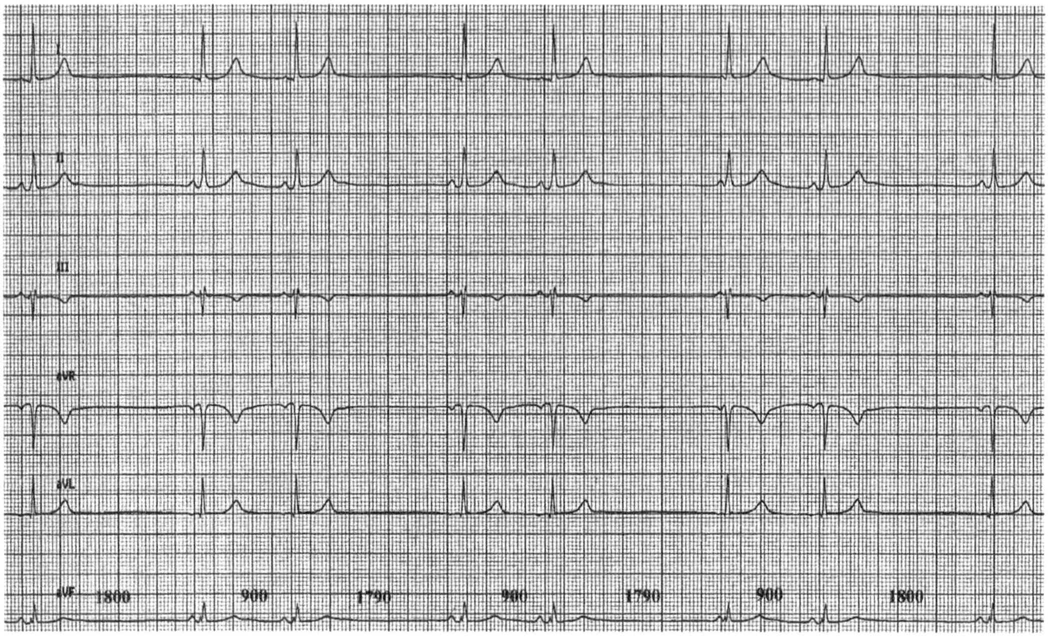

Fig. 14.3 Second degree sinoatrial exit block, 2:1 type. Numbers indicate the duration of the PP intervals in milliseconds

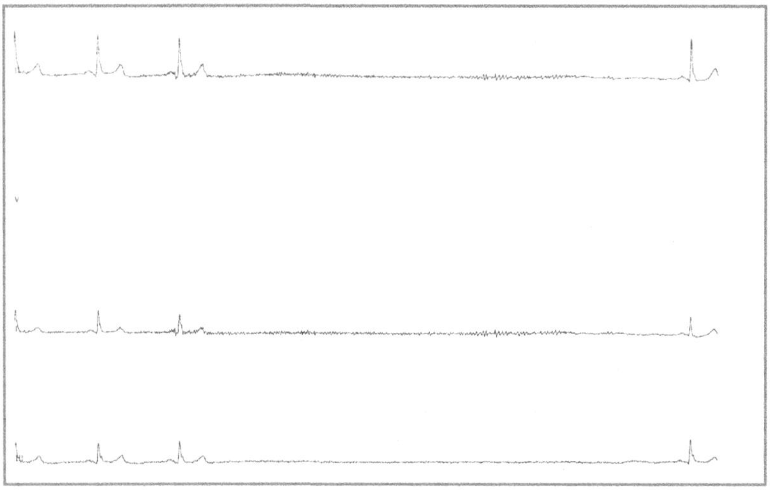

Fig. 14.4 Asystole caused by sinus arrest or third degree sinoatrial exit block. Telemetric ECG monitoring

Ischemic, inflammatory or, more frequently, degenerative conditions can cause this syndrome.

Pathological alterations may be confined to the sinus node, or involve both atria and the AV node, with AV conduction defects. Symptoms of sick sinus syndrome are usually due to very low HR or to long pauses. In the presence of significant sinus bradyarrhythmias, escape rhythms from atrial or junctional subsidiary pacemakers often emerge and drive cardiac activity. In absence of these escape rhythms, the patient may experience prolonged asystolic periods with a marked reduction of cardiac output and symptoms due to cerebral hypoperfusion: lipothymia, syncope, which may be associated with tonic-clonic seizures and sphincter incontinence (Morgagni-Adam-Stokes syndrome), cardio-respiratory arrest leading to death or, in case of effective resuscitation, irreversible residual neurologic impairment (up to a vegetative state).

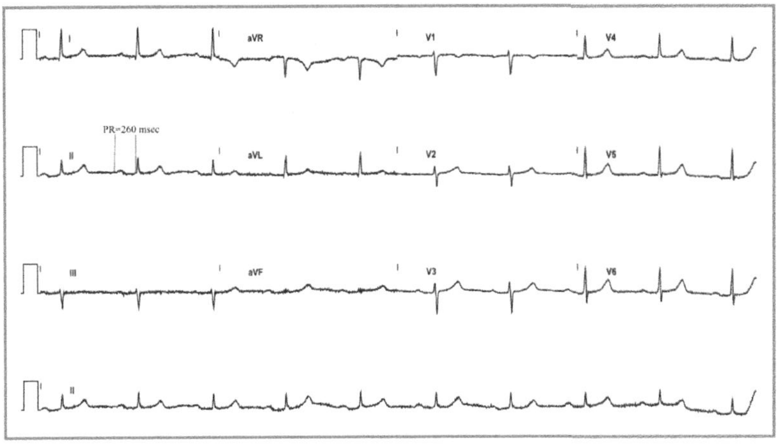

Fig. 14.5 Sinus rhythm with first degree atrioventricular block

In the case of bradycardia-tachycardia syndrome, in addition to the presence of symptoms related to bradyarrhythmias, the patients may experience symptoms due to the presence of supraventricular tachyarrhythmias (typically palpitations). The management of sick sinus syndrome requires the treatment of its specific manifestations, as previously reported.

14.2.6 Wandering Pacemaker

The term *wandering pacemaker* refers to a continuous change of the dominant pacemaker from the sinus node to other latent pacemakers located in different areas of the atrial myocardium or the AV junction. The change occurs gradually, over several beats and each beat is produced by a single pacemaker. P waves have different morphologies and are associated to slight variations of PR and RR intervals. This phenomenon may be considered physiological and occurs very often in young athletes because of an increased vagal tone. Treatment is frequently not needed; when indicated, it is identical to that of sinus bradycardia.

14.2.7 Atrioventricular Blocks

Atrioventricular blocks consist in conduction disturbances from the atria to the ventricles, in the atrioventricular node or in the His-Purkinje system.

As for sinoatrial blocks, we can distinguish three degrees of AV block on the basis of the severity of the conduction disorder.

The term *first degree AV block* is considered by some authors as a misnomer, because it is characterized by a prolonged PR interval, exceeding 200 ms, with a normal morphology and duration of the QRS complex and with maintenance of 1:1 AV conduction, without blocked P waves (Fig. 14.5).

In the *second degree AV block* some atrial impulses are not conducted to the ventricles. It may be divided, in turn, in type 1 (Wenckebach or Mobitz 1), type 2 (proper Mobitz or Mobitz 2) and AV block with 2:1 conduction ratio.

Mobitz 1 AV block is characterized by progressively increasing PR intervals, until a P wave is not conducted. The PR interval elongation is maximum in the beat following the first conducted P and progressively decreases while getting closer to the blocked P wave: as a result we see a progressive shortening of the RR intervals before the pause. Mobitz 1 AV block is usually located in the AV node, therefore it may improve with atropine and physical exercise and worsen during carotid sinus massage. This type of block is very common in trained athletes, especially during the night, because of increased vagal tone and reduced sympathetic tone, and in this case it has a benign nature. It may also appear in patients with inferior myocardial infarction (12-20%); in this case it is associated with an increased mortality because it is an indirect sign of occlusion of the proximal right coronary artery with involvement of the right ventricle. Early myocardial revascularization is

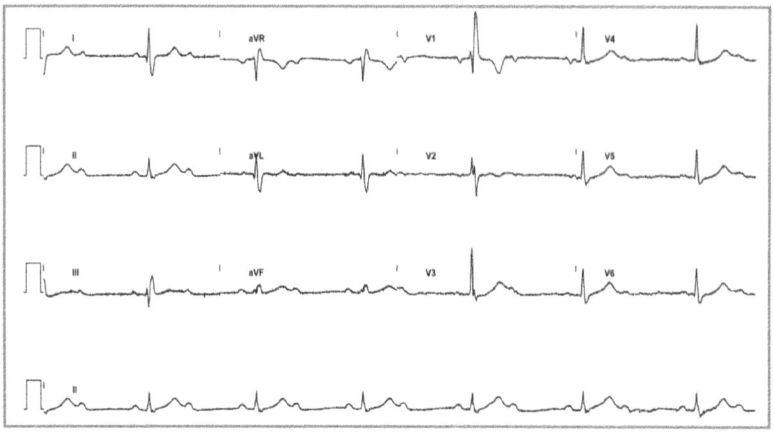

Fig. 14.6 Second degree atrioventricular block with 2:1 atrioventricular conduction ratio

usually followed by AV block resolution (as a reperfusion sign). In case of progression to complete AV block associated to heart failure, bradycardia-induced ventricular arrhythmias, cardiogenic shock, the implantation of a temporary pacemaker may be necessary. Permanent pacemaker implantation is indicated if II or III degree AV block persists after the infarction.

Mobitz 2 AV block is characterized by abrupt AV conduction failure with constant PR intervals in the conducted beats. Different P/QRS ratios are possible, thus identifying different types of Mobitz 2 AV blocks (3:2, 4:3, 3:1, etc.). Mobitz 2 AV block is generally due to an infra-hisian lesion and it may be associated with a wide QRS complex. Therefore, atropine administration can apparently worsen AV conduction because of an increase of sinus node firing rate, while carotid sinus massage may paradoxically improve it for the opposite reason. This type of block often abruptly progresses to complete AV block, thus requiring pacemaker implantation. The most frequent cause of Mobitz 2 AV block is a fibrotic degeneration of the myocardial conduction tissue associated to advanced age. It is never a physiological finding in young athletes. Its appearance in the presence of anterior myocardial infarction indicates a proximal occlusion of left anterior descending coronary artery and it is associated to high mortality.

Second degree AV block with 2:1 conduction (Fig. 14.6) cannot be defined either as Mobitz 1 or as Mobitz 2 AV block because it is not possible to assess the presence or absence of lengthening of the PR interval in the conducted beats. The dysfunction can be nodal, intra-hisian or infra-hisian. Treatment depends on the presence of symptoms and the site of block, which can be determined through non-invasive tests (atropine, exercise, carotid sinus massage) or invasive tests (intracardiac electrophysiological study).

Advanced AV block implies the presence of two or more consecutive P waves not followed by QRS complexes. In *third degree or complete AV block* no P wave is conducted to the ventricles. It is one of the causes of AV dissociation: there is no relationship between P waves and QRS complexes, and ventricular activation (if present) is due to junctional or idioventricular escape rhythm with HR generally less than 50 bpm. (Fig. 14.7). In most cases, third degree AV block is an emergency situation that requires pacemaker implantation. However, when a narrow-QRS escape rhythm presents, it is possible to wait, to determine the cause of block and in some cases, for example in the case of congenital AV block, to follow its clinical course over time. Furthermore, complete AV block during a myocardial infarction, although requiring a temporary pacemaker implantation in the acute phase, may disappear after coronary revascularization.

Paroxysmal AV block is a particular type of AV block, in which a 1:1 AV conduction suddenly changes in complete AV block. It generally occurs as result of a critical PP interval elongation, such as the pause following a atrial premature beat, which causes a block in phase 4 of conduction cells (usually below the AV node). This phase 4 block is not

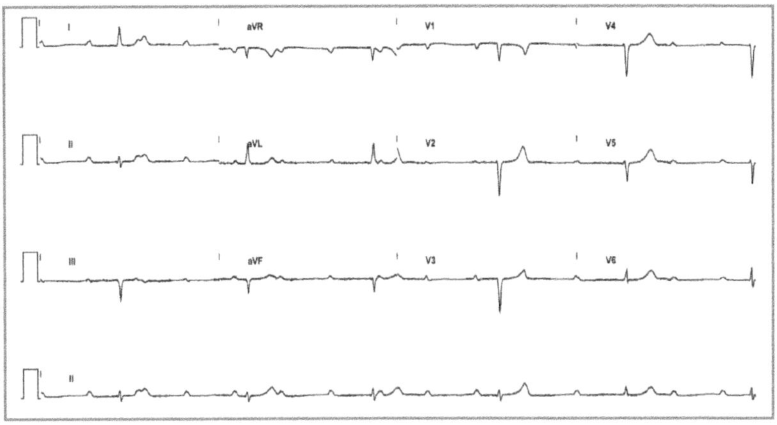

Fig. 14.7 Third degree atrioventricular block with junctional escape rhythm

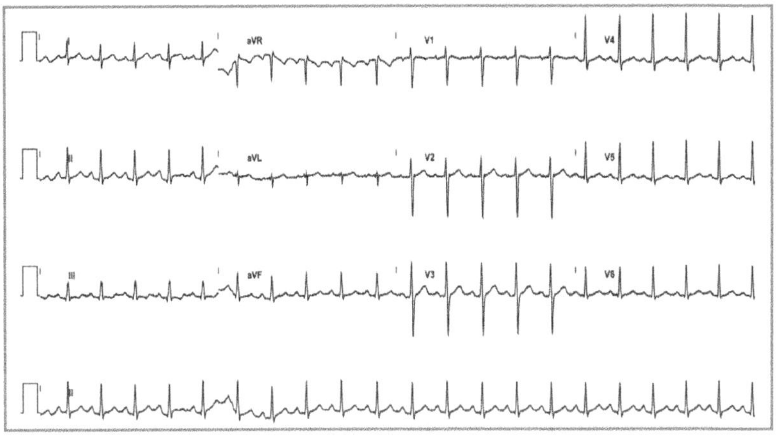

Fig. 14.8 Sinus tachycardia

a physiological mechanism, but it is often associated with a significant underlying organic disease. Paroxysmal AV block is potentially life-threatening because escape rhythms are generally unstable, also leading to sudden death. Furthermore, its diagnosis is very difficult because of its paroxysmal appearance and the absence of conduction disturbances apart from the episodes of block. Patients with this type of AV block should be treated with a permanent pacemaker [1].

14.3 Tachyarrhythmias

14.3.1 Sinus Tachycardia

Sinus tachycardia (Fig. 14.8) is characterized by an acceleration of the sinus rhythm above 100 bpm. It is usually a normal response to physiological conditions (physical exercise, emotional stress) or pathological conditions (fever, anemia, low blood pressure, hyperthyroidism, heart failure) that directly or indirectly increase the adrenergic activity. At the ECG, P waves of normal morphology are regularly followed by QRS complexes after normal PR intervals. Vagal manoeuvres only lead to a slight and transient decrease in the HR. Sinus tachycardia begins and ends gradually. It has no clinical significance, and does not need any therapy but the identification and treatment of underlying pathological conditions. In rare cases sinus tachycardia may be persistent, exacerbated by exercise but present even at rest, without any underlying pathology: in this case, it is called *inappropriate sinus tachycardia*. The causes of this type of sinus tachycardia are unclear. It is often found in young women and, when symptomatic, it can be treated with beta-blockers, calcium channel blockers or ivabradine (cases of si-

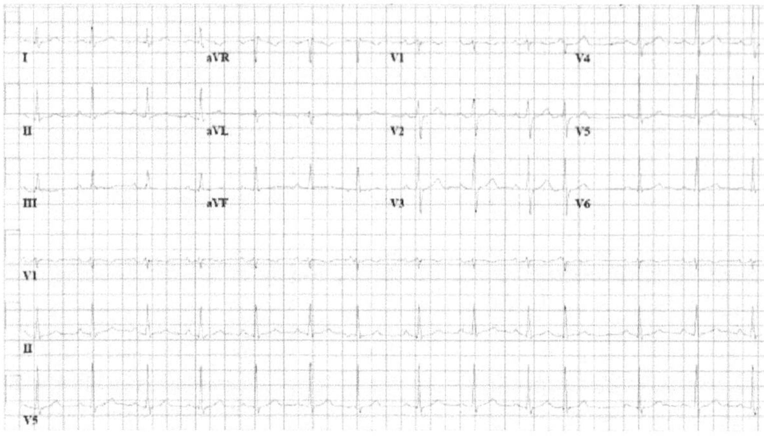

Fig. 14.9 Supraventricular premature beats (7th and 11th QRS complex)

nus node modulation through percutaneous radiofrequency ablation have also been reported) [2].

14.3.2 Sinoatrial Re-entrant Tachycardia

It is a rare condition, due to a re-entry circuit located in the perinodal tissues. It is characterized by P waves identical to sinus rhythm, with a heart rate of 120-130 bpm. Its onset is sudden, usually triggered by extrasystoles. It is generally well tolerated. Class II and class IV antiarrhythmic agents (beta-blockers and calcium channel blockers) may be employed for its treatment.

14.3.3 Supraventricular Premature Beats

Supraventricular premature beats (or extrasystoles) are depolarizations that occur earlier than the expected normal sinoatrial activation wavefront and are generated by atrial or AV junction cells (Fig. 14.9). *Atrial premature beats* (APBs) may originate anywhere in the atria or in the surrounding venous structures, such as caval and pulmonary veins, whose walls may contain muscle tissue spurs with automatic activity. Premature complexes commonly arise in structurally normal hearts, although they are more often associated with structural heart disease and with ageing. Electrocardiographically, they appear as premature P waves followed or not by QRS complexes (in the second case they are defined as blocked atrial extrasystoles) (Fig. 14.10). P wave morphology is generally different from that of sinus ones because of the different atrial activation sequence, and it varies depending on the origin site; atrial activation is generally eccentric, different from atrial activation due to retrograde propagation of the impulse through the normal nodal-hisian conduction pathway. Ventricular activation follows the normal conduction system, and QRS complexes may be similar to basal ones or aberrant, with bundle branch block or hemiblock morphology. Premature P wave may be followed by a compensatory pause (twice the basal PP interval; common in the case of very early APBs), or, more frequently, by a non-compensatory pause. APBs are seldom interpolated (included in a normal PP interval) or followed by a more-than-compensatory pause (more than twice the basal PP interval; more frequent in presence of sick sinus syndrome).

Junctional premature beats (JPBs) are generated in the AV junction or in the His bundle. Electrocardiographically, they appear as premature QRS complexes, with the same morphology of the baseline QRS complexes. If present, P wave may precede, follow or overlap with the QRS complex (in the last case it is not evident); it is typically negative in the inferior leads, positive and narrow in V1 because of a concentric retrograde atrial activation.

Supraventricular extrasystoles may be isolated or organized in repetitive form, i.e. in succession of two (pairs) or three or more beats (runs). Sometimes they arise rhythmically after a fixed number of sinus

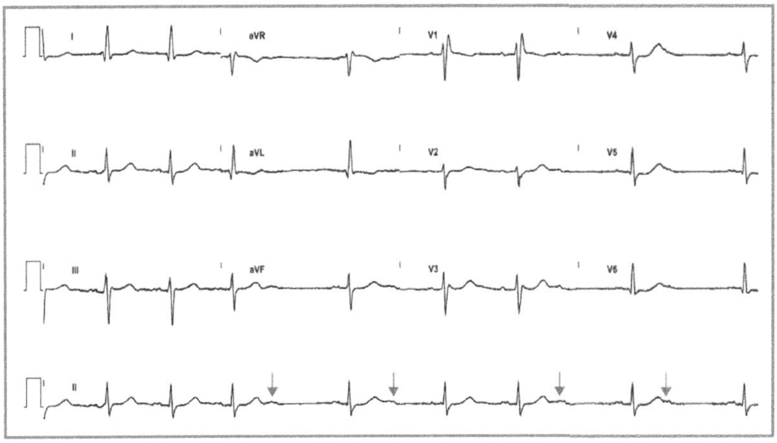

Fig. 14.10 Blocked atrial extrasystoles (*arrows*)

beats, and in these cases they are called bigemine (if they occur after each sinus beat), trigemine (if occurring after every second sinus beat), and so on. The interval between the premature beat and the previous sinus beat is the copula (or coupling interval), and in many cases it is constant. Supraventricular premature beats may occur in different clinical situations, such as inflammation, myocardial ischemia, infections, or they may be triggered by drugs, emotional stress, tobacco, caffeine. They do not require a specific treatment unless they are highly symptomatic or trigger more complex tachycardias. In these cases, the most used drugs are beta-blockers and calcium channel blockers, but sometimes other anti-arrhythmic agents may be required.

14.3.4 Parasystole

Parasystole is a rhythm disorder caused by a peculiar automatic focus that works in parallel with the SA node. It has its own firing rate and is protected from depolarization by the sinus node by an entrance block [3]. This focus, which can be atrial, junctional or ventricular, competes with the dominant rhythm for the depolarization of a certain cardiac chamber, and it is able to excite the myocardium whenever this is not refractory; inter-ectopic intervals are usually multiple of the baseline focus cycle. It has been shown that the dominant rhythm, whether not able to penetrate into the focus, can influence it, accelerating or slowing it down. The diagnosis of parasystole is based on three criteria:

- ectopic beats coupling interval is generally variable;
- intervals between the ectopic beats are multiples of a common denominator (which represents the intrinsic focus firing cycle);
- fusion beats can be present (atrial or ventricular; the former are very difficult to recognize on the basis of P wave morphology).

This particular type of arrhythmia has generally no clinical relevance and does not require any treatment, except for rare cases of very high firing rate generating a so-called *parasystolic tachycardia.*

14.3.5 Atrial Tachycardia

Atrial tachycardia is defined by three or more atrial ectopic beats with an atrial rate between 100 and 240 bpm (Fig. 14.11). As premature beats, atrial tachycardia can originate from any part of the atria, although there are preferential sites, such as the crista terminalis, the origin of pulmonary veins, the base of the left atrial appendage. Underlying mechanisms may be different: enhanced automatism, triggered activity or re-entry [4]. ECG is not useful in order to determinate the mechanism on the basis of the arrhythmia, while P wave morphology may be helpful in the identification of the site of origin. When arrhythmias are due to an increased automaticity, the first P wave is generally equal to the following ones and gradual heart rate acceleration is present at the beginning of the tachycardia (*warm-*

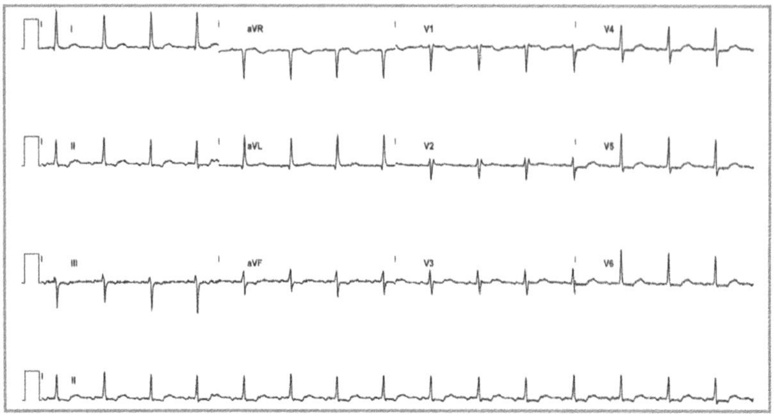

Fig. 14.11 Atrial tachycardia with 2:1 atrioventricular conduction ratio

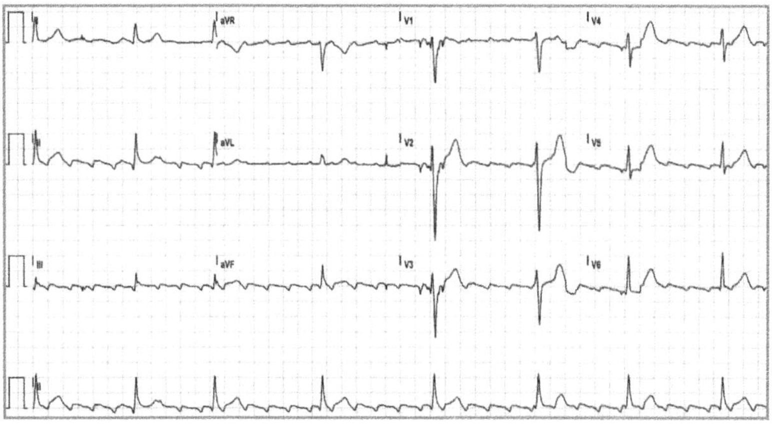

Fig. 14.12 Typical counter-clockwise atrial flutter with moderate ventricular response (74 bpm)

up phenomenon), while in re-entrant forms the P wave triggering the arrhythmia is different from the following ones and the warm-up phenomenon is not present. During tachycardia, the P waves may be conducted to the ventricles with varying degree of block (this is the case of sleep apnoea syndrome and digitalis intoxication).

Paroxysmal atrial tachycardia is the most common form of atrial tachycardia: it is characterized by abrupt onset and termination and it is caused by re-entry or triggered mechanisms. The incessant or permanent form, in which the arrhythmia is present for more than 50% of time, is much more rare but potentially dangerous, as it can lead to a tachycardia-induced cardiomyopathy (tachycardiomyopathy) due to a constant high ventricular response. In these cases, the location of the tachycardia site of origin (which is often due to increased automatism) and its elimination by catheter ablation may lead to a regression of the left ventricular dysfunction. A particular type of tachycardia is *chaotic or multifocal atrial tachycardia*, caused by multiple atrial foci firing independently from each other, thus irregularly depolarising the atria. P waves show different morphologies and the heartbeat is completely irregular. This arrhythmia often precedes the onset of atrial fibrillation.

14.3.6 Atrial Flutter

Atrial flutter (Fig. 14.12) is a fast (> 240 bpm) atrial tachycardia, supported by a macro-re-entry circuit involving one of the two atria (usually the right one). The re-entry circuit is generally delimited by anatomical barriers or surgical or post-ablation scars. In the past years different and contrasting terms were proposed for atrial flutter classification, until in 2001 a consensus statement was published in order to establish a universally accepted nomenclature [5]. According to this paper, atrial flutter can be defined as typical or atypical.

Typical atrial flutter is a right atrial tachycardia whose macro-re-entry circuit includes the cavo-tricuspid isthmus as an area of compelled passage and critical conduction deceleration. Typical atrial flutter is further divided into two subtypes, known as *counterclockwise*, in which the loop is crossed by the wavefront in a counterclockwise direction (when evaluated in an oblique left anterior projection), and *clockwise* (10% of all cases of typical atrial flutter), in which the loop is crossed in a clockwise direction.

Atypical atrial flutter is sustained by macro-reentry circuits which can be located in the right or left atrium and do not include the cavo-tricuspid isthmus; these circuits are often generated by surgical or post-ablation scars (a common example is left atrial flutter occurring after pulmonary veins isolation for catheter ablation of atrial fibrillation).

A particular type of atrial flutter is the so-called *lower loop atrial flutter* in which re-entry circuit is located around the inferior vena cava, therefore it includes the cavo-tricuspid isthmus.

Atrial flutter is frequent in conditions characterized by atrial dilation, such as pulmonary embolism, atrial septal defects, mitral or tricuspid valve disease, heart failure; although rarely, it may occur in the absence of any structural heart disease. Other conditions such as thyrotoxicosis, alcohol intoxication and pericarditis may cause atrial flutter.

In counterclockwise atrial flutter, atrial waves (F waves) in the inferior leads (II, III, aVF) have an initial ascending branch (typically steep) followed by a descending terminal portion (slow and frequently broken) without an isoelectric line between consecutive F waves, giving rise to the characteristic *saw-tooth* morphology. Sometimes it is possible to identify the isoelectric line in V1. Atrial rate, typically around 300 bpm, may be slowed by administration of class IC antiarrhythmic drugs. Ventricular response can be of three types:

- regular, with a fixed AV conduction ratio (1:1, 2:1, 4:1 and so on);
- irregular, with a grouping of QRS complexes (group beating), due to a Wenckebach conduction (decremental);
- irregular, in the absence of a fixed pattern (variable AV conduction).

Clockwise flutter waves have typically symmetrical branches and prevalent positivity in the inferior leads.

One-to-one AV conduction ratio is quite rare in atrial flutter, but it can be observed during administration of class IC antiarrhythmic drugs that, reducing the flutter atrial rate, may allow AV *synchronization* with an increase of the ventricular rate and a clinical deterioration of the patient. Atypical flutter does not have peculiar electrocardiographic characteristics: atrial waves morphology is variable according to the circuit site and atrial rate is included between 240 and 350 bpm. In patients with atrial flutter, the treatment of choice is catheter ablation, which is performed by creating a line of block between the tricuspid annulus and the inferior vena cava in cases of typical atrial flutter and by eliminating other targets in the case of atypical atrial flutter.

In some cases, pharmacological treatment may be useful for the prevention of recurrences (class IC antiarrhythmic drugs, amiodarone, dronedarone) or for ventricular rate control (beta-blockers, calcium channel blockers, digoxin). Treatment of acute episodes is represented by pharmacological cardioversion (particularly ibutilide, that has the highest efficacy, around 60-90%) or electrical cardioversion. Transesophageal overdrive pacing may represent an alternative strategy.

14.3.7 Atrial Fibrillation

Atrial fibrillation (AF) (Fig. 14.13) is a very common rhythm disorder characterized by chaotic and disorganized atrial electrical activity with an atrial rate faster than 350 and up to 600 bpm in the absence of atrial mechanical contraction. The currently used classification identifies the following types of AF [6]:

- *new onset* (or *first detected*), in the case of the first episode of AF;
- *paroxysmal*, characterized by spontaneous arrhythmia termination within 7 days (usually within 24 hours);
- *persistent*, if the arrhythmia does not stop spontaneously within 7 days, or it is interrupted by an external intervention (pharmacological or electrical cardioversion); it includes *long-standing persistent AF* (arrhythmia duration was

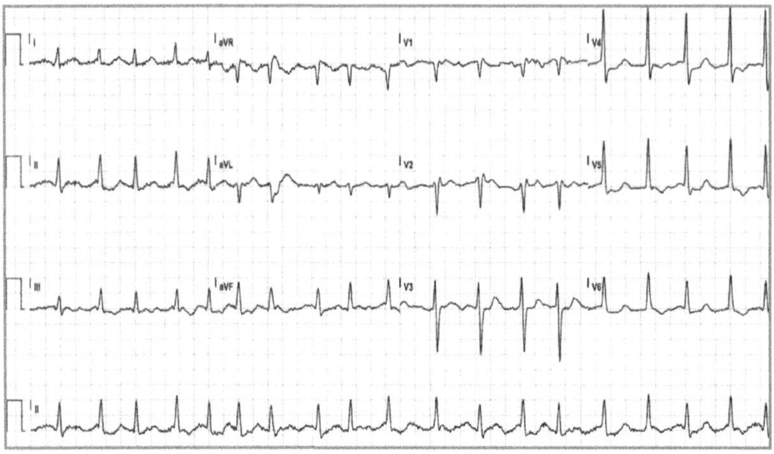

Fig. 14.13 Atrial fibrillation

more than one year when it was decided to adopt a rhythm control strategy);

- *permanent*: attempts to terminate the arrhythmia were ineffective or were not conducted.

Multiple mechanisms have been implied in AF induction and maintenance. To explain the heterogeneity of this arrhythmia, Allessie and his team theorized that AF is the final result of complex electrophysiological mechanisms in which three fundamental elements must be identified: main triggers, initiator and perpetuator [7]. *Triggers* are variable, they may be represented by various types of tachycardia or by automatic foci located in the pulmonary veins. In order to initiate the arrhythmia, triggers need an electrophysiological substrate (*initiator*) favouring a re-entry mechanism. The initiator may be represented by areas of refractoriness dispersion or depressed conduction. Experimental studies also indicate the Bachmann bundle (which connects the two atria at atrial roof level) and the interatrial septum as potential initiators. *Perpetuators* are fundamental to give clinical relevancy to the arrhythmia. Otherwise, after a few seconds or a few minutes, the arrhythmia would spontaneously terminate. Several factors may act as perpetuators, such as atrial enlargement, muscle anatomical damage, atrial electrical and structural remodeling due to continuous recurrences. The pathogenetic importance of these three factors (triggers, initiators, perpetuators) is different in the various forms of AF. In paroxysmal AF (typical of healthy or near-healthy hearts), trigger plays a dominant role, while initiator and perpetuator are less important. In persistent AF, perpetuator has growing importance, which becomes maximal in permanent AF.

AF is the most common cardiac arrhythmia; its incidence increases with age. The Framingham Heart Study showed that the risk of AF onset during a lifetime is 26% after 40 years of age. Like atrial flutter, AF is more frequent in the presence of structural heart disease (dilated cardiomyopathy of different etiologies, mitral valve disease, etc.) or other disorders such as thyrotoxicosis. However, it can also occur in the absence of cardiac or extracardiac disease, especially in younger subjects (lone atrial fibrillation). AF worsens morbidity and mortality by increasing the risk of heart failure, death and embolic phenomena including stroke.

Electrocardiographically, AF is characterized by the absence of P waves (a high frequency oscillation of isoelectric line, determining deflections called *f waves*, is sometimes present) and irregularly irregular ventricular activity, usually at high rate. The number of atrial impulses that reach the AV node is very high, but they are variously blocked in the AV node itself, thus limiting the ventricular rate.

Clinical presentation may be extremely variable. In some cases AF is completely asymptomatic (silent AF). When present, the most common symptoms are represented by irregular palpitations (especially on arrhythmia onset), wheezing, worsening heart failure due to loss of atrial contribution to ventricular filling and/or to reduced diastole duration (diastolic heart failure), or more rarely chest pain (especially in presence of pre-existing coronary artery disease).

In addition to the prevention of thromboembolic phenomena, the goals of treatment are:

- sinus rhythm restoration and maintenance;
- heart rate control.

Arrhythmia interruption may be obtained by administration of antiarrhythmic drugs, particularly class IC (propafenone, flecainide) or class IA (quinidine, disopyramide) drugs, and amiodarone, or by electrical cardioversion. Both pharmacological and electrical cardioversion are contraindicated when the arrhythmia is lasting for more than 48 hours, due to an increased risk of thromboembolic phenomena, unless it causes acute heart failure or transesophageal echocardiography has excluded the presence of atrial thrombi. During AF, in fact, blood stasis in the atrial chambers favours the formation of thrombi, and recovery of atrial contractility (during the transition from AF to sinus rhythm) is associated to high risk of systemic embolization, particularly in brain areas. In these cases, a ventricular rate control strategy (with target average heart rate preferably below 100 bpm) should be adopted, together with effective oral anticoagulation (INR value between 2 and 3) administering vitamin K antagonists for at least 4 weeks, before proceeding to sinus rhythm restoration by electrical cardioversion. Successful pharmacological cardioversion is dramatically reduced in long-lasting AF.

Sometimes sinus rhythm restoration is not achievable or not deemed useful: in these cases a definitive rate control and anticoagulation strategy is adopted.

The same drugs used for cardioversion can be used to prevent arrhythmia recurrences as well. Amiodarone is slightly superior to other agents, but it presents a significant number of long term side effects. Some of these effects could be avoided with the use of a new drug, dronedarone, but it is contraindicated in patients with class IV heart failure or in patients who have had a recent episode of decompensated heart failure, especially if they have depressed left ventricular function. When a rate control strategy is indicated, the drugs of choice are beta-blockers, non-dihydropyridine calcium channel blockers (diltiazem and verapamil) and, in patients with heart failure, digoxin.

Several clinical studies have concluded that there is no difference between maintenance of sinus rhythm with antiarrhythmic drugs and heart rate control in terms of mortality, morbidity and quality of life [8-9]. However, the major limitation of these studies is represented by the therapeutic tools used to maintain the sinus rhythm, i.e. antiarrhythmic drugs. On the other hand, a post-hoc analysis of the AFFIRM trial [10] showed that maintenance of the sinus rhythm, when obtained without antiarrhythmic drugs, improves survival, while antiarrhythmic drug use reduces it. Therefore, antiarrhythmic drug therapy is not an optimal therapeutic option since it has limited effectiveness in maintaining sinus rhythm and it is associated to numerous cardiac and extracardiac side effects which may counterbalance the potential benefits associated with sinus rhythm persistence. Other strategies for the treatment of AF are:

- radiofrequency catheter ablation, based on electrical isolation of the pulmonary veins from the rest of the left atrium and the eventual creation of other lesions involving a more or less extensive portion of both atria;
- surgical ablation, usually (but not exclusively) performed during cardiac surgery for other indications [11];
- pacemaker therapy: performed when antiarrhythmic drug therapy causes episodes of marked bradycardia and/or pathological pauses (for example, patients with bradycardia/tachycardia syndrome), or when AV node ablation is necessary;
- AV node ablation or modulation, which is the last chance when it is not possible to achieve adequate heart rate control with drugs.

In patients with significant thromboembolic risk, treatment with oral anticoagulants is indispensable. These patients primarily include those with AF and a prosthetic valve. Additional factors to take into account in the thromboembolic risk evaluation are a previous ischemic episode, heart failure, hypertension, diabetes mellitus and advanced age.

14.3.8 Atrioventricular Nodal Re-entrant Tachycardia (AVNRT)

Atrioventricular nodal re-entrant tachycardia (AVNRT) is the most common form (more than 50% of cases) of paroxysmal supraventricular

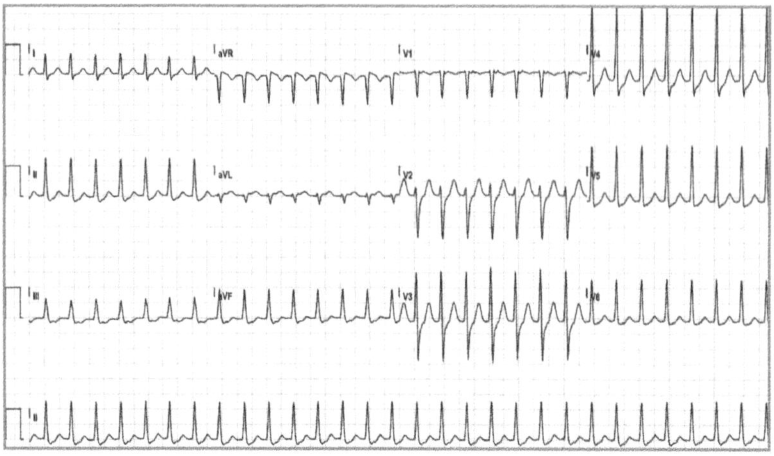

Fig. 14.14 Paroxysmal supraventricular tachycardia with short RP interval, suggesting typical atrioventricular nodal re-entrant tachycardia

tachycardia in the adults. It is more common in women, less common in children and adolescents.

In subjects with this arrhythmia, AV node has two connections with the surrounding atrium: a *fast pathway*, located upstream the His bundle, and a *slow pathway*, located near the ostium of the coronary sinus [12]. There is great evidence supporting the presence of two conduction pathways between the atria and the ventricles in subjects with AVNRT episodes (*dual nodal physiology*), since these two pathways differ from each other in terms of conduction velocity and refractoriness, therefore their presence can be demonstrated during an electrophysiological study. However, an anatomical substrate of the two ways has not been demonstrated yet. AVNRT is sustained by a re-entry circuit involving the AV node and its connections with the atrium. According to the wavefront direction in the re-entry circuit, two major forms of AVNRT can be distinguished. In typical AVNRT (*slow-fast*), the re-entry circuit uses the slow pathway as antegrade branch and the fast pathway and the perinodal atrial tissue as retrograde pathway. In atypical AVNRT (*fast-slow*), the re-entry circuit is crossed in the opposite direction. There is another form of atypical AVNRT (*slow-slow type*) in which both branches of the circuit are represented by slow pathways, one of them serving as anterograde branch and the other as retrograde branch. Finally, in some subjects fast-slow and slow-slow AVNRT may coexist at different times, suggesting the possibility of multiple connections between the AV node and surrounding atrium [13].

Electrocardiogram during sinus rhythm does not show peculiar features; sometimes, when the fast pathway is only capable of antegrade conduction, a very long PR interval (more than 300 ms) may be present. Typical AVNRT (Fig. 14.14) electrocardiographically appears as a regular narrow QRS rhythm (with the exception of the presence of aberrant conduction), with fast heart rate (sometimes over 200 bpm), in which P waves are not well recognisable because they are often included in the QRS complexes, or they may be represented as a small notch at the end of QRS: this feature suggests almost synchronous depolarization of the atria and the ventricles). The retrograde P wave is narrow (simultaneous activation of the two atria from the septal region), negative in the inferior leads (II, III, aVF) and positive in V1, where it may simulate a right bundle branch block because it is positioned at the end of the QRS complex (pseudo-r'). RP interval is typically short, shorter than PR interval. Exactly the opposite (PR<RP) occurs in the fast-slow AVNRT, since the antegrade conduction time is significantly longer than retrograde conduction time through the fast pathway. In the slow-slow form, the P wave is approximately located in an intermediate position between two consecutive QRS complexes.

Tachycardia is frequently triggered by premature atrial beats (rarely by ventricular beats), that in typical AVNRT have a PR interval longer than the baseline PR due to a *jump* of the antegrade conduction from the fast to the slow pathway.

Because of the type of circuit involved in the arrhythmia, AV conduction ratio is usually 1:1; in rare cases it may be different (for example 2:1) because of a conduction block below the re-entry circuit. This event is so rare that when it occurs it is important, first of all, to exclude an atrial tachycardia. AVNRT is usually a paroxysmal, self-limiting and not life-threatening arrhythmia. It is more frequent in healthy hearts. Symptoms are usually represented by regular palpitations with sudden onset. Vagal manoeuvres, such as carotid sinus massage or Valsalva manoeuvre, and intravenous administration of adenosine, may interrupt the arrhythmia. A pharmacological approach with beta-blockers, calcium channel blockers or other antiarrhythmic agents (flecainide, propaphenone) may be attempted to prevent recurrences, but the definitive treatment is represented by catheter ablation of one of the two pathways (generally the slow pathway). This technique has a very high success rate, more than 90%, and rather low complication rate, but carries the risk of complete AV block with the need of permanent pacemaker implantation [14].

14.3.9 Atrioventricular Reciprocating Tachycardia Due to Accessory Pathways and Ventricular Preexcitation Syndrome (Wolff-Parkinson-White Syndrome)

Wolff-Parkinson-White syndrome is a condition of ventricular preexcitation, sustained by an AV accessory pathway with all-or-nothing conduction, which manifests with atrioventricular circus-movement tachycardias. It is described in detail in Chapter 15.

14.3.10 Supraventricular Tachycardias Sustained by Accessory Pathways with Decremental Conduction

Two rare types of tachycardia use accessory pathways characterized by decremental conduction (conduction velocity is inversely related to impulse frequency).

The first one is the *tachycardia mediated by atriofascicular (Mahaim fibre) accessory pathways*, which is an antidromic reciprocating tachycardia. *Mahaim* fibres are atrio-fascicular or nodo-fascicular bundles, composed by cells with AV nodal-like electrophysiological properties (not very short conduction time; decremental conduction). They are generally located at or near the lateral, antero-lateral or postero-lateral tricuspid annulus, and usually connect the right atrium to the final portion of the right bundle branch. Of note, these pathways only allow antegrade impulse conduction. Antidromic reciprocating tachycardia uses the accessory pathway antegradely and the normal conduction system retrogradely. During sinus rhythm, the electrocardiogram is generally normal; in rare cases peculiar features, such as minimal preexcitation with left bundle branch block morphology, have been described. Tachycardia is typically preexcited with left bundle branch block morphology [15].

The second form of re-entrant tachycardia due to an accessory pathway with decremental conduction properties is *permanent junctional reciprocating tachycardia (PJRT) or Coumel-type tachycardia*. The accessory pathway underlying this arrhythmia is characterized by a prevalent retrograde conduction capability (it is believed to be able to conduct antegradely with a very low velocity). During sinus rhythm there is no evidence of preexcitation. The tachycardia is typically incessant (lasting usually more than 12 hours daily), with long tachycardia episodes spaced out by few sinus beats. P waves are typically large and inverted in II, III and aVF leads; PR interval is slightly shorter than RP interval. Arrhythmia re-entry circuit is formed by a postero-septal accessory pathway with slow and decremental conduction as the retrograde branch and the nodo-hisian system as the antegrade branch.

14.3.11 Accelerated Junctional Rhythm and Idiopathic Junctional Tachycardia

Accelerated junctional rhythm and *idiopathic junctional tachycardia* are arrhythmias from sub-

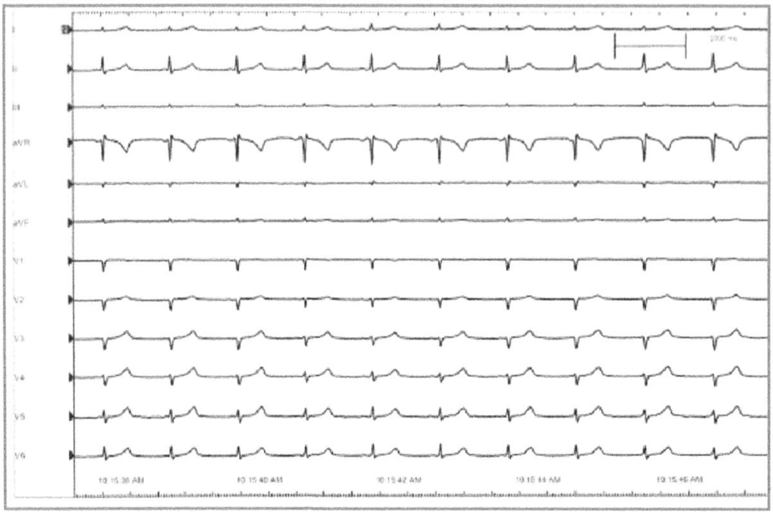

Fig. 14.15 Accelerated junctional rhythm with sinus activation of the atria, causing isorhythmic atrioventricular dissociation. P waves are evident in leads II and aVR

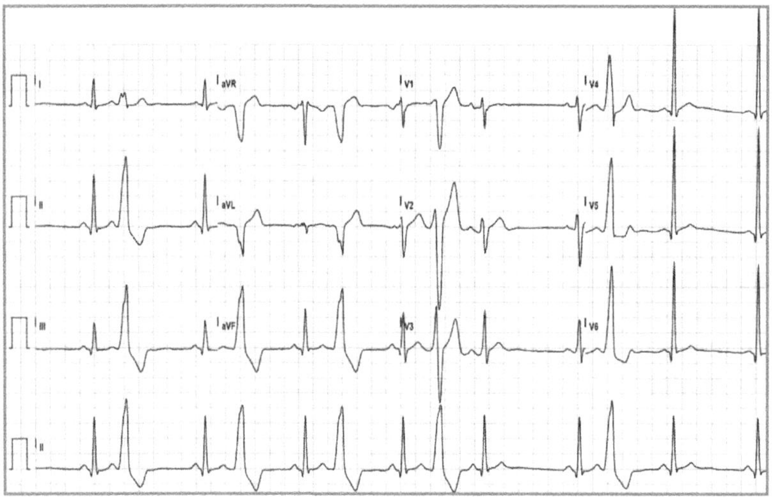

Fig. 14.16 Ventricular premature beats

sidiary pacemakers in the AV node and the His bundle that, because of an enhanced automatism, take over the physiological sinus node activation as the dominant cardiac pacemaker. The resultant arrhythmia is classified as accelerated junctional rhythm if the HR is less than 100 bpm, and automatic junctional tachycardia if the HR is equal or more than 100 bpm.

During these rhythm disorders, ECG shows a regular succession of QRS complexes, with the same morphology as QRS during located at or near the lateral, antero-lateral, or posterolateral tricuspid annulus rhythm, not preceded by sinus P waves. Atria may be retrogradely activated by the AV node (with a P wave morphology typical of concentric retrograde conduction), or may be normally activated by the sinus node. In the latter case, P waves have a normal morphology, but they are dissociated by QRS complexes. Sometimes atrial and ventricular activity have a similar frequency, thus mimicking a 1:1 AV conduction ratio, although the two electrical activities are in fact totally disconnected from each other (*isorhythmic AV dissociation*; Fig 14.15). These arrhythmias are relatively common in patients with digitalis toxicity or inferior myocardial infarction, but they can also occur in healthy subjects. Junctional firing rate increases with exercise, while it can be slowed by carotid sinus massage. Accelerated junctional rhythm is usually asymptomatic and it rarely requires a specific therapy. The treatment of junctional tachycardia is based on calcium channel blockers and beta-blockers.

14.3.12 Ventricular Premature Beats

Ventricular premature beats (VPBs) are anticipated ventricular depolarizations that may start from any ventricular area. They may be isolated or organized in repetitive forms (couples or runs of three or more beats; bigeminy, trigeminy and so on). In the same patient, VPBs may have only one or more than one morphology (monomorphic and polymorphic extrasystoles, respectively), depending on whether their origin is unifocal or multifocal. Electrocardiographically, a VPB appears as an early QRS complex with abnormal morphology and prolonged duration (typically more than 120 ms and longer than the sinus QRS complex), followed by a T wave with opposite polarity. If present, P wave usually origins from the sinus node and it is dissociated from the ectopic QRS complex; sometimes it is produced by atrial retrograde activation and follows the QRS complex. If atrial retrograde activation is associated with sinus node reset, the pause following VPB is *not compensatory*; however, in the case of VPBs, post-ectopic pauses are more frequently *compensatory* because the premature beat is often not so precocious to reset the sinus node. VPBs may also be *interpolated*: in this case it may not produce any pause or it may sometimes produce a *postponed compensatory pause*. This is a compensatory pause that appears after the first sinus beat following the VPB: the interpolated VPB prolongs the PR interval of the first post-ectopic beat so that the following P wave finds the AV node refractory and it cannot reach the ventricles. A distinction between VPBs and SVPBs with aberrant conduction is not always possible with the surface ECG.

Ventricular premature beats are very common in the general population, both in the presence and in the absence of structural heart disease. In the absence of underlying cardiopathies, predisposing factors are the same described for atrial extrasystoles. Among heart diseases, ischemic heart disease and heart failure are most frequently associated to VPBs.

The clinical relevance of VPBs is mainly related to the underlying pathology. However, some ECG criteria suggest a potentially increased risk:

- occurrence of more than 10 VPBs per hour;
- organization into more complex forms (couples, runs of non sustained ventricular tachycardia);
- presence of different morphologies;
- marked precocity, with occurrence of the ectopic beat in correspondence of the apex or descending branch of the T wave from the previous sinus beat (*R on T phenomenon*), a period in which ventricles are more vulnerable to ventricular arrhythmias.

Extrasystole suppression by physical exertion cannot always be considered a certain marker of benignity because it was also observed in cases of VPBs associated to coronary artery disease. In patients with structurally and functionally normal heart, the risk of major arrhythmic events is very low. On the other hand, in some cardiopathies, VPBs suggest a relevant risk of potentially life-threatening arrhythmic events. For example, in patients with acute myocardial infarction, VPBs may trigger potentially life-threatening arrhythmias. Like supraventricular extrasystoles, in most cases VPBs are asymptomatic. The most frequent symptoms are represented by palpitations, *chest thump* sensation due to the cardiac output increase in the post-ectopic beat, feeling of a missing beat due to the post-ectopic pause, *heart in throat* sensation. If frequent, VPBs may be perceived as heart rhythm irregularities.

Ventricular extrasystoles usually do not require a specific treatment apart from the removal of any underlying cause (myocardial ischemia, electrolyte disturbances, caffeine abuse, etc.), especially in normal hearts. Treatment is usually based on the presence and extent of related symptoms. The drugs of choice are beta-blockers. Class IC antyarrhythmic drugs are quite effective in reducing VPBs, but their use is contraindicated in the presence of structural heart disease, in this case amiodarone may be safer. In exceptional cases, for example very frequent drug-refractory VPBs causing or worsening left ventricular dysfunction, treatment by catheter ablation may be considered.

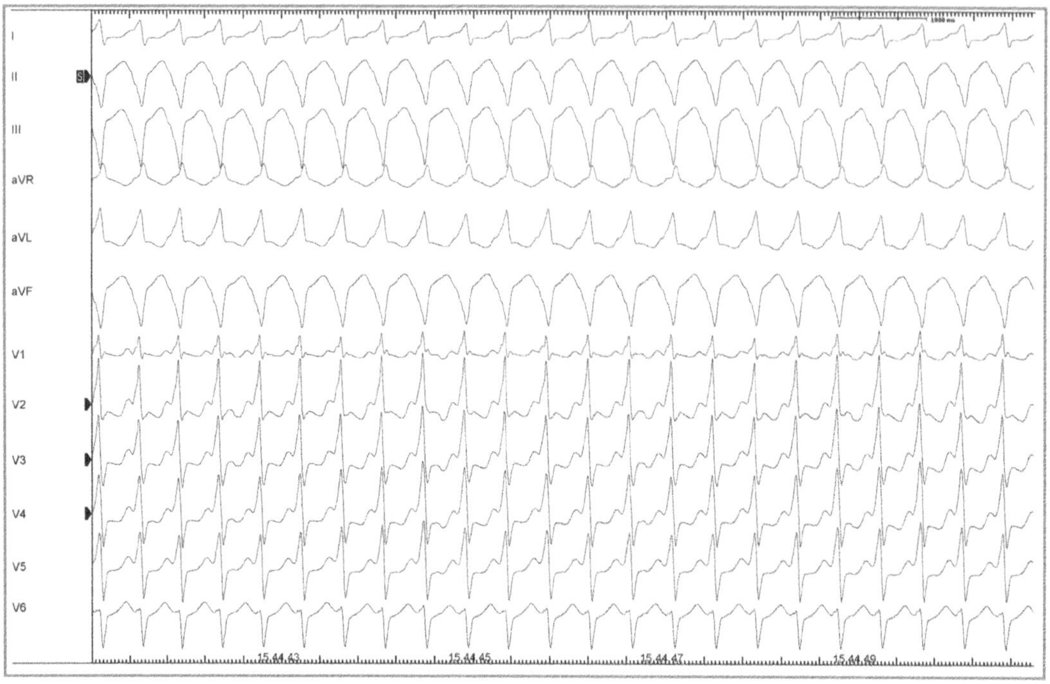

Fig. 14.17 Ventricular tachycardia in a patient with ischemic heart disease

14.3.13 Accelerated Idioventricular Rhythm

Accelerated idioventricular rhythm (AIVR) is caused by enhanced automatism of a pacemaker located in the conduction tissue, distal to the His bundle, depolarizing the ventricles at 60-110 bpm. QRS complexes, because of their ventricular origin, last more than 120 ms; P waves dissociated by the QRS complexes and fusion beats are often present. Sometimes there is a competition between the AIVR and sinus rhythm, causing an alternation of these two rhythms during electrocardiographic recording. AIVR is frequently observed in patients with myocardial infarction after thrombolysis or percutaneous revascularization, during hypokalemia or digitalis intoxication. It is usually asymptomatic, has a good prognosis and do not require treatment, apart from elimination of underlying causes. Acceleration of the sinus rhythm by atropine administration or atrial pacing may be useful when accelerated idioventricular rhythm causes symptomatic AV dissociation, which is quite rare.

14.3.14 Ventricular Tachycardias

Ventricular tachycardias (VTs) are consist of three or more VPBs, frequently at more than 110 bpm, arising in the ventricles or in the conduction system distal to the His bundle bifurcation. They can be caused by re-entry mechanisms (especially in the context of structural heart disease, such as ischemic heart disease), by enhanced automatism or by triggered activity. A VT lasting less than 30 seconds is defined as *not sustained*, a VT lasting more than 30 seconds or causing hemodynamic compromise (for example syncope) or requiring an external intervention is defined as *sustained*.

Ventricular tachycardias frequently occur in the presence of structural heart disease (ischemic heart disease, dilated or hypertrophic cardiomyopathy, right ventricular arrhythmogenic cardiomyopathy). Many hereditary diseases due to genetic defects involving membrane ion channels can predispose to VT development: Brugada syndrome, congenital long QT syndrome, short QT syndrome, catecholaminergic polymorphic VT.

Electrocardiographically (Fig. 14.17) VT presents as a wide (> 120 ms) QRS complex tachycardia with abnormal morphology, usually (but not always) regular, with a frequency between 110 and 250 bpm. ST-T segment has an opposite polarity as compared to QRS. During tachycardia, QRS morphology may be stable (*monomorphic VT*), may randomly vary (*polymorphic VT*), or it may show a beat-to-beat alternation in the frontal axis (*bidirectional VT*). Atrial activation may be retrograde with different VA conduction ratios (1:1 or different degrees of retrograde block such as 2:1, 3:1 or Wenckebach periodism), or a sinus atrial activation with AV (or VA) dissociation may be present. Electrocardiographic distinction between VT and supraventricular tachycardia with aberrant conduction can be particularly complex; sometimes a definite diagnosis is not possible on the basis of the surface ECG alone.

Some elements may point towards a diagnosis of VT:

- previous myocardial infarction or history of coronary artery disease;
- QRS duration > 140 ms;
- abnormal morphology of the QRS complex, quite different from a typical bundle branch block;
- negative correlation of QRS complexes in the precordial leads;
- AV dissociation or AV ratio < 1:1;
- fusion or capture beats.

As a general rule the management, prognosis and treatment of VTs depend on the presence or absence of underlying heart disease: except for inherited arrhythmogenic syndromes (Brugada, long QT etc.), the prognosis is usually benign in the absence of structural abnormalities. Symptoms occurring during VT are mainly related to low cardiac output (dyspnea, syncope, dizziness) or to coronary blood flow reduction (angina). Sometimes, especially if the arrhythmia is not fast, the patient may only experience palpitations or even be asymptomatic.

Nevertheless, the diagnosis ventricular tachycardia implies an emergency treatment, since this arrhythmia may provoke rapid hemodynamic deterioration or degenerate into ventricular fibrillation with cardiac arrest. General treatment of the acute episode is represented by removal of underlying causes (ischemia, electrolyte disturbances), intravenous administration of antiarrhythmic or other drugs (amiodarone, lidocaine, procainamide, magnesium sulphate, propofol) and, in drug-refractory cases or in the presence of hemodynamic deterioration, synchronized electrical cardioversion (or defibrillation in the case of cardiac arrest). In some cases overdrive pacing can represent a valid alternative to a pharmacological treatment. Strategies for the primary or secondary prevention of VTs in patients at risk are mainly represented by cardioverter-defibrillator implantation and, in selected cases, by catheter ablation (often in patients with frequent ICD shocks). Drug treatment has not proved any efficacy in the prevention of sudden cardiac death, but it may reduce the number of ICD shocks. However, VT management vary depending on the different types of VTs, each one having different characteristics and prognosis.

14.3.14.1 Idiopathic Ventricular Tachycardia

It can be paroxysmal or repetitive. It is monomorphic and often associated to numerous monomorphic ventricular extrasystoles. It has a focal origin: triggered activity due to late post-depolarizations is the pathogenetic mechanism.

It is frequently observed in young patients with a normal heart. The prognosis is good. Palpitations are the main symptom. In some cases this arrhythmia can lead to syncope. Physical effort, emotive stress or isoprenaline infusion may favour this arrhythmia. It can be interrupted by vagal manoeuvres and adenosine.

Beta blockers and verapamil can be adopted in the treatment of this arrhythmia. Catheter ablation can also be considered. Idiopathic ventricular tachycardia can typically originate in the:

- right ventricular outflow tract: left bundle branch block morphology and inferior axis, no R waves in V1-V2 (Fig. 14.18) [16];
- left ventricle ouflow tract: right bundle branch block morphology, early R wave transition, S wave in D1;
- aortic cusps, mitro-aortic continuity, mitral annulus [17].

14.3.14.2 Fascicular Tachycardia

This arrhythmia starts in one of the two fascicles of the left bundle branch, generally the left poste-

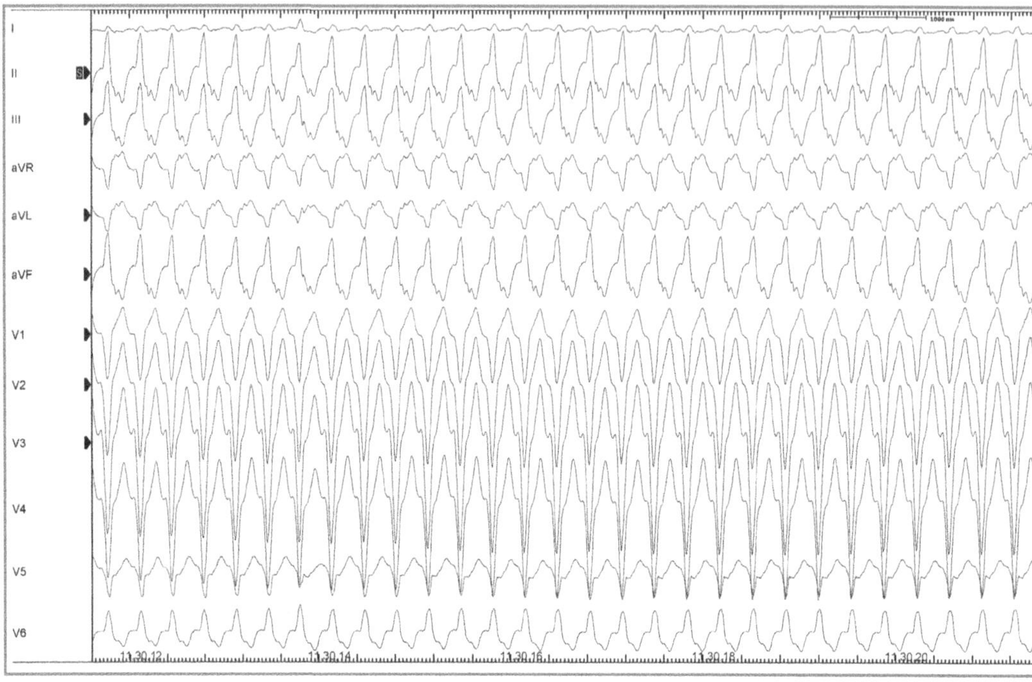

Fig. 14.18 Idiopathic ventricular tachycardia originating from the right ventricular outflow tract

rior fascicle. It has a right bundle branch block with left anterior fascicle block morphology with a not very large QRS complex (Fig. 14.19). This arrhythmia often occurs in young healthy subjects and has a good prognosis. It is caused by a re-entry mechanism including the His-Purkinje system on the left side of the posterior interventricular septum (but triggered activity has also been proposed as a possible pathogenetic mechanism).

This arrhythmia can be interrupted by verapamil (or diltiazem) and, in a lower percentage of cases, by adenosine. Catheter ablation may be an option in symptomatic cases after failure of the pharmacological treatment [18].

14.3.14.3 Bundle Branch Re-entrant Ventricular Tachycardia

This type of monorphic VT features a re-entry circuit including the right bundle branch, the interventricular septum, the left bundle branch and the His bundle. It can occur in patients with dilatative cardiomyopathy, neuromuscular disorders (such as type 1 myotonic dystrophy) and with very large baseline QRS complex. During VT, the QRS has a left bundle branch block morphology, since retrograde conduction takes place in the left bundle branch. However, the right bundle branch or the left anterior or left posterior fascicles can represent the retrograde portion of the re-entry circuit as well.

In the acute phase, rapid ventricular stimulation can often terminate the arrhythmia. Catheter ablation can prevent recurrences, but an implantable cardioverter-defibrillator is usually needed, especially in the case of patients with a cardiomyopathy.

14.3.14.4 Torsades de Pointes (TdP)

This is a polymorphic VT with 200-250 bpm ventricular rate, featuring a progressive change of QRS complex electric axis around an ideal baseline, with a continuous change from one polarity to the opposite in the same lead. It is correct to refer as TdP only in patients with a significantly long QT interval during sinus rhythm (at least in the beat preceding the beginning of the TdP), in all the other cases the arrhythmia should be mentioned as *polimorphic ventricular tachycardia*. TdP usually takes place during severe bradycardia, electrolyte imbalance (especially hypokalemia or hypomag-

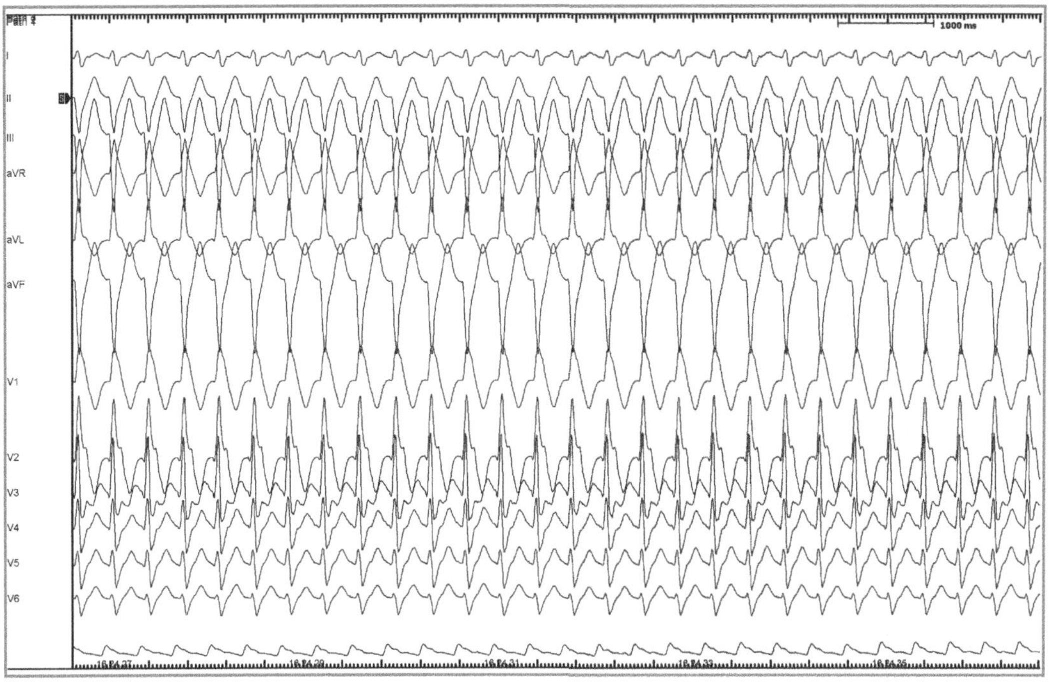

Fig. 14.19 Fascicular tachycardia

nesemia) or drug toxicity, and it is often triggered by ventricular ectopic beats leading to a long cycle-short cycle sequence. TdP pathophysiology is still not fully understood. Transmural re-entry, triggered activity and abnormal automatism have been thought as possible pathogenetic mechanisms. The hypothesis of trasmural re-entry is the most accredited to date.

TdP can spontaneously end, sometimes after an increase of the arrhythmia cycle length, on the other hand it can also cause syncope and it can turn into ventricular fibrillation and cardiac arrest if an effective treatment is not early carried out.

Therapy consists in correcting electrolyte imbalance (intravenous potassium and magnesium administration), temporary overdrive pacing or isoproterenol infusion (in order to avoid bradycardia-induced recurrences). Secondary causes leading to QT interval prolongation should be recognized and treated. Class IA, IC and III antiarrhythmic drugs should be avoided. Lydocaine, mexiletin and phenytoin could be safely used.

When TdP occurs in the presence of a normal QT interval, treatment is similar to that of VT. Beta-blockers, surgical sympathectomy and implantable cardioverter-defibrillator therapy can be adopted to prevent recurrences.

14.3.14.5 Ventricular Flutter

Ventricular flutter is a regular ventricular tachycardia with a very high rate (200-300 bpm). ST segment and T wave identification is very hard. QRS complexes follow each other at very high rate with a typical sinusoid shape. Ventricular flutter rapidly leads to hemodynamic compromise, syncope and, if not promptly interrupted, to ventricular fibrillation or cardiac arrest. Therapy consists of synchronized cardioversion or defibrillation if ventricular flutter has changed into ventricular fibrillation.

14.3.15 Ventricular Fibrillation

Ventricular fibrillation (VF) consists of a chaotic and disarranged ventricular electric activity. Both ventricles are simultaneously activated by multiple and disarranged wavelets. No QRS complex, ST segment or T wave can be detected at ECG

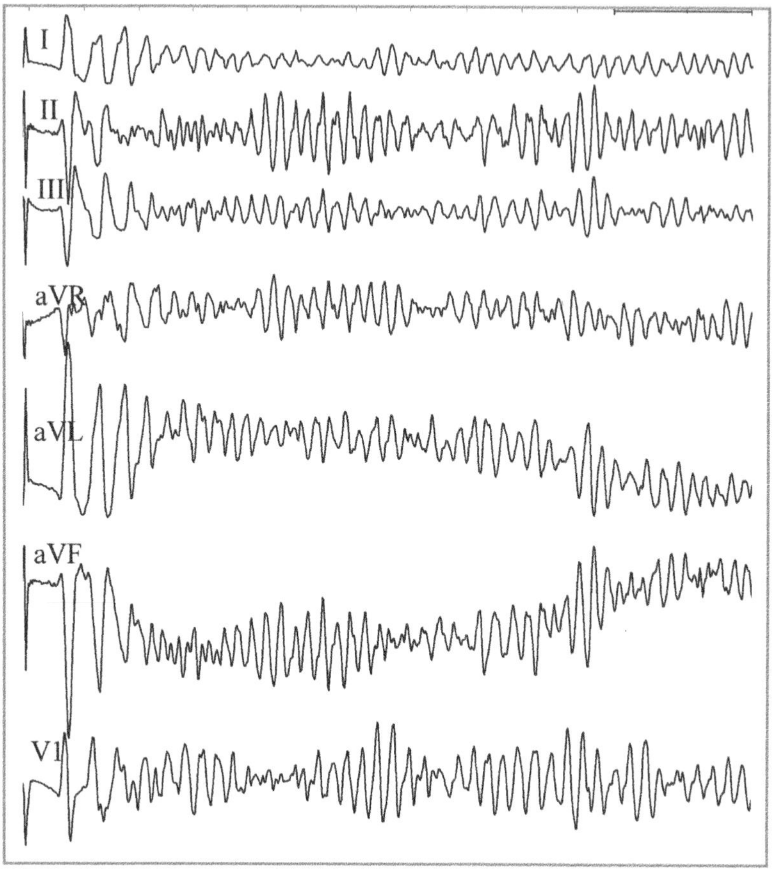

Fig. 14.20 Ventricular fibrillation

(Fig. 14.20). VF can take place in several situations, such as acute myocardial infarction or arrhythmogenic cardiomyopathies, and it invariably leads to cardiac arrest [19]. A less common cause of VF in younger people is atrial fibrillation with high ventricular response in the presence of an accessory pathway in patients with Wolff-Parkinson-White syndrome. Moreover, *idiopathic VF* should be mentioned, but this issue will be described in detail elsewhere in this book [20].

The only suitable treatment for VF is represented by cardio-pulmonary resuscitation and early defibrillation. However, chances to restore spontaneous circulation progressively decrease over time, approaching zero few minutes after VF onset, hence VF-related mortality, especially in the case of out-of-hospital VF, is still extremely high. Secondary prevention with an implantable cardioverter-defibrillator should be considered in all VF survivors, if a reversible cause has not been detected.

References

1. Lee S, Wellens HJJ, Josephson ME (2009) Paroxysmal atrioventricular block. Heart Rhythm 6:1229-1234
2. Yusuf S, Camm AJ (2005) The sinus tachycardias. Nat Clin Pract Cardiovasc Med 2:44-52
3. Chung EK (1968) Parasystole. Prog Cardiovasc Dis 11:64-81
4. Patel A, Markowitz SM (2008) Atrial tachycardia: mechanisms and management. Expert Rev Cardiovasc Ther 6:811-22
5. Saoudi N, Cosio F, Waldo A et al (2001) Classification of atrial flutter and regular atrial tachycardia according to electrophysiologic mechanism and anatomic bases: a statement from a joint expert group from the Working Group of Arrhythmias of the European Society of Cardiology and the North American Society of Pacing and Electrophysiology. J Cardiovasc Electrophysiol 12:852-866
6. Camm AJ, Kirchhof P, Lip GY et al (2010) Guidelines for the management of atrial fibrillation: the Task Force for the Management of Atrial Fibrillation of the European Society of Cardiology (ESC). Europace 12:1360-1420
7. Allessie MA, Konings K, Kirchhof C, Wijffels M

(1996) Electrophysiologic mechanisms of perpetuation of atrial fibrillation. Am J Cardiol 77:10A-23A
8. Wyse DG, Waldo AL, DiMarco JP et al (2002) The Atrial Fibrillation Follow-up Investigation of Rhythm Management (AFFIRM) Investigators. A comparison of rate control and rhythm control in patients with atrial fibrillation. N Engl J Med 347:1825-1833
9. Hohnloser SH, Kuck KH, Lilienthal J (2000) Rhythm or rate control in atrial fibrillation -Pharmacological Intervention in Atrial Fibrillation (PIAF): a randomized trial. Lancet 356:1789-1794
10. The AFFIRM Investigators (2004) Relationship between sinus rhythm, treatment and survival in the atrial fibrillation follow-up investigation of rhythm management (AFFIRM) study. Circulation 109:1509-1513
11. Calkins H, Brugada J, Packer D et al (2007) HRS/EHRA/ECAS Expert consensus statement on catheter and surgical ablation of atrial fibrillation: recommendations for personnel, policy, procedures and follow-up. Heart Rhythm 4:816-861
12. Lee PC, Chen SA, Hwang B (2009) Atrioventricular node anatomy and physiology: implications for ablation of atrioventricular nodal re-entrant tachycardia. Curr Opin Cardiol 24:105-112
13. Pasquié JL, Gervasoni R, Macia JC et al (2003) Atypical forms of atrioventricular nodal re-entrant tachycardia. Arch Mal Coeur Vaiss 96(Spec):54-60
14. Blomström-Lundqvist C, Scheinman MM, Aliot EM et al (2003) ACC/AHA/ESC guidelines for the management of patients with supraventricular arrhythmias - executive summary. A report of the American college of cardiology/American heart association task force on practice guidelines and the European society of cardiology committee for practice guidelines (writing committee to develop guidelines for the management of patients with supraventricular arrhythmias) developed in collaboration with NASPE-Heart Rhythm Society. J Am Coll Cardiol 42:1493-531
15. Aliot E, de Chillou C, Revault d'Allones et al (1998) Mahaim tachycardias. Eur Heart J 19(Suppl E):E25-31, E52-53
16. Cole CR, Marrouche NF, Natale A (2002) Evaluation and management of ventricular outflow tract tachycardias. Card Electrophysiol Rev 6:442-447
17. Storey J, Iwasa A, Feld GK (2002) Left ventricular outflow tract tachycardia originating from the right coronary cusp: Identification of location of origin by endocardial noncontact activation mapping from the right ventricular outflow tract. J Cardiovasc Electrophysiol 13:1050
18. Chiarandà G, Di Guardo G, Gulizia M et al (2001) Fascicular ventricular tachycardia. Ital Heart J Suppl 2:1181-1186
19. Srivathsan K, Ng DW, Mookadam F (2009) Ventricular tachycardia and ventricular fibrillation. Expert Rev Cardiovasc Ther 7:801-809
20. Tilz RR, Fedele L, Satomi K et al (2007) Idiopathic ventricular fibrillation. Herz 32:233-239

Pre-excitation Syndrome

15

Caterina Bisceglia and Augusto Mazzetti

Pre-excitation is an electrocardiographic pattern due to the presence of an accessory conducting pathway (AP) between the atrium and ventricle, so that, after atrial events all or part of the ventricular muscle can be activated sooner than if traveling only by the normal conduction system. In most cases, a direct AV by-pass tract with Kent properties is present [1].

The AV by-pass tracts have different anatomic locations and specific electrophysiological properties; they represent the cornerstone of Wolff-Parkinson-White syndrome, a miscellaneous group of associated arrhythmias, mostly AV re-entrant tachycardia or atrial fibrillation. Unlike the A-V node cells, whose potential is calcium-dependent, fibers of AV by-pass tracts are sodium-dependent, so conduction over these connections runs fast and usually in an all-or-nothing fashion. This explains the typical electrophysiological behavior of these connections, with the atrial impulse conducting without delay until sudden block, instead of a progressive conduction delay along the AV node in response to faster rates. Moreover, they can be capable of antegrade conduction (from the atrium to the ventricle, then producing the typical ECG pattern of pre-excitation) and retrograde conduction (from the ventricle to the atrium, mostly during tachycardia); alternatively, they exhibit only retrograde conduction, so ECG abnormalities are not recognizable (concealed AP). Because they represent developmental defects of the heart, it is not unusual for the same patient to have multiple types of AP.

During embryonic development, atria and ventricles are first connected by muscle bands that disappear after AV groove insertion; APs are fibers that survive after the fibrous skeleton has been completed.

15.1 Diagnosis

Electrocardiographic diagnosis of pre-excitation is comprised of:

- short PR interval (<120 msec);
- presence of δ wave (slurring of the initial portion of the QRS complex);
- abnormalities of the ST-segment and T-wave.

The fast conduction along APs explains the short PR interval, because the part of the ventricle near the connection is activated earlier than the rest. The 12-lead ECG sign of such activation is represented by the initial slurring of the QRS (Fig. 15.1), which

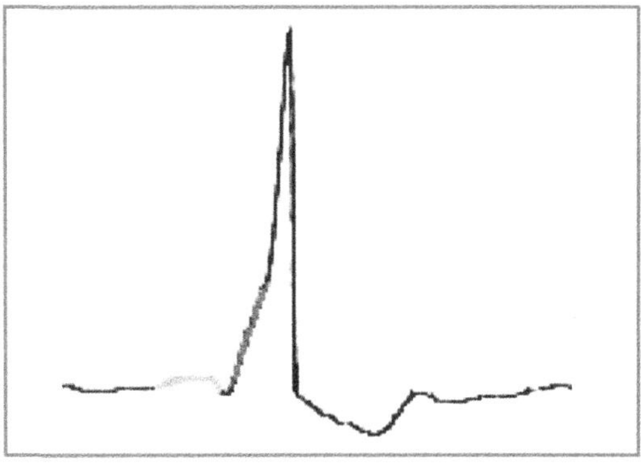

Fig. 15.1 ECG lead showing pre-excitation. Note the short interval between the P-wave (green) and the initial portion of the QRS, that is δ-wave (red). Repolarization abnormalities are also shown (ST depression and biphasic T-wave)

C. Bisceglia (✉)
Electrophysiology Department
"San Raffaele" University Hospital, Milan, Italy

M. Fioranelli and G. Frajese (eds.), *Sports Cardiology*,
DOI: 10.1007/978-88-470-2775-6_15, © Springer-Verlag Italia 2012

Table 15.1 The most frequent accessory conducting pathways among the population

Site	Incidence
Left free-wall	46%
Infero-paraseptal	26%
Right free-wall	18%
Supero-paraseptal	10%

normally disappears after the impulse penetrates the AV node and runs along the normal conducting system. APs deeply change repolarization events, so abnormalities of the ST-segment and T-wave inversion in leads facing the AP insertion are the rule; T-wave polarity is generally opposite to delta-wave.

Different algorithms for ECG localization of APs have been published, but their systematic explanation is outside the scope of this text. Briefly, they analyze the QRS polarity in inferior leads and V1 or the δ-wave duration and morphology [5,6].

The incidence of different APs is listed in Table 15.1. They can theoretically be found everywhere along the course of the AV sulcum except for the mitro-aortic continuity.

Septal connections have generally been classified as antero-septal and postero-septal pathways, the former being localized at the apex of the koch triangle, in the hisian region, and the latter along the coronary sinus ostium. Actually they are distinct in the supero-paraseptal, because there is no interatrial septum after the His bundle, and the postero-paraseptal, since the ostium of the coronary sinus is the posterior portion of the right atrium [7].

If the AP is capable only of retrograde conduction, pre-excitation signs are not present (concealed pathway). In patients with paroxysmal supraventricular tachycardia, the diagnosis and localization of connections is performed during the EPS (electrophysiological study), that generally precedes the catheter ablation of the AP.

15.2 Clinical features

ECG pattern in patients with pre-excitation can erroneously lead to a diagnosis of myocardial infarction or bundle branch block, mostly due to the presence of repolarization abnormalities and QRS-widening. The clinical relevance of pre-excitation relies on the high incidence of paroxysmal supraventricular tachycardia, named atrio-ventricular reciprocating tachycardia (AVRT); more than 80% of patients with APs had palpitations and regular QRS tachycardia, with abrupt onset and termination. Arrhythmias involve a re-entrant circuit between the normal conduction system and AP. In orthodromic AVRT, there is an antegrade conduction down to the AV node and His-Purkinje system and a retrograde up to the AP, making a

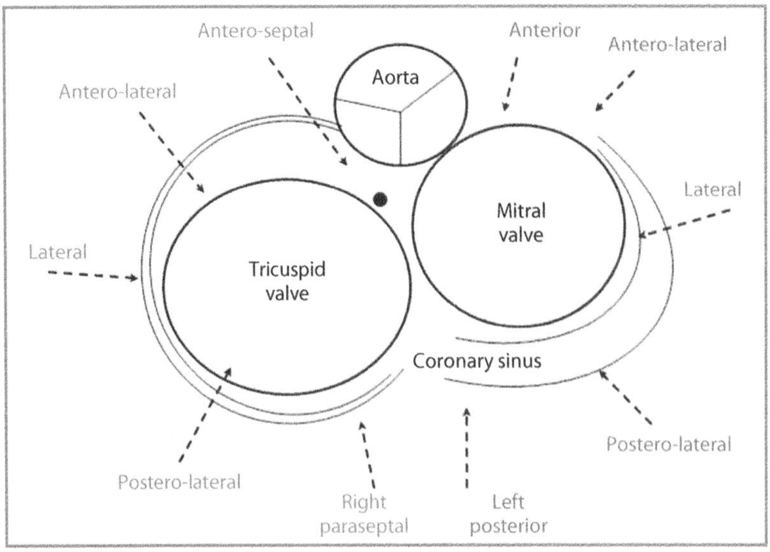

Fig. 15.2 Schematic representation of AP localization. Left-sided APs are indicated in *red*, left-sided in *blue*.

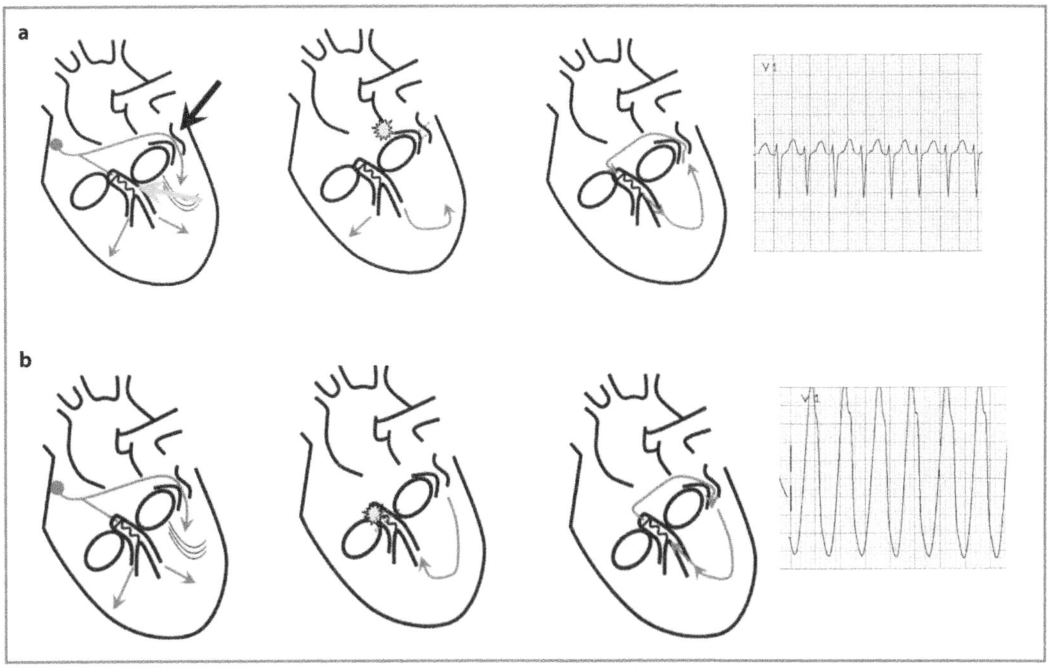

Fig. 15.3 Schematic diagrams of AVRT. a Representation of orthodromic tachycardia. *On the left*, conducting wavefront travels over AV node (*red arrow*) and AP (*black arrow*); *middle*: a premature beat blocks along AP, so conduction passes only through the AV node and is able to enter the AP retrogradely (*on the right*), thus beginning the reciprocating tachycardia. b Representation of antidromic tachycardia: in this case (*middle*), premature beat blocks along normal conducting system, so the impulse passes through AP and is able to enter the AV node retrogradely (*on the right*). Next to the strips, 12-lead ECG of orthodromic (*upper right corner*) and antidromic (*lower corner*) AVRT. Note the difference in QRS duration between these two types of supraventicular arrhythmia

typical ECG pattern of regular, narrow-QRS tachycardia (see the figure below). If the impulse travels in the opposite direction, a regular, wide-QRS tachycardia is recorded by ECG, because antegrade conduction is due solely to the AP: the enhanced δ-wave led to a broad QRS complex and a differential diagnosis with ventricular tachycardia has to be performed (Fig. 15.3 a,b).

During paroxysmal tachycardia, patients generally complained of palpitations with abrupt onset and termination. Heart rate during tachycardia may even exceed 250 bpm, so faintness episodes or syncope are not rare.

Atrial flutter and atrial fibrillation are present in more than 20% of patients with APs, and the reciprocating tachycardia is often the trigger of such arrhythmias. In patients with overt APs showing ERP <230 msec, AF is a feared event and is rarely associated with sudden cardiac death. As previously described, APs are capable of causing conduction to the ventricles even at highest rates (as opposed to AV node), so atrial fibrillation can degenerate into ventricular fibrillation leading to cardiac arrest. All patients with pre-excitation need at least a non-invasive assessment of the clinical risk (see below), including an exercise stress test and ECG Holter monitoring.

15.3 Prognosis and Therapy

The natural history of patients with WPW-syndrome has dramatically changed since percutaneous catheter ablation of the accessory pathways became available. The very high success rate of this technique (up to 90% of patients) has made this curative treatment the first line therapy in symptomatic patients, especially those suffering an aborted sudden death (Fig. 15.4). Catheter ablation is also supported in asymptomatic patients with

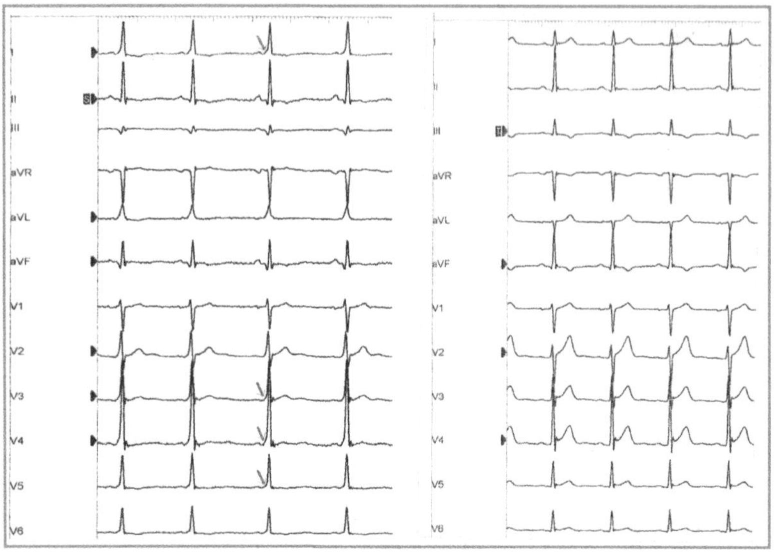

Fig. 15.4 *On the left*: 12-lead ECG of a non-competitive athlete (runner) with pre-exciation due to left posteriorAP (red arrows show the delta-wave); *on the right*: 12-ECG of the same patient after the ablation procedure

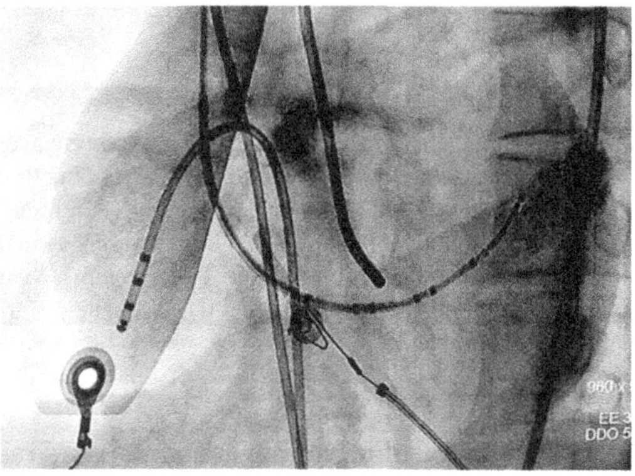

Fig. 15.5 Fluoroscopic view (LAO projection) during ablation of a left posterior AP. The red arrow marks the tip of the ablation catheter; the yellow shadow outlines the course of a decapolar catheter placed in the coronary sinus; the blue shadow is dragged along the catheter placed into the right ventricle apex

high-risk APs, in athletes and other specific categories (airline pilots, drivers).

Ablation of left-sided free-wall APs has the highest success rate (>90%), but needs anticoagulation to be performed during the procedure and for a short period after ablation; moreover, transeptal puncture may be required to overcome difficult cases. The right-sided APs, generally approached by the venous femoral route, are associated with a higher recurrence rate (Fig. 15.5).

The risks of catheter ablation are to be reviewed in specific settings, such as AV block during ablation of supero-paraseptal APs, close to the AV compact node and His bundle. Some authors reports the safety of cryoablation for these cases, because of the reversible cryomapping and increased catheter stability.

Medical therapy is generally limited to class I or III anti-arrhythmic drugs (AAD). They prevent the induction of paroxysmal tachycardia by modifying the electrical properties of APs and reducing the reentry phenomena, even if efficacy is limited over time. Class I AADs are also effective in preventing atrial fibrillation and eventually in reducing fast conduction to the ventricles during AF.

The prognosis of patients with pre-excitation is generally good, because this condition is rarely associated with a structural cardiomyopathy. An association between right-sided APs and Ebstein's anomaly has been described.

The risk of sudden death is extremely low and is strictly dependent of the antegrade refractory period of the AP [12,13].

The non-invasive diagnostic work-up includes exercise tests, Holter monitoring and 2D-echocardiography; the first provides helpful insight because several studies have shown that the loss of pre-excitation during exercise correlates with low-risk AP. Intermittent pre-excitation or conduction block along the AP during challenging pharmacological tests (ajmaline, procainamide) is useful as well. Holter monitoring may show a pattern of intermittent pre-excitation or asymptomatic atrial fibrillation. 2D echo is performed to rule out a structural cardiomyopathy that may raise issues about the safety of AADs, but is not a contraindication to catheter ablation. A complete cardiological work-up may include EPS (see chapter 12), which generally precedes the ablation attempt. If the refractory period of AP is less than 230 msec, it is considered to be a high-risk AP, and catheter ablation is supported even in asymptomatic patients.

During EPS, it is also useful to check the shortest RR interval exhibiting pre-excitation during atrial fibrillation, and if it is less than 200 msec, the patient is considered to be at *high risk* [9-11]. Sudden death due to ventricular fibrillation is, however, a rare complication of the syndrome, even in high-risk patients, although it may represent the first clinical event [15].

These clinical considerations and the prevalence of pre-excitation explain the attention of cardiologists and sport physicians to WPW syndrome. Screening of athletes with AP requires additional considerations, because exercise enhances the conduction capabilities of these pathways [8].

Actually, the eligibility is possible only in the following cases:

1. No structural cardiomyopathy;
2. Asymptomatic patients if:
   - Pre-excited atrial fibrillation with shortest R-R interval > 240 msec at rest and >200 msec during effort;
   - Afib /AVRT not inducible and/or antegrade effective refractory period of AP >240 msec at rest and >200 msec during exercise.

After catheter ablation, patients may usually start competing again after 1 month, if no recurrence has been documented and cardiomyopathy has been ruled out [16].

References

1. Yee R, Klein GJ, Guiraudon GM (1995) The Wolff-Parkinson-White syndrome. In Zipes DP, Jalife J (eds) Cardiac Electrophysiology: From Cell to Bedside. WB Saunders, Philadelphia, pp 1199-1214
2. Wolff L, Parkinson J, White PD (1930) Bundle-branch block with short PR interval in healthy people prone to paroxysmal tachycardia. Am Heart J 5:685-704
3. Leitch J, Klein GJ, Yee R, Murdoch C (1990) New concepts on nodoventricular accessory pathways. J Cardiovasc Electrophysiol 1:220-230
4. Anderson RH, Becker AE (1990) Anathomy of the conduction tissues and accessory atrioventricular connections. In Zipes DP, Jalife J (eds) Cardiac Electrophysiology: From Cell to Bedside. WB Saunders, Philadelphia, pp. 240-248
5. Arruda MS, McClelland JH et al (1998) Development and validation of an ECG algorithm for identifying accessory pathway ablation site in Wolff-Parkinson-White syndrome. J Cardiovasc Electrophysiol 9:2-12
6. Fitzpatrick AP, Gonzales RP et al (1994) New algorithm for the localization of accessory atrioventricular connections using a baseline electrocardiogram. Am Coll Cardiol 23:107-16
7. Davis LM, Byth K et al (1991) Dimensions of the human posterior septal space and coronary sinus. Am J Cardiol 68:621-625
8. Jonathan CP, Dwyn D et al (1995) Effect of exercise on ventricular response to atrial fibrillation in Wolff-Parkinson-White syndrome. Br Heart J 54:80-85
9. Levy S, Broustet JP (1979) Syndrome de Wolff Parkinson White. Correlation entre l'exploration electrophysiologique et l'effet de l'epreuve d'effort sur l'aspect electrocardiographique de pre-excitation. Arch Mal Coeur 72:634-640
10. Bricker JT, Porter CBJ et al (1985) Exercise testing in children with Wolff-Parkinson-White syndrome. Am J Cardiol 55:1001-1004
11. Strasberg B, Ashley WW et al (1980) Treadmill exercise testing in the Wolff-Parkinson-White syndrome. Am J Cardiol 45:742-748
12. Dreyfus LS, Haiat R, Watanabe Y (1971) Ventricular fibrillation: a possible mechanism of sudden death in patients with Wolff-Parkinson-White syndrome. Circulation. 43:520-527
13. Klein GJ, Bashore TM et al (1979) Ventricular fibrillation in the Wolff-Parkinson-White syndrome. N Engl J Med 15:1080-1085
14. Fukatani M, Tanigawa M et al (1990) Prediction of a fatal atrial fibrillation in patients with asymptomatic Wolff-Parkinson-White pattern. Jpn Circ J 54:1331-1339
15. Timmermans C, Smeets JLRM et al (1995) Aborted sudden death in the Wolff-Parkinson-White syndrome. Am J Cardiol 76:492-494
16. Protocolli cardiologici per il giudizio di idoneità allo sport agonistico 2009 (2010) Med Sport Vol 1

Electrophysiological Studies in Athletes 16

Luigi Sciarra, Antonella Sette, Annamaria Martino,
Alessandro Fagagnini, Lucia de Luca, Ermenegildo de Ruvo,
Claudia Tota, Marco Rebecchi, Fabio Sperandii,
Emanuele Guerra, Gennaro Alfano, Fabrizio Guarracini,
Fabio Pigozzi and Leonardo Calò

16.1 Introduction

Electrophysiological studies are instrumental methods enabling the registration of electric endocavitary cardiac signals relative to the various phases of the cardiac cycle. Registration is carried out through unipolar or bipolar electrocatheters, which also allow electrical stimulation of the heart. Stimulation of the cardiac chambers is an extremely useful method for accurately measuring intervals and/or pauses and for reproducing in the laboratory arrhythmias that patients may experience clinically (arrhythmic inducibility test). Electrophysiological evaluations can be performed via the transesophageal or endocavitary pathways. All the material used both for endocavitary and transesophageal electrophysiological studies is sterile and for single use.

A transesophageal electrophysiological study is conducted by inserting an electrocatheter through the nasal cavity and into the esophagus. The posterior wall of the left atrium is in strict proximity with the esophagus and therefore with the electrocatheter it is possible to register the signals emanating from the left atrium, as well as performing programmed atrial stimulations. The theoretical advantages of this method are reduced invasiveness compared to an endocavitary study and the possibility of registrations and/or stipulations even during physical exertion (bed-ergometer) [1]. Limits include the scarcity of electrical information (registration only of atrial signals) compared to a complete endocavitary study, the possibility of stimulating only the atrial cavity and not the ventricular cavity, potentially low patient tolerability (painful stimulations), the need to consider an eventual ablative intervention in another context, which, in case of an endocavitary study, can be carried out at the same time.

An *endocavitary electrophysiological study* is conducted by inserting electrocatheters (generally between one and four) directly into the cardiac cavities. The procedure is carried out with local anesthesia and the catheters are inserted through venous and/or, more rarely, arterial vascular access points. The insertion of the catheters into the vascular system towards the heart and, subsequently, their positioning in the various anatomical segments of the heart, is not painful and is performed under a fluoroscopic guide (Fig. 16.1). The electrocatheters (see also Chapter 17) are positioned in certain anatomically determined areas of the heart (for example the lateral wall of the right atrium, bundle of His, coronary sinus, right ventricle apex). The registration of electric signals in these areas enables the accurate reconstruction of the sequence of endocavitary activation of a particular cardiac rhythm. A precise endocavitary electrogram of the heartbeat is therefore reconstructed allowing accurate diagnosis of the electrophysiological genesis of cardiac arrhythmias. Through the electrocatheters, as previously mentioned, programmed stimulations of the cardiac cavities can be carried out. These enable further measurements of intervals and/or pauses, artificial initiation of cardiac arrhythmias (Fig. 16.2) leading to possible clinical arrhythmic episodes in a patient.

L. Calò (✉)
Electrophysiology Department
Policlinico Casilino, Rome, Italy

M. Fioranelli and G. Frajese (eds.), *Sports Cardiology*,
DOI: 10.1007/978-88-470-2775-6_16, © Springer-Verlag Italia 2012

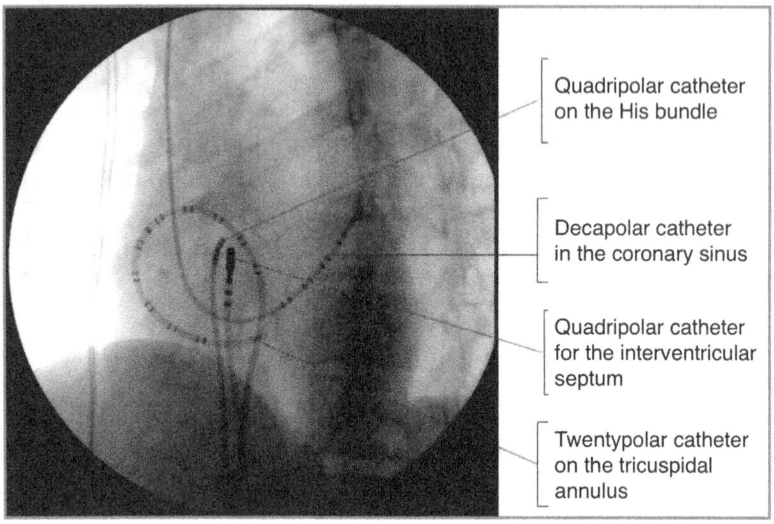

Fig. 16.1 Example of fluoroscopic visualization of electrocatheters positioned in the heart during an electrophysiological endocavitary study (lateral anterior oblique view)

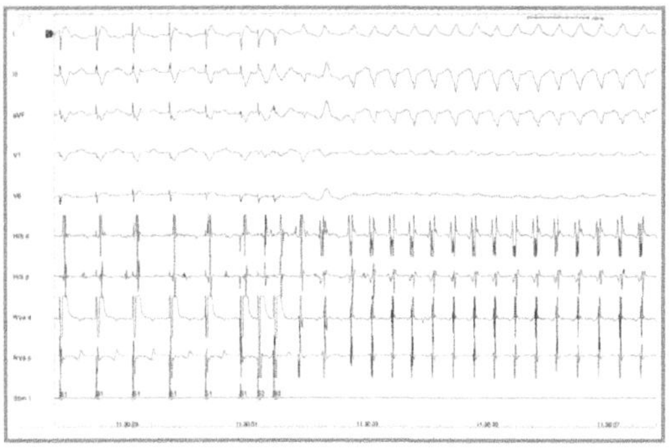

Fig. 16.2 Example of ventricular tachycardia induction using programmed ventricular stimulation. The pacing catheter is positioned in the right ventricular apex and the recorded signal is identified by RV. From this site, programmed ventricular stimulation has been performed, consisting of the paced train of extrastimulus (S1) and two premature beats (S2 and S3) that induced the rapid monomorphic ventricular tachycardia with initial hemodynamic compromise. It has been promptly interrupted by using ventricular stimulation in overdrive, i.e. the frequency of ventricular pacing is higher than the frequency of tachycardia

16.2 Clinical Evaluation of Arrhythmia in Patients: General Principles

Sporadic arrhythmias of benign prognostic significance can be present even in perfectly normal subjects. The athlete can also manifest rhythm disorders connected to the intensified vagal tone caused by physical exercise or by adrenergic hypertone during intense physical activity. Establishing a limit between normality and disease is not always simple. For this reason the clinical evaluation of arrhythmia in an athlete needs to be accurate and takes advantage of opportune instrumental diagnostic principals, from the most simple to the most complex, which may become necessary.

As specified in the COCIS protocol (Organizational Cardiac Committee for Suitability to Practice Sport) in 2009 [2], the connection of suitability for competitive sport activity has to include:

- suspected or demonstrated arrhythmias;
- heart diseases that are predisposing factors for malign arrhythmias;
- arrhythmias treated with transcatheter ablation, pacemaker implantation or defibrillators.

The clinical evaluation of arrhythmia in an athlete has to be based on three levels for an adequate identification of competitive suitability. Accurate gathering of the patient's medical history, an objective examination, and a 12-lead electrocardiogram at rest and after a step test are the *first level* of evaluation during a medical examination to establish competitive suitability. The *second level* of evaluation must also include non-invasive assessments, such as mono- and bi-dimensional echocardiography studies and color-Doppler analysis, a maximum ergometric test, and the 24-hour Holter monitor. The latter must include a workout session during registration, in the absence of any contraindications, and a nycthemeral cycle. If necessary during this level, biohumoral examinations can be included (hemochromocytometric tests, thyroid hormone tests, and possibly infectiology tests and other indicated tests).

Based on the type of arrhythmia documented and on the symptoms reported by the athlete, it could be necessary to pass to a *third level* of evaluation that includes invasive and non-invasive studies. Third-level tests are: the tilt test, pharmacological tests (atropine, isoproterenol, flecainide etc.), the investigation of ventricular late potentials with the *signal averaging* method, the variability of cardiac frequency study, the alternance of T-wave study, the transesophageal electrophysiology study at rest and under stress, and the endocavitary electrophysiology study.

16.3 Indications for Electrophysiological Studies in Athletes

An electrophysiology study is part of the third level of the evaluation of an athlete. It may be indicated based on the symptoms reported by the subject and the arrhythmias found during the second-level tests, in particular surface ECG, Holter ECG and the maximum stress test. The symptoms most often reported by athletes include palpitation at rest and under stress, and occasionally pre-syncopal and/or syncopal episodes. All symptoms, however, need a high degree of attention and diagnostic accuracy.

As for the selection criteria for an electrophysiological endocavitary study, the usual indications for this exam must be valid both for athletes and sedentary subjects. However, in athletes, other indications for an electrophysiological endocavitary study are more closely related to arrhythmic risk tests in connection with sport, e.g. with Wolff-Parkinson-White (WPW) syndrome. Furthermore, it includes not only the diagnostic results but also the possible therapeutic results. In other words, invasive electrophysiological studies are certainly indicated in athletes when there is also an indication for ablative treatment of a certain arrhythmia (see Chapter 17).

Based on a subject's symptoms it is possible to propose an invasive electrophysiological evaluation in the presence of: recurrent syncopal episodes associated with palpitations [3] (suspected presence of tachyarrhythmias); syncopal episodes in presence of heart disease that is not the cause of non-suitability or familiarity with sudden death, following second-level assessments; paroxysmal palpitations and/or hemodynamic compromise; palpitations with a strong suspicion of supraventricular tachycardia; palpitation in subjects with heart disease or suspected ventricular tachycardia.

On the other hand, an electrophysiological study can be indicated even if specific arrhythmias or arrhythmogenic conditions are found during the first- and/or second-level assessments. Obviously, even in this situation, a possible indication for a more in-depth invasive electrophysiological study cannot involve clinical elements and the patient's medical history, which provide a clinical classification of the arrhythmic problem in the subject, ruling out or confirming, for example, the presence of a potential underlying structural cardiopathy.

As for bradyarrhythmias, an electrophysiological study can be taken into consideration with the objective of studying supra-Hisian, infra-Hisian and sub-Hisian atrioventricular conduction, only in the presence of any type of atrioventricular block, only if these are associated with delays in intra-ventricular conduction, and in the rare cases in which second-degree atrioventricular block with narrow QRS is found during physical exertion [4,5].

In patients with supraventricular tachycardia, electrophysiological studies can be indicated in the case of: paroxysmal forms in which re-entrant tachycardia is suspected (nodal tachycardia, atrioventricular re-entrant tachycardia); paroxystic supraventricular tachycardia in the absence of WPW syndrome during surface ECG to investigate whether arrhythmias induced during the electrophysiological study do not have a high frequency; iterative and persistent supraventricular tachycardia (for example inappropriate sinusal tachycardia, re-entrant tachycardia through a slow decremental accessory pathway, *Coumel* tachycardia and focal atrial tachycardia resulting from increased automaticity); identification of possible triggers the paroxystic atrial fibrillation, such as nodal re-entrant tachycardia or an accessory pathway, pulmonary venous foci with the related possibility of ablation; asymptomatic subjects affected by WPW syndrome and in absence of underlying heart disease (with the exception of children under 12 years of age since, according to the COCIS, the stratification of risk can be envisaged beyond this age).

A separate and in-depth consideration needs be reserved for the value of the electrophysiological study in ventricular pre-excitation syndrome, and more precisely in WPW syndrome. Physical activity, as is known, promotes the trigger of certain cardiac arrhythmias, and this is true even in ventricular preexcitation. In WPW syndrome a theoretical risk of sudden death exists, albeit very low. This risk is directly connected to the presence of atrial fibrillation (generally, even if not exclusively, triggered by atrioventricular re-entrant tachycardia) and by an accessory pathway with an elevated anterograde conductive capacity from the atria to the ventricles. The arrhythmic risk is not deducible by non-invasive clinical and structural parameters and can occur even in a completely asymptomatic subject. All risk parameters connected to the syndrome are, however, easily identifiable in the course of the electrophysiological study. Therefore, this study is generally indicated in competitive subjects with ventricular preexcitation and can be carried out via both the transesophageal and endocavitary pathways (see above). According to the judgment of experts at the COCIS, the invasive electrophysiological evaluation can be delayed in asymptomatic subjects below 12 years of age, due to the almost virtual risk of atrial fibrillation and sudden death. On the basis of the parameters of the electrophysiological study, suitability to perform competitive activities can be conceded in asymptomatic subjects and those without heart disease: atrial preexcitation fibrillation inducibility with a minimum R-R interval > 240 ms (baseline conditions) and > 200 ms (under stress); non inducibility of atrial fibrillation and/or atrioventricular re-entrant tachycardia at rest and under stress, and an anterograde effective refractory period of the accessory pathway > 240 ms at rest and > 200 ms under stress [6,7].

Ventricular tachycardias in the presence of asserted organic heart disease are not covered by the present study, as they occur in subjects for whom the problem of competitive suitability cannot be taken into consideration. Nonetheless, electrophysiological endocavitary studies can be useful in certain forms of ventricular tachycardia which are supposedly *benign*, namely in subjects without significant structural heart disease. These arrhythmic forms mainly include: fascicular ventricular tachycardia, ectopic idiopathic ventricular tachycardia originating from the right and, more rarely, left ventricular outflow tract. Even for these arrhythmias the idea that an electrophysiological study is still indicated when an ablative indication also subsists is valid. Furthermore, in certain cases, it may be difficult to conduct a differential diagnosis based on first- and second-level studies, between ventricular tachycardia of the right ventricular outflow tract and ventricular tachycardia of the right ventricular outflow tract in the context of arrhythmogenic myocardiopathy of the right ventricle. Electrophysiological endocavitary studies can provide useful data for the differential diagnosis. In fact, in arrhythmic cardiopathy, ventricular stimulation easily tends to induce sustained ventricular tachycardia based on the re-entry mechanism (presence of the phenomenon of concealed entrainment). Instead, in idiopathic ventricular tachycardias, often only the stimulation after infusion of isoproterenol is capable of reproducing such arrhythmias (catecholamine-mediated tachycardia resulting from an intensified automatism). Ventricular fascicular tachycardia, in some cases, can be confused with paroxystic supraventricular tachycardias conducted with aberration. In these cases, electrophysiological study results are extremely useful for clear differential diagnosis [8-10].

16.4 Possible New Areas of Application

Electrophysiological endocavitary studies can be carried out with specific catheters that allow three-dimensional mapping of the cardiac chambers, providing both electric and anatomic (electroanatomic maps) information. This is made possible by increasingly accurate mapping systems and three-dimensional non-fluoroscopic navigation. These systems enable the localization of the

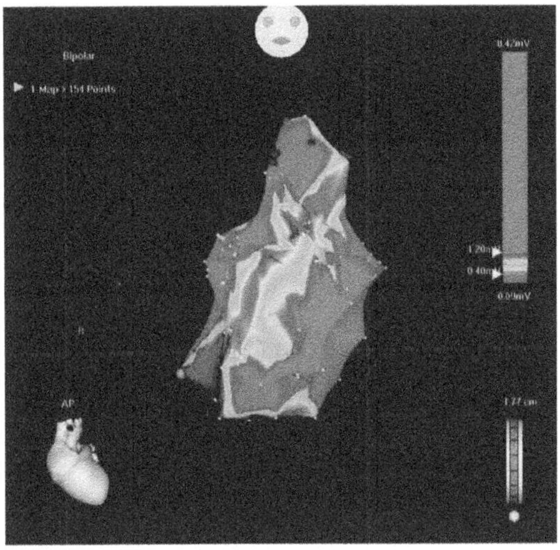

Fig. 16.3 Example of the bipolar voltage map of the right ventricle reconstructed by the three-dimensional electroanatomical mapping system (CARTO®, Biosense Webster). The anteroposterior view shows a wide low-voltage area (red regions) in the right ventricular free wall, a peritricuspid area and basal region of the right ventricular outflow tract. Scar areas (red) are surrounded by low-voltage areas (yellow-blue). Purple areas identify normal myocardial tissue. The patient is an athlete with a *Brugada type* ECG pattern. As is well known, Brugada is a syndrome that affects patients with a structurally normal heart. The electroanatomical mapping has shown structural abnormalities of the right ventricle. The subject is obviously not suitable for practicing sport

electrocatheters through the emission of magnetic fields and/or the use of electric impedance. Maps of this kind are certainly more useful for supporting ablative interventions of complex arrhythmias. Furthermore, some of these three-dimensional maps can also enable adequate measurement of the voltage of endocavitary signals registered by the electrocatheter [11,12]. It is intuitive to see how, in case of an eventual scar area on the ventricular muscle, or an area substituted by fibrous or fibroadipose tissue, the catheter positioned in these regions can register very low signals or signals that are completely absent (Fig. 16.3). This type of reconstruction has proven to be very useful, for example, as published by the Italian group of Corrado, in the diagnosis of the arrhythmogenic cardiopathy of the right ventricle [13]. It is also possible to predict that this method could be used even in the diagnostic course of athletes with malignant ventricular arrhythmias, helping to identify or rule out the presence of potential underlying structural heart disease.

References

1. Vergara G, Furlanello F, Disertori M et al (1988) Induction of supraventricular tachyarrhythmia at rest and during exercise with transesophageal atrial pacing in the electrophysiological evaluation of asymptomatic athletes with Wolff-Parkinson-White syndrome. Eur Heart J 9:1119-1125
2. Comitato Organizzativo Cardiologico per l'Idoneità allo Sport ANCE-ANMCO-FMSI-SIC-SIC SPORT (2009) Protocolli cardiologici per il giudizio di idoneità allo sport agonistico 2009. Cesi Casa Editrice Scientifica Internazionale, Roma
3. Lawless CE, Briner W et al (2008) Palpitations in athletes. Sports Med 38:687-702
4. Zeppilli P, Fenici R, Sassara M et al (1980) Wenckebach second-degree A-V block in top-ranking athletes: an old problem revisited. Am Heart J 100:281-294
5. Alboni P, Pirani R, Paparella N et al (1985) Electrophysiology of normal anterograde atrio-ventricular conduction with and without autonomic blockade. Eur Heart J 6:602-698
6. Delise P, Sciarra L. et al (2007) Asymptomatic Wolff-Parkinson-White: what to do. Extensive ablation or not? J Cardiovasc Med 8:668
7. Brembilla-Perrot B, Ghawi R et al (1993) Electrophysiological characteristics of asymptomatic Wolff-Parkinson-White syndrome. Eur Heart J 14:511-515
8. Heidbüchel H, Hoogsteen J, Fagard R et al (2003) High prevalence of right ventricular involvement in endurance athletes with ventricular arrhythmias. Role of an electrophysiologic study in risk stratification. Eur Heart J 24:1473-1480
9. Biffi A, Ansalone G, Verdile L et al (1996) Ventricular arrhythmias and athletes heart Role of signal-averaged electrocardiography. Eur Heart J 17:557-563
10. Furlanello F, Bettini R, Bertoldi A et al (1989) Arrhythmia patterns in athletes with arrhythmogenic right ventricular dysplasia. Eur Heart J 10 Suppl D:16-19
11. L. Sciarra, E. Marras, E. De Ruvo et al (2008) Right ventricular voltage mapping. In Brugada Syndrome: always an electrical disease in structurally normal hearts? Heart Rhythm:S74
12. Corrado D, Basso C, Leoni L et al (2005) Three-dimensional electroanatomic voltage mapping increases accuracy of diagnosing arrhythmogenic right ventricular cardiomyopathy/displasia. Circulation 111:3042-3050
13. Corrado D, Basso C, Leoni L et al (2008) Three-dimensional electroanatomical voltage mapping and histologic evaluation of myocardial substrate in right ventricular outflow tract tachycardia. J Am Coll Cardiol 51:731-739

Transcatheter Ablation in Athletes 17

Luigi Sciarra, Marco Rebecchi, Annamaria Martino, Ermenegildo de Ruvo, Lucia de Luca, Claudia Tota, Fabio Sperandii, Emanuele Guerra, Fabrizio Guarracini, Fabio Pigozzi and Leonardo Calò

17.1 Introduction

The natural history of arrhythmias has suffered an epochal change after the advent of transcatheter ablation. It is a minimally invasive procedure that enables the elimination of additional electric circuits or foci that are responsible for supraventricular and ventricular arrhythmias. In most cases it is carried out under local anesthesia, for which the patient, who is perfectly conscious or possibly mildly sedated, follows the operations and cooperates actively in the procedure and can at any moment communicate with the medical team. The catheters are inserted through venous and/or, more rarely, arterial vascular access points and are moved painlessly and under radioscopic guidance towards the heart. All the material used is completely sterile and for single use. The electrocatheters are positioned in certain anatomically defined areas of the heart, and the electric signals corresponding to cardiac activity are registered. An intracardiac electrocardiogram is thus performed, enabling the analysis and precise reconstruction of a particular cardiac rhythm. Through the electrocatheters it is also possible to perform both atrial and ventricular programmed stimulations that provoke the trigger of arrhythmic phenomena. Once a particular arrhythmia is triggered, it is possible to accurately study its characteristics by analysing particular parameters such as the method of induction, the behaviour of arrhythmia in response to particular manoeuvres of pacing or vagal stimulation, the interruption methods, the intramyocardial activation sequence, and many other parameters. All this enables an accurate reconstruction of the precise electrophysiological mechanisms that underline a particular arrhythmia. As well as guaranteeing diagnostic functions like all the others, one of the catheters used is also able to deliver radiofrequency. The resulting effect is localized tissue damage with the elimination of the arrhythmic substratum that underlies a particular arrhythmia. Furthermore, a temperature sensor is embedded in the ablation catheter to monitor the temperature of the tip of the catheter during ablation, thus avoiding possible excessive tissue damage.

In addition to radiofrequency it is possible to use many other forms of energy to induce permanent ablative damage. Certainly radiofrequency is by far the form of energy most widely employed, followed by cold application. Cryoenergy is also widespread in certain ablations where the arrhythmic substratum is located in particularly delicate areas, such as in close proximity to the normal conduction tissue. In this case, diffuse tissue damage could destroy both the tissue responsible for arrhythmia and the normal conduction tissue. Cold offers the possibility of creating a reversible tissue damage, and thus of observing whether delivery may lead to potential damage that could be resolved. Once such damage is ruled out, it is possible to lower the temperature of cold application even further, causing permanent damage. In the transcatheter ablation of arrhythmic substrates, for example in proximity to the bundle of His, the use of cryoenergy is preferred. This has even more relevance in young subjects, who are likely to carry out physical activity.

There are certain more complex forms of ar-

L. Calò (✉)
Electrophysiology Department
Policlinico Casilino, Rome, Italy

M. Fioranelli and G. Frajese (eds.), *Sports Cardiology*,
DOI: 10.1007/978-88-470-2775-6_17,

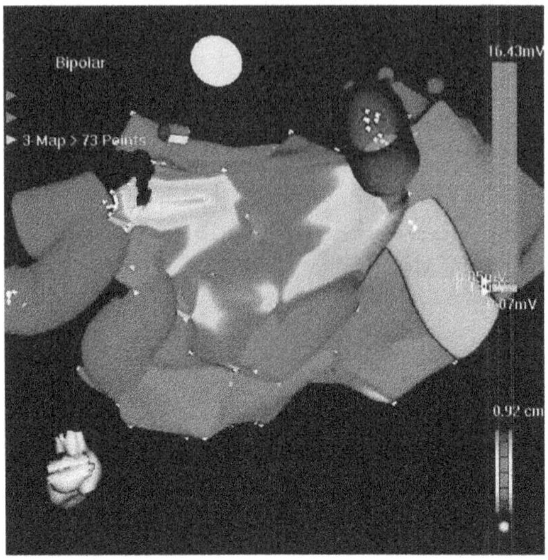

Fig. 17.1 Example of three-dimensional electroanatomical reconstruction of the cardiac chamber by CARTO® system (Biosense Webster). Tubes represent pulmonary venous branches. The red area represents the site of origin of arrhythmia, located near the ostium of the left superior pulmonary vein (blue tube). Radiofrequency applications in this site (red tags) determine the interruption of arrhythmia

rhythmia that require more anatomic accuracy in the positioning of the catheter, modern mapping systems that enable navigation of catheters without the aid of a fluoroscope, and the precise reconstruction of the anatomic or, even better, the electroanatomic map (Fig. 17.1) of the heart. Three-dimensional mapping systems today allow for increased safety and precision for ablations of even the most complex cardiac arrhythmias by reducing, among other things, patients', doctors', technicians' and nurses' exposure to radiations [1].

17.2 Results of Transcatheter Ablation

The ablative technique of focal or re-entrant cardiac arrhythmias today leads to very high success rates. In particular, in cardiac arrhythmias such as common and uncommon atrioventricular nodal re-entry tachycardias, focal ectopic atrial tachycardias, or re-entrant tachycardias through concealed or manifest atrioventricular accessory pathways (Fig. 17.2), transcatheter ablation is to be considered a therapeutic method of choice, due to the very favourable risk/benefit relationship [2-6]. Success rates for ablation are also very high in cases of arrhythmia such as common and uncommon atrial flutter, with a very low complication rate. In atrial fibrillation, this is slightly different. Ablative techniques today do not guarantee the high success rates of the other arrhythmic forms mentioned above, and the complication rate is not as negligible as in the other cases [7, 8]. This is due to the fact that the degree of complexity of the ablative intervention for atrial fibrillation is not insignificant, with the need, for example, for a transeptal puncture in the heart in order to access the left atrial cavity and execute circular lesions around the pulmonary veins, causing electric isolation [9-11] (Fig. 17.3). According to international reports, the risk of important complications is around 3%. It also needs to be stated that the growing experience of invasive electrophysiological centres and the constant and continuous technological progress with materials that are always better in quality, is guaranteeing results that are ever more favourable, and a complication rate that is always lower even in arrhythmias such as atrial fibrillation.

Certainly, a fundamental element to keep in mind, especially in young physically active subjects, is the opportunity to plan ablative procedures that are the most selective possible [12-14]. In order to operate in this way, it is necessary to reconstruct the precise electrophysiological mechanism of the arrhythmia in a single patient trying to eliminate only the pathologic substrate, thus avoiding excessively extended lesions. This assumes particular relevance in physically active subjects with healthy hearts: in this case it is highly probable that there is a precise arrhythmic mechanism, such as underlying supraventricular tachycardia or an isolated ectopic arrhythmogenic focus that triggers fibrillation [15-19]. In these cases the elimination of a peak of the arrhythmogenic substrate, with much lower risks, can guarantee elevated success rates even in terms of recurrence of atrial fibrillation. The research possibilities in this field are numerous. For example, it is known that physically active subjects can have a form of atrial fibrillation that is particularly connected with the vagal hypertone. Many groups, including ours, are evaluating

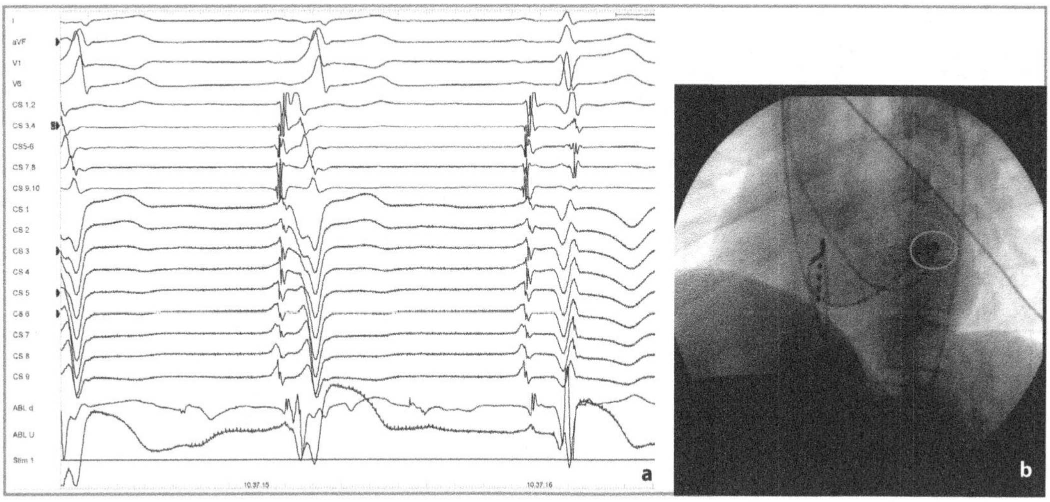

Fig. 17.2 Example of transcatheter ablation of manifest accessory pathway (left lateral origin). a Surface ECG leads and electrograms recorded by intracavitary catheters. b Left anterior oblique view. The first four signals in a represent four surface ECG recordings and the first two beats show ventricular pre-excitation as confirmed by short PR and delta wave. The signal CS1-2, recorded by distal dipole of multielectrodes catheter positioned in coronary sinus (*red circle* in b), shows nearly fused atrial and ventricular electrograms, not present on the other signals recorded by the coronary sinus catheter. The positioning of the ablation catheter in this site (*red circle* in b) through a retrograde approach allows for the radiofrequency lesions deployment and the preexcitation disappearance. In fact, the last beat on four surface ECG recordings in a is characterized by PR prolongation and the disappearance of the delta wave, and intracardiac recordings show separation of atrial and ventricular electrograms, thus confirming the effective ablation of the accessory pathway

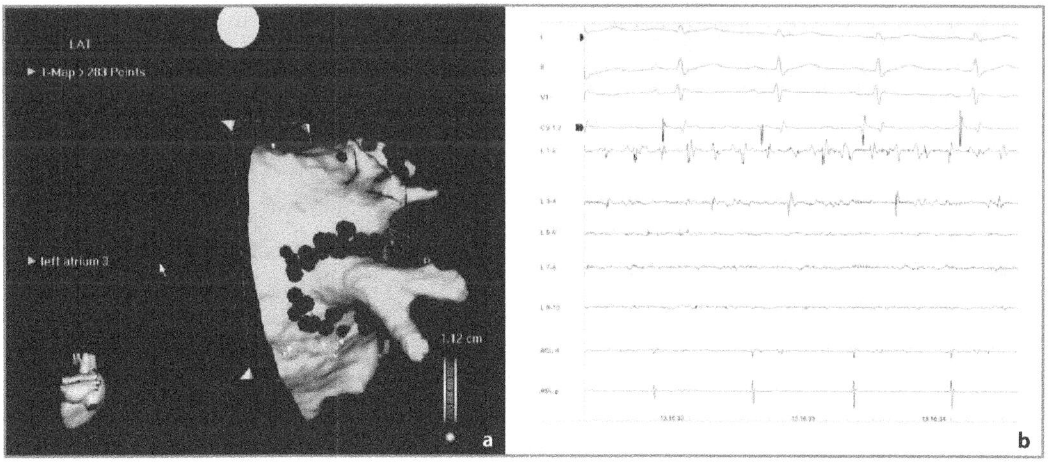

Fig. 17.3 Example of transcatheter ablation of atrial fibrillation and pulmonary venous electrical disconnection. a Three-dimensional electroanatomical reconstruction of the left atrium based on computed tomography (CT) imaging imported into the electroanatomical system. The CT image has been selected to allow endoscopic views. Red tags represent radiofrequency lesions and a circumferential ablation lesion around right inferior pulmonary vein is shown in the posterior-anterior view. b Three ECG recordings show sinus rhythm. The LS1-2 signal is recorded by one dipole of the multielectrode catheter positioned in the right inferior pulmonary vein. It is interesting to note that atrial fibrillation is present inside the vein while the atrium is in sinus rhythm, thus confirming the obtained electrical disconnection of the vein

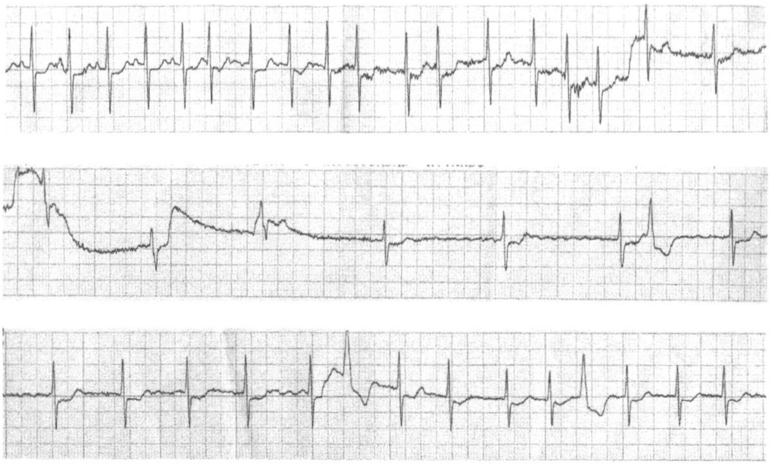

Fig. 17.4 Example of atrial fibrillation with vagal trigger. The ECG signal has been recorded during carotid sinus massage in a young, physically active subject with recurring paroxysmal atrial fibrillation during sleep or after a large meal. Vagal stimulation represents the atrial fibrillation trigger. The ablative approach based on vagal denervation has determined the interruption of atrial fibrillation episodes

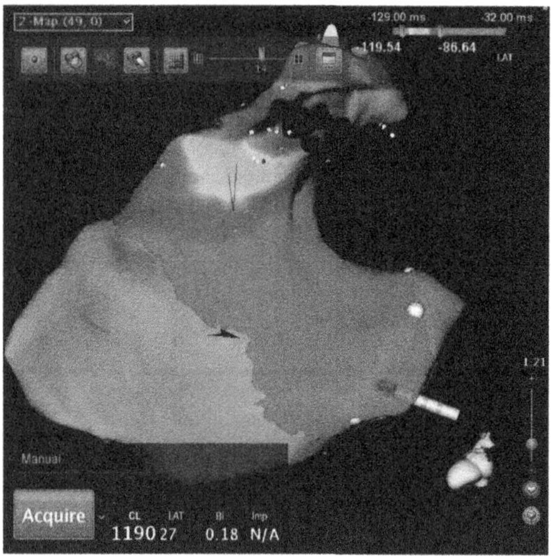

Fig. 17.5 Example of transcatheter ablation of frequent and highly symptomatic premature ventricular beats, originating from the right ventricular outflow tract. The image represents the electroanatomical reconstruction of the right ventricle in left lateral view performed using the new CARTO® system (Biosense Webster). The map shows the earliest activation are (in red) corresponding to the septal portion of the outflow tract, below the pulmonary annulus. Radiofrequency applications in this site (*red tags*) have determined the irritation and subsequent disappearance of focal activity

study protocols with the aim of carrying out ablative procedures in areas of the atrial myocardium where parasympathetic lymph node reflexes are found, both in the right and left atrium. It is possible to hypothesize that in cases of atrial fibrillation with a particular parasympathomimetic trigger (Fig. 17.4) an ablative approach of this kind could be indicated. Further studies could in the future provide more precise answers to these questions.

Even certain ventricular arrhythmias can effectively be eliminated with transcatheter ablation. The best results are obtained in subjects with ventricular arrhythmic forms in structurally normal hearts. Such kinds of arrhythmia, which are encountered most frequently in clinical practice, especially in physically actives subjects, are tachycardia or the common ventricular extrasystoles from the right ventricular outflow tract (Fig. 17.5) and more rarely the left, as well as fascicular tachycardia.

Other ventricular tachycardias, for example post-infarct forms, are not covered by this chapter, as they require much more complex ablative interventions and generally affect populations who do not practise sport competitively.

17.3 Indications for Ablation in Athletes

In this paragraph, the indications for transcatheter ablation of cardiac arrhythmias in athletes are reported according to the guidelines of the 2009 COCIS (Cardiologic Organizational Committee for the Suitability to practice Sport) protocol [20]. First it is necessary to state that the indications for ablative therapy in a physically active subject with arrhythmia differ from those intended for the general population. In fact, the objectives of transcatheter ablation include: elimination of the risk of sudden death, elimination of invalidating symptoms, and the possibility of re-admitting athletes with potential arrhythmogenic conditions to competitive events. On the basis of this necessary premise, ablation is indicated as a form of therapy with a favourable cost/benefit relationship in these conditions:

- paroxysmal re-entrant tachycardia (in the absence of WPW [Wolf-Parkinson-Wright syndrome]), except in cases with rare and unsustained crises and those in which the heart rate is similar or lower than the maximum sinusal rate for their age;
- incessant or iterative atrial tachycardia, with the exception of cases with low frequency crises;
- symptomatic WPW;
- asymptomatic WPW with *borderline* or *at risk* electrophysiological aspects;
- right atrial isthmus-dependent atrial flutter;
- fascicular tachycardia and symptomatic ventricular tachycardia of the outflow tract;
- ventricular ectopic heartbeats that are frequent and heavily symptomatic or the cause of depression of the pump function.

17.4 Resumption of Physical Activity After Transcatheter Ablation

After the ablative procedure, intense physical activity is not recommended for a few days in order to avoid possible hemorrhagic complications related to vascular access sites, in particular for arterial access. In most cases the athletes subjected to ablative treatment can be considered suitable for agonistic activity after having undertaken simple assessments such as an echocardiogram and Holter ECG for 24 hours on condition that:

- there is no cardiopathic cause of non-suitability;
- at least one month has passed since the ablation intervention;
- the ECG does not show signs of ventricular pre-excitation in cases of WPW;
- the subject is asymptomatic, without evidence of arrhythmic recurrences;
- in cases in which there remains a doubt about the result of the ablative intervention, the COCIC protocol suggests the practice of an electrophysiological study, which is otherwise not considered mandatory.

This differs from the case of ablation of atrial fibrillation, a procedure for which the resumption of physical activity is suggested after a period of 3-6 months during which the presence of arrhythmic recurrence is ruled out. In any case, the resumption of competitive activity remains determined by the suspension of antiarrhythmic and oral anticoagulant therapy.

References

1. Sciarra L, Allocca G, Calò L (2008) Use of electroanatomic mapping in the assessment of atrial tachycardia aetiology. J Cardiovasc Med 9:1280-1281
2. Sauer WH, Alonso C, Zado E et al (2006) Atrioventricular nodal re-entrant tachycardia in patients referred for AF ablation. Response to ablation that incorporates slow-pathway modification. Circulation 114:191-195
3. Jackman WM, Beckman KJ, McClelland JH et al (1992) Treatment of supraventricular tachycardia due to atrioventricular nodal re-entry by radiofrequency catheter ablation of slow pathway conduction. N Eng J Med 327:313-318
4. Haissaguerre M, Gaita F, Fischer B et al (1992) Elimination of atrioventricular nodal re-entrant tachycardia using discrete slow potentials to guide application of radiofrequency energy. Circulation 85:2162-2175
5. Chen X, Borggrefe M, Shenasa M et al (1992) Characteristics of local electrogram predicting successful transcatheter radiofrequency ablation of left sided accessory pathways. J Am Coll Cardiol 20:656-665
6. Kistler PM, Roberts-Thomson KC, Haqqani HM et al (2006) P-wave morphology in focal atrial tachycardia: development of an algorithm to predict the anatomic site of origin. J Am Coll Cardiol 48:1010-1017
7. Haissaguerre M, Gencel L, Fischer B et al (1994) Successful catheter ablation of atrial fibrillation. J Cardiovasc Electrophysiol 5:1045-1052
8. Cappato R, Calkins H, Chen SA et al (2005) Worldwide survey on the methods, efficacy and safety of catheter ablation for human atrial fibrillation. Circulation 111:1100-1105
9. Haissaguerre M, Jais P, Shah DC et al (1996) Right and left atrial radiofrequency catheter therapy of paroxysmal AF. J Cardiovasc Electrophysiol 7:1132-1144
10. Pappone C, Rosanio S, Oreto G et al (2000) Circumferential radiofrequency ablation of pulmonary vein ostia. A new anatomic approach for curing atrial fibrillation. Circulation 102:2619-2628
11. Calò L, Lamberti F, Loricchio ML et al (2006) Left atrial ablation versus biatrial ablation for persistent and permanent atrial fibrillation: a prospective and randomized study. J Am Coll Cardiol 47:2504-2512
12. Link MS, Homoud MK, Wang PJ (2001) Cardiac arrhythmias in the athlete. Cardiol Rev 9:21-30

13. Link MS, Homoud MK, Wang PJ et al (2002) Cardiac arrhythmias in the athlete: the evolving role of electrophysiology. Curr Sports Med Rep 1:75-85
14. Furlanello F, Bertoldi A, Inama G et al (1995) Catheter ablation in competitive athletes: indication. J Interv Cardiol 8:837-840
15. Gerstenfeld EP, Callans DJ, Dixit S et al (2003) Incidence and location of focal atrial fibrillation triggers in patients undergoing repeat pulmonary vein isolation: implication for ablation strategies. J Cardiovasc Electrophysiol 13:685-690
16. Calvo N, Mont L, Tamborero D et al (2010) Efficacy of circumferential pulmonary vein ablation of atrial fibrillation in endurance athletes. Europace 12:30-36
17. Furlanello F, Lupo P, Pittalis M et al (2008) Radiofrequency catheter ablation of atrial fibrillation in athletes referred for disabling symptoms preventing usual training schedule and sport competition. J Cardiovasc Electrophysiol 19:457-462
18. Lampert R et al (2008) Atrial fibrillation in athletes: toward more effective therapy and better understanding. J Cardiovasc Electrophysiol 19:463-465
19. Heidbüchel H, Anné W, Willems R et al (2006) Endurance sports is a risk factor for atrial fibrillation after ablation for atrial flutter. Int J Cardiol 107:67-72
20. Comitato Organizzativo Cardiologico per l'Idoneità allo Sport (2009) ANCE-ANMCO-FMSI-SIC-SIC SPORT. Protocolli cardiologici per il giudizio di idoneità allo sport agonistico 2009. Cesi Casa Editrice Scientifica Internazionale, Roma

Valvulopathies in Young Athletes 18

Enrica Mariano, Armando Passeri and Massimo Fioranelli

18.1 Introduction

Considerable mass-media attention to tragic events that involve young athletes awakens public opinion and interest in cardiovascular diseases as a cause of sudden death [1]. The significance of this issue raises problems related not only to forensic scientific work but also to ethical features of the medical profession in general. In comparison with the USA where no medical certification is obligatory in order to evaluate fitness for competitive sport activity [2] and athletes assume responsibility for participating in potentially risky sporting competitions, in Italy there is a mandatory medical certification for sports physicians. Even in cases where athletes report injury following this authorization, the doctor is presumed to be directly responsible.

Evaluation of the state of health or physical ability is made by a sports physician concerning competitive activity and pediatricians for non-competitive activity.

18.1.1 Classification of Physical Activities

Physical activity provides cardiovascular system overload that in patients affected by heart diseases may induce worsening of the illness and increase the risk of sudden cardiac death.

E. Mariano (✉)
Interventional Cardiology Unit
"Tor Vergata" University, Rome, Italy

Physical activities may be classified in accordance with the type (dynamic or static) and strength of exercise (low, mild or high). Dynamic exercise leads to changes in muscle fibre length, osteoarticular movements, with rhythmic contractions that develop relatively small muscle strength. Static exercise develops high muscle strength with reduced variations in muscle length and osteoarticular movement (Table 18.1). These two types of exercises are to be considered as the extremes of a continuous series because physical activities normally have both of the components. Typical examples are represented by marathon, with a high dynamic component and low static component, and weight lifting, with a low dynamic component and high static component. Both of the two components produce different parameter variations such as oxygen consumption, heart rate, wall stress and contractility.

18.1.2 Effects of Physical Activity on Cardiovascular Hemodynamics

Dynamic exercise produces a strong increase of oxygen consumption, systolic stroke, cardiac index, systolic pressure, with slight rise in average pressure, a decrease in diastolic pressure and peripheral resistance.

On the other hand, static exercise induces a slight rise in oxygen consumption, cardiac index and heart rate without alterations to systolic stroke, with a consequent increase in systolic, diastolic and average pressures, without significant variations in peripheral resistance values (Fig. 18.1).

M. Fioranelli and G. Frajese (eds.), *Sports Cardiology*,
DOI: 10.1007/978-88-470-2775-6_18, © Springer-Verlag Italia 2012

Table 18.1 Type and intensity of exercise in some sports

	A. Dynamic (low strength)	B. Dynamic (mild strength)	C. Dynamic (high strength)
I. Static (low strength)	Billiards Bowling Bowls Golf Rifle-shooting	Baseball Softball Table tennis Tennis (doubles) Volleyball	Cross-country skiing Lawn hockey Speed-walking Water polo Distance running Football Tennis (singles)
II. Static (mild strength)	Archery Motor racing Diving Horse racing Motorcycling	Fencing Jumping Skating Quick racing Synchronized swimming	Basketball Ice hockey Racing (medium distance) Swimming Handball
III. Static (high strength)	Shot Put, throwing the hammer Karate/Judo Mountain climbing Water skiing Weight lifting Windsurf	Body-Building Downhill skiing Cycling	Boxing Canoeing/Kayak Floor exercises Decathlon Racing Skating (speed)

18.1.3 Effects on Cardiac Hypertrophy

Any kind of physical activity produces specific effects on the cardiac muscle. Exercises characterized by a strong dynamic component induce heart hypertrophy associated with dilatation of left ventricle (eccentric hypertrophy), which normally develops gradually and is correlated with maximum oxygen consumption [3].

Exercises characterized by strong static components induce heart hypertrophy that is not associated with left chamber dilatation (concentric hypertrophy) which does not correlate with maximum oxygen consumption. Sports such as skiing, which provides both of these components, lead to eccentric and concentric hypertrophy.

18.1.4 Guidelines

Data in the literature provide some specific guidelines on evaluation criteria for physical fitness assessment during non-competitive activity in athletes affected by congenital and valvular heart disease after cardiac surgery [4].

18.1.5 Fitness for Competitive Sport

With the term *fitness for competitive sport* we mean the ability to participate in official competitive activities [5,6] organized by sports authorities and organizations that have the obligation of certifying competitive ability according the suggestions of *Cardiology protocols for the evaluation of ability to competitive sport* (COCIS).

With the term *fitness for recreational-instructional activity* we mean the ability to participate in non-competitive sporting activities, for which a general fitness certification is required, which is generally issued by pediatricians or general practitioners.

In clinical practice, general indications concerning judgements on fitness for competitive sport have to be applied to any specific heart disease, considering its effects on every patient. A careful evaluation of young athletes allows for establishing a crucial balance to be made between the immediate physical, social and psychological benefits of physical activity and long-term worsening of heart diseases.

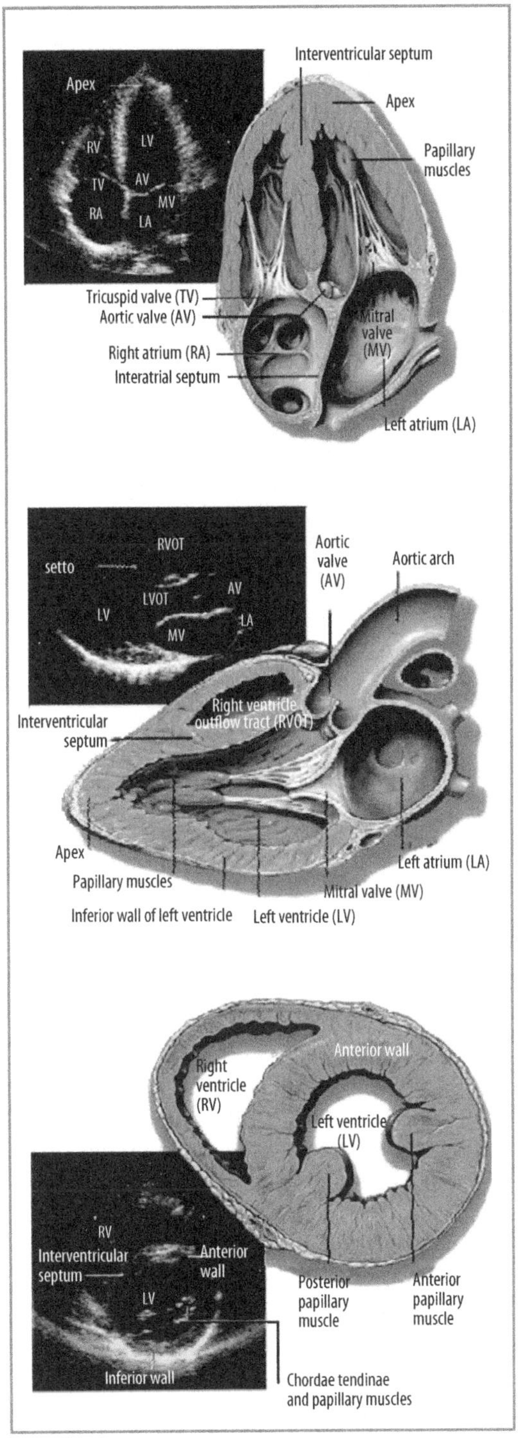

Fig. 18.1 Cardiac adaptations in *athlete's heart* are typical in athletes used to high competitive activities, in whom strenuous training causes dilatation of the left heart chambers, thickening of the interventricular septum, increased cardiac mass and variations in the valvular apparatus

18.2 Atrioventricular Valves Anomalies

18.2.1 Mitral Stenosis

The most common etiopathogenesis of mitral stenosis is rheumatic disease whose incidence is, nowadays, largely decreased. Anatomical obstruction at the level of the left ventricle inflow leads to an increase in left atrial and pulmonary capillary wedge pressures at rest and especially during exercise because of a heart rate increase (which provokes reduction in cardiac filling and the cardiac index). An independent risk factor is peripheral embolization.

The hemodynamic seriousness of mitral stenosis may be evaluated with adequate reliability with the integration of various non-invasive parameters such as clinical examination, ECG and especially echocardiography [7-8]. Doubtful cases may be studied with transesophageal echocardiography too.

Mitral stenosis is universally considered mild if the estimated valvular area is >1.5 cm^2; moderate if the estimated valvular area is between 1 and 1.5 cm^2, and severe if the estimated valvular area <1 cm^2 (Table 18.2).

18.2.1.1 Sports Competition Ability

All competitive activity is contraindicated in moderate and severe forms and in any case of persistent atrial fibrillation.

In mild cases and selected patients affected by moderate mitral stenosis ability for group A, sports may be considered, when a normal effort tolerance, a slight increase in average atrioventricular gradient (<15 mmHg) and systolic pulmonary artery pressure (< 60 mmHg) during echo stress tests, and the absence of mayor arrhythmias during Holter ECG monitoring and ergometric tests are clearly detected.

Fitness for selected sports in A groups and B may be granted to athletes who have undergone open heart surgery or valvuloplasty, six months after the intervention, in the absence of significant pulmonary hypertension (systolic pulmonary artery pressure < 30 mmHg) and considerable valve incontinency with a valve area equal to or greater than 1.5 cm^2.

Table 18.2 Classification of the seriousness of valvulopathies

Parameter	Mild	Moderate	Severe
Mitral stenosis			
Average atrioventricular gradient (mmHg)	<5	5-10	>10
Systolic pulmonary artery pressure (mmHg)	<30	30-50	>50
Estimated valvular area (cm^2)	>1.5	1.0-1.5	<1.0
Mitral insufficiency			
Color-Doppler jet area (cm^2)	<4	4-8	>8
Left atrium area	<20%	20-40%	40%
Vena contracta (mm)	<3	3-6.9	≥7
Regurgitant orifice area (cm^2)	<0.2	0.2-0.39	≥0.4
Left atrial diameter	normal	mildly increased	moderately increased
Left ventricle volumes	normal	mildly increased	moderately increased
Left ventricle ejection fraction	normal	normal	decreased
Aortic stenosis			
Doppler peak velocity (m/s)	<3.0	3.0-4.0	>4
Average left ventricle-aorta gradient (mmHg)	<25	25-40	>40
Estimated valvular area (cm^2)	>1.5	1.0-1.5	<1.0
Valvular area indexed for BSA (cm^2/m^2)			<0.6
Aortic insufficiency			
Color-Doppler jet area (diameter left ventricle outflow)	<25%	25-65%	>65%
Vena contracta (mm)	<3	3-6	>6
Pressure half time (m/s)	<400	>400	
Regurgitant orifice area (cm^2)	<0.1	0.1-0.29	≥0.3
Left ventricle volumes	normal	mildly increased	moderately increased
Left ventricle ejection fraction	normal	normal	decreased

BSA, Body Surface Area.

18.2.2 Mitral Insufficiency

The high prevalence of tricuspid valve insufficiency (up to 90%) in young athletes is the direct consequence of physiological right heart volume overload while the detection of left valve insufficiency in these subjects has to be interpreted with accuracy and requires the ruling out of morphological alterations and valve diseases.

Left valve insufficiency is defined as *physiological* if it is mild (central jet, a few centimetres below the valve plane) and structural alterations of the valvular leaflets are absent [9]. Mitral insufficiency etiologies are multiple: rheumatic disease in rare cases, the congenital presence of a *cleft* in the anterior leaflet (see *atrioventricular channel*), degenerative because of mitral valve prolapse, annular and posterior leaflet calcification and infective endocarditis.

In the classification of the seriousness of mitral insufficiency for certifying fitness for sporting competitions, the first element of judgment is the etiology:

- in secondary forms (i.e. Marfan syndrome) judgement is conditioned by the expression of the primary illness;
- in primitive forms (rheumatic or degenerative) judgement is to be formulated according to the hemodynamic status of the athlete, assessed by left atrial and ventricular volumes (ECG and echocardiography), the change in ejection fraction at rest and during exercise (stress echocardiography or radioisotope ventriculography) and finally the presence of arrhythmias detected by Holter monitoring and ergometric tests during a regular session of physical training.

For practical purposes mitral insufficiency is considered:

- mild if documented only by an acoustic finding, confirmed by a slight jet with echocardiography in the absence of ECG alterations and atrial or

ventricular dilatation with transthoracic echocardiography (Table 18.2);
- moderate when a moderate color-Doppler jet is associated with a slight increase in left ventricular volume, indexed for BSA and normal ejection fraction at rest and during exercise;
- severe in all other cases.

18.2.2.1 Sports Competition Fitness

Young athletes affected by mild mitral insufficiency are able to practise A and B sporting activities, while in selected cases the ability for other kinds of sports characterized by higher efforts may be considered, by strictly monitoring left ventricle dimensions and contractility and by re-evaluating fitness for sport every six months. Any kind of competitive activity is contraindicated for all subjects affected by severe mitral insufficiency and moderate insufficiency, except for A and B group activities in the latter cohort.

In subjects with severe insufficiency, no sporting activity is permitted.

In young athletes who have undergone open heart surgery, COCIS requires the judgement of ability to participate in sporting competitions to be accurately reviewed by experienced healthcare workers, based upon evaluation of certain critical features such as a potential course for primary disease, valve function and hemodynamics, left ventricle dimensions and contractility and the presence of major arrhythmias, during Holter monitoring and ergometric test, after cardiac surgery.

18.2.3 Aortic Stenosis

The same considerations expressed for the congenital form are valid for acquired aortic stenosis (see Chapter 24) which, except for some rare cases associated with rheumatic disease, is generally the expression of a degenerative calcification process that sometimes occurs in congenitally malformed aortic valves, especially the bicuspid aortic valve.

18.2.4 Aortic Insufficiency

The principal etiopathogenic factors of aortic insufficiency are: bicuspid aortic valve, rheumatic disease and infective endocarditis secondary to Marfan syndrome. General hemodynamic aspects described for mitral insufficiency may be applied to aortic insufficiency, while in severe forms a relative coronary insufficiency may occur during exercise. Nevertheless, in general, the effort-related hemodynamic status of aortic insufficiency is more favourable in comparison with mitral insufficiency, because diastolic shortening and reduction of peripheral resistance tends to decrease regurgitant blood volume.

For practical purposes aortic insufficiency is considered:

- mild if a slight regurgitant jet is present with echocardiography in the absence of ventricular dilatation or decreased ejection fraction with transthoracic echocardiography or radiosotope ventriculography; moreover, no peripheral signs of aortic insufficiency such as raized differential pressure or *pulsus celere* are present;
- moderate when a moderate color-Doppler regurgitant jet is associated with peripheral signs of aortic insufficiency, a slight increase in left ventricular dimensions and normal ejection fraction at rest and after exercise;
- severe in all other cases (Table 18.2).

18.2.4.1 Fitness for Competitive Sport

Young athletes affected by mild aortic insufficiency are able to practise A and B sporting activities, while in selected cases the ability for other kinds of sports characterized by higher efforts may be considered, by strictly monitoring left ventricular dimensions and contractility and by re-evaluating fitness for sports every six months. Any kind of competitive activity is contraindicated for all subjects affected by severe mitral insufficiency and moderate insufficiency, except for A and B group activities [10] in the latter cohort.

18.2.5 Valve Prosthesis

Specialists agree not to grant fitness to sporting competitions to young athletes with mechanical valve prostheses receiving chronic anticoagulant drugs.

On the other hand, it is reasonable to hypothesize that in selected cases of mechanical prostheses and especially in biological prostheses, fitness for sporting competitions may be granted for group A sports if normal function of the prostheses at rest and during exercise (echo-stress test), good ventricular function and the absence of major arrhythmias are clearly demonstrated during a regular training session.

18.2.6 Mitral Valve Prolapse

Mitral valve prolapse (MVP) is defined as the protrusion of one or both mitral leaflets above the valvular annulus towards left atrium, during the systolic phase. In most of the patients this disease is due to myxomatous degeneration of the valve and subvalvular apparatus. Acoustic findings are characterized by mesotelesystolic clicks and heart murmurs that can be heard at the heart apex. Echocardiography plays a crucial role in the diagnostic evaluation of the seriousness of MVP and association with other anomalies (other valve prolapses, aortic dilatation). Morphological criteria for distinguishing *true* MVP in the long axis parasternal view are represented by:

1. leaflet redundancy (*billowing*), which is disproportionately large in comparison with left heart chambers;
2. valvular thickening, when at least one of the leaflets has a thickness > 5 mm (maximum thickening of medium portion of leaflets);
3. posterior systolic displacement > 2 mm in respect to the valvular plane of at least one valvular leaflet;
4. possible regurgitant jet with color-Doppler, which depends on loss of the leaflet coaptation line.

Other suggestive features are marphanoid phenotype, familiar tendency, atypical chest pain, constitutional and orthostatic hypotension and thrilling. On the other hand, MVP is frequently associated with tachyarrhythmias or bradyarrhythmias.

An adequate evaluation of a young athlete affected by MVP requires a careful personal and family medical history, performance of transthoracic echocardiography, maximal ergometric tests (METs), and electrophysiological tests with endocavitary mapping (EM). The seriousness spectrum of the disease oscillates between severe and mild forms, with no or slight mitral insufficiency.

The following subjects must be considered *at risk* of MVP and thus excluded from competitive activity:

- those with inexplicable syncope, family tendency for sudden death, long QT;
- those with moderate or severe mitral insufficiency;
- those with recurrent supraventricular tachyarrhythmias or complex ventricular arrhythmias at rest or during effort.

18.2.6.1 Fitness for Competitive Sport

Ability for sporting competitions (groups B1 and B2, competitive and non-competitive group A) may be allowed for subjects with at least one clearly myxomatous leaflet but only slight mitral regurgitation. Yearly checks are necessary, considering the risk of worsening of myxomatous degeneration, chordae tendinae ruptures and infective endocarditis, especially in cases of bicuspid aortas. In any case, preventive antibiotic prophylaxis is always recommended in these subjects.

The simultaneous presence of tricuspid valve prolapse does not modify the criteria stated for mitral valve prolapse [11], while more caution is to be reserved in the presence of aortic cusp prolapse or aortic arch dilatation even if not associated with Marfan syndrome.

18.2.7 Obstructions to Left Ventricle Inflow

Congenital anomalies of left ventricle inflow are rare and may be divided into three large subgroups: isolated obstructions of pulmonary veins, supravalvular obstructions (cor triatriatum and mitral supravalvular membrane) and congenital mitral stenosis.

Isolated obstructions of pulmonary veins are very rare and its prognosis is generally inauspicious. Cor triatriatum and mitral supravalvular membrane are very similar anomalies, characterized by a membrane covering the left atrium that separates the portion that surrounds the pulmonary veins from that related to the mitral valve. In supravalvular membranes, the membrane itself is adherent to the mitral valve while in cor triatriatum it is far away from the valve plane, usually associated with interatrial defects (the membrane is situated upstream or downstream of the defect).

The membrane is necessarily perforated and raized in a wedged position between the pulmonary artery and right ventricle, with pressure depending on the dimensions of the perforations.

Congenital mitral valve anomalies may involve valve annulus, leaflets, the subvalvalvular apparatus and papillary muscles. Generally these valves are dysplasic and present a mixed contribution of two different hemodynamic components of stenosis and insufficiency. Anatomical and functional assessment of left ventricle inflow obstructions may be non-invasively obtained with the careful integration of clinical parameters, ECG, transthoracic and transesophageal echocardiographic data (average atrioventricular gradient, pulmonary hypertension).

18.2.8 Valvulopathies with Left Ventricle Outflow Obstruction

Pulmonary valve stenosis and *subvalvular pulmonary stenosis* are treated in Chapter 24.

18.2.9 Pulmonary Artery and Branch Stenosis

Congenital pulmonary artery stenosis, isolated or in association with other cardiac defects, represents 2-3% of all congenital cardiopathies. These valvulopathies are frequently associated with other cardiac anomalies such as pulmonary valve stenosis, septal defects and the tetralogy of Fallot. In one third of the cases they are isolated and are the expression of extracardiac malformations such as systemic vascular dysplasia (Marfan and Ehler-Danlos syndromes), embryopathies (rubeola, rosolia) and complex genetic syndromes (Williams Beurens and Alagille syndromes).

Acquired stenosis is normally subsequent to surgical complications of the correction of intracardiac malformations, simple or complex. A common pathophysiological background is a rise in systolic pressure in the right ventricle and pulmonary artery, upstream the stenosis.

Echocardiographic evaluation usually documents right ventricle dilatation and some turbulent zones in the distal tract of the pulmonary arteries, if a good acoustic view makes it possible to detect these features.

Judgement for competitive sport fitness is made by high qualification centres, considering the rarity and complexity of clinical presentations and instrumental diagnostic tools necessary before and after surgical treatment.

18.2.10 Aortic Congenital Stenosis

Congenital aortic valvular stenosis is generally due to the absence/malformation of one of the valvular cusps; the most frequent malformation is *bicuspid aorta* (BA).

BA has to be suspected when ejective clicks associated with systolic sound in aortic or neck points are detected during routine visits in young athletes [12]. Transthoracic echocardiography is feasible for the diagnosis and estimation of the seriousness of valve stenosis or insufficiency.

For practical purposes, aortic valve stenosis is defined as hemodynamically insignificant if the average gradient at rest is < 25 mmHg.

BA is actually the most common cardiac anomaly detected in the general population (prevalence 1-2%); it is due to the altered development of aortic buttons that leads to the formation of a valve with only two cusps and a systolic eccentric oval-shaped orifice. Valve closure lines appear transversal in the diastolic phase while a rafe (a remnant of the non-division of cusps) may be present on one of the cusps that can lead erroneously to false diagnosis of tricuspid valve.

BA frequently is associated with aortic coarctation, ascending aorta dilatation with a higher risk of aortic insufficiency, and dissection. These athletes undergo periodical checks because of the progressive nature of their disease, with possible calcium deposits and a higher risk of endocarditis. Non-complicated bicuspid aorta is defined when not significant stenosis or insufficiency are detected, associated with normal dimensions of the bulbus and ascending aorta.

18.2.10.1 Fitness for Competitive Sport

Subjects affected by mild aortic stenosis and non-complicated BA [13] can participate in every kind of sport, as long as these criteria are respected:

- absence of left ventricle hypertrophy (ECG and echocardiography data);
- normal values of ejection fraction in left and right ventricle;
- normal dimensions of the aortic root [14] and ascending aorta (the evaluation of this is a crucial aspect that is assessed by echocardiography and, in some cases, by MRI, because of the risk of developing aorta ascending and thoracic aneurysms);
- normal ergometric test (MET) that is defined as a normal increase in systolic pressure and an absence of ECG alterations during effort;
- absence of major arrhythmias at rest and during exercise (MET and EM).

Subjects with hemodynamically significant aortic valvular stenosis (average gradient >20 mmHg) cannot participate in competitions and have to be directed to cardiac surgery, if indicated by clinical and instrumental parameters.

Fitness for agonistic competition sports (B2 and some types of group B1, such as horseracing and sailing) and non-competitive group A sports may be allowed after valvuloplasty correction with a favourable prognosis (residual average gradient < 20 mmHg, non-significant aortic insufficiency, absence of ECG alterations and major arrhythmias on MET and EM) with an obligation of six-month checks. The same criteria may be adopted for subjects carrying homografts or well- functioning biological prostheses. On the other hand, athletes subjected to Ross operations (aortic valve replacement with pulmonary autografts, coronary artery reimplantation, pulmonary homograft placement) showed, frequently, mild residual defects.

Fitness for sporting competitions (B2 and some types of group B1, such as horseracing and sailing, and non-competitive group A sports) may be considered in this cohort of patients in some cases, with an obligation for six-month checks:

- normal ventricular dimensions and ejection fraction;
- right ventricle-pulmonary artery average gradient < 20 mmHg;
- absence of significant aortic insufficiency;
- absence of ECG alterations and major arrhythmias on MET and EM.

In *membrane subvalvular aortic stenosis* [15], we normally use the same criteria adopted for the valvular form. In subjects with subvalvular aortic stenosis, six months after the intervention, fitness for any kind of sport may be allowed in the absence of major atrioventricular conduction alterations and ventricular activation disorders, in the absence of significant aortic insufficiency, if ventricular dimensions and the ejection fraction are normal and if the residual average gradient is < 20 mmHg.

Moreover, a normal rise in systolic pressure, the absence of significant ST alterations during ergometric tests, the absence of major arrhythmias at rest and during ergometric tests and Holter monitoring have to be documented. Supravalvular stenosis has to be carefully studied because of the possible anomalies in peripheral and coronary circulation, aortic arch-associated pathology and complex malformations and congenital syndromes (Williams syndrome) etc.

18.2.11 Aortic Coarctation

This condition is largely studied in Chapter 26.

18.2.12 Physiological Insufficiency

A frequent finding in young athletes is the presence of a physiological insufficiency of cardiac valves, which is usually not hemodynamically significant. Prevalence is generally correlated with training time and physiological heart chamber dilatation [19-20]. An expert sonographer safely distinguishes between physiological and pathological insufficiency.

In physiological insufficiency, transthoracic echocardiography detects:

- no structural valvular alteration;

- no turbulence and aliasing phenomenon with color-Doppler;
- a regurgitant area limited to the central subvalvular zone, up to a maximum of 1-2 cm from the valvular plane.

Physical examination documented a mesosystolic or holosystolic murmur, (1-2/6) that can be detected in up to 50% of young athletes and normally diminished with the transition from supine to orthostatic position. This finding is probably a consequence of non-laminar flux through aortic and pulmonary valves because of increased systolic stroke.

References

1. Maron BJ (2003) Sudden death in young athletes. N Engl J Med 349:1064-1075
2. Mitchell JH, Maron BJ, Epstein SE (1985) 16th Bethesda conference: cardiovascular abnormalities in the athlete: recommendations regarding eligibility for competition. October 3-5, 1984. J Am Coll Cardiol 6:1186-1232
3. Toraa M, Pouillard F, Merlet P, Friemel F (1999) Cardiac hypertrophy and coronary reserve in endurance athletes. Cam J Appl Physio 24:87-95
4. Cheitlin MD, Douglas PS, Parmley WW (1994) 26th Bethesda conference: recommendations for determining eligibility for competition in athletes with cardiovascular abnormalities. Task Force 2: acquired valvular heart disease. Med Sci Sports Exerc 26:S254-260
5. Maron BJ, Chaitman BR, Ackerman MJ, Bayés de Luna A for the Working Groups of the American Heart Association Committee on Exercise, Cardiac Rehabilitation, and Prevention; Councils on Clinical Cardiology and Cardiovascular Disease in the Young (2004) Recommendations for physical activity and recreational sports participation for young patients with genetic cardiovascular diseases. Circulation 8:2807-2816 6. Lawless CE (2009) Return-to-play decisions in athletes with cardiac conditions. Phys Sportsmed 37:80-91
7. Abergel E, Oblak A (2006) Echocardiography in athletes. Arch Mal Coeur Vaiss 99:969-974
8. Vasconcelos DF, Junqueira Júnior LF, Sanchez Osella OF (1993) Doppler echocardiographic comparison of valvular dynamics in bicycling, running, and football athletes, and sedentary subjects. Arq Bras Cardiol 61:161-164
9. Stout M (2008) Athletes heart and echocardiography: athletes' heart. Echocardiography 25:749-754
10. Mellwig KP, van Buuren F, Gohlke-Baerwolf C, Bjørnstad HH (2008) Recommendations for the management of individuals with acquired valvular heart diseases who are involved in leisure-time physical activities or competitive sports. Eur J Cardiovasc Prev Rehabil 15:95-103
11. Thompson PD (1999) Evaluating and managing athletes with valvular heart disease. Conn Med 63:665-675
12. Doyle EF, Arumugham P, Lara E et al (1974) Sudden death in young patients with congenital aortic stenosis. Pediatrics 53:481-489
13. Spataro A, Pelliccia A, Rizzo M et al (2008) The natural course of bicuspid aortic valve in athletes. In J Sports Med 29:81-85
14. D'Andrea A, Cocchia R, Riegler L et al (2010) Aortic root dimensions in elite athletes. Am J Cardiol 105:1629-1634
15. Thompson PD (2002) Aortic valvular disease in active patients: overcoming diagnostic and management challenges. Phys Sportsmed 30:19-35
16. Pelech AN, Kartodihardjo W, Balfe JA et al (1986) Exercise in children before and after coarctectomy: hemodynamic, echocardiographic, and biochemical assessment. Am Heart J 112:1263-1270
17. Gojanovic B, Feihl F, Gremion G, Waeber B (2007) Sudden death in young athletes. Praxis (Bern 1994) 96:189-198
18. Fishbein MC (2010) Cardiac disease and risk of sudden death in the young: the burden of the phenomenon. Cardiovasc Pathol 19:326-328
19. Douglas PS, Berman GO, O'Toole ML (1989) Prevalence of multivalvular regurgitation in athletes. Am J Cardiol 64:209-212
20. Assanelli D, Marconi M, Corsini C et al (1992) Noninvasive evaluation of asymptomatic athletes with cardiac murmur. Acta Cardiol 47:71-75

Cardiomyopathies in the Athlete

19

Caterina Bisceglia and Maddalena Piro

Hypertrophic cardiomyopathy (HCM) and arrhythmogenic right ventricular cardiomyopathy (ARVD) are two important causes of sudden death in young athletes. Preparticipation screening in healthy general athlete populations may raise the suspicion of HCM or ARVD, and ultimately lead to definitive diagnosis. However, controversy has recently arisen regarding the most effective and practical strategy for the screening of athletes. European investigators have promoted routine 12-lead ECGs as part of a national mandatory program distinct from the customary practice in the US which is limited to patient history and physical examinations. Consensus criteria and recommendations for eligibility and disqualification of athletes with HCM or ARVD have proved useful to the practising community.

19.1 Hypertrophic Cardiomyopathy

HCM is a complex and relatively common genetic cardiac disease that has been the subject of intense scrutiny and investigation for more than 40 years. Hypertrophic cardiomyopathy is an important cause of disability and death in patients of all ages, although sudden and unexpected death in young people is perhaps the most devastating component of its natural history. Because of marked heterogeneity in clinical expression, natural history, and prognosis HCM often represents a dilemma to primary care clinicians and cardiovascular specialists, even to those for whom this disease is a focus of their investigative careers. Controversy abounds with regard to diagnostic criteria, clinical course, and management for which difficult questions often arise, particularly among practitioners infrequently engaged in the evaluation of HCM patients. Consequently, it is timely to place in perspective and clarify many of these relevant clinical issues and profile the rapidly evolving concepts regarding HCM.

In the United States of America, Hypertrophic Cardiomyopathy (HCM) represents the first cause of sudden death in young athletes (36% of total). It's a familial and primitive cardiomyopathy, characterized by a marked heterogeneity in clinical expression, natural history and prognosis [1]. Therefore, HCM is the most common genetic cardiovascular disease, with a prevalence in the adult general population of about 0.2% (1: 500).

Hypertrophic cardiomyopathy is inherited as a mendelian autosomal dominant trait and caused by mutations in any 1 of 10 genes, each encoding proteins of the cardiac sarcomere (components of thick or thin filaments with contractile, structural, or regulatory functions).

Three of the HCM-causing mutant genes predominate, namely, b-myosin heavy chain (the first identified), cardiac troponin T, and myosin-binding protein C. The other genes each account for a minority of HCM cases, namely, cardiac troponin I, regulatory and essential myosin light chains, titin, α-tropomyosin, α-actin, and α-myosin heavy chain [2]. This diversity is compounded by intragenic heterogeneity, with more than 150 mutations identified, most of which are missense with a single amino acid residue substituted with another.

M. Piro (✉)
Heart Center
Casa di Cura Mater Dei, Rome, Italy

M. Fioranelli and G. Frajese (eds.), *Sports Cardiology*,
DOI: 10.1007/978-88-470-2775-6_19, © Springer-Verlag Italia 2012

Table 19.1 Genetic of HCM

Gene	Abbr.	Locus
β-Myosin heavy chain	MYH7	14q12
α-Myosin heavy chain	MYH6	14q12
Regulatory myosin light chain	MYL2	12q23-q24
Essential myosin light chain	MYL3	3p21
Myosin binding protein C	MYBPC3	11p11.2
Troponin T	TNNT2	1q32
Troponin I	TNNI3	19q13.4
α-Tropomyosin	TPM1	15q22.1
Protein-kinase 2	PRKAG2	7q36
Muscle LIM proteins	CSRP3	11p15.1
Titin (connectin)	TTN	2q24.3
Actin	ACTC1	15q14
Troponin C	TNNC1	3p21-p14
Troponin C	TNNC1	3p21-p14

Molecular defects responsible for HCM are usually different in unrelated individuals, and many other genes and mutations, each accounting for a small proportion of familial HCM, remain to be identified (Table 19.1).

19.1.1 Diagnosis

The clinical diagnosis is based on the echocardiographic definition of the typical features of the disease (Fig. 19.1):

- asymmetric hypertrophy of the left ventricle (LVH), in association with a normal endocavitary dimensions;
- absence of another cardiac or systemic disease (e.g., hypertension or aortic stenosis) capable of producing the magnitude of hypertrophy;

Given that most patients do not have LV outflow tract obstruction at rest and most of the well-documented physical findings (e.g., loud systolic heart murmur and bifid arterial pulse) are limited to patients with outflow gradients, the signs suggestive of a dynamic LVOT obstruction, such as a systolic heart murmur, a *Systolic Anterior Motion (SAM)* of the mitral valve or a premature closure of the aortic valve, do not represent diagnostic criteria.

LVH, which represents an independent risk factor for the sudden death in young people affected by HCM, is variable in distribution and extension [1,2].

Although many patients show diffusely distributed LVH, almost one third have mild wall thickening localized to a single segment (interventricular septum, apex, antero-lateral and posterior wall), including the apical form, that appears most commonly in the Japanese population. In clinically diagnosed patients, increased LV wall thicknesses range widely from mild (13-15 mm) to massive (30 mm [normal, 12 mm]), up to 60 mm.

In trained athletes, modest segmental wall thickening (i.e., 13-15 mm) raises the differential diagnosis between extreme physiologic LVH (i.e., athlete's heart) and mild morphologic expressions of HCM, without outflow obstruction.

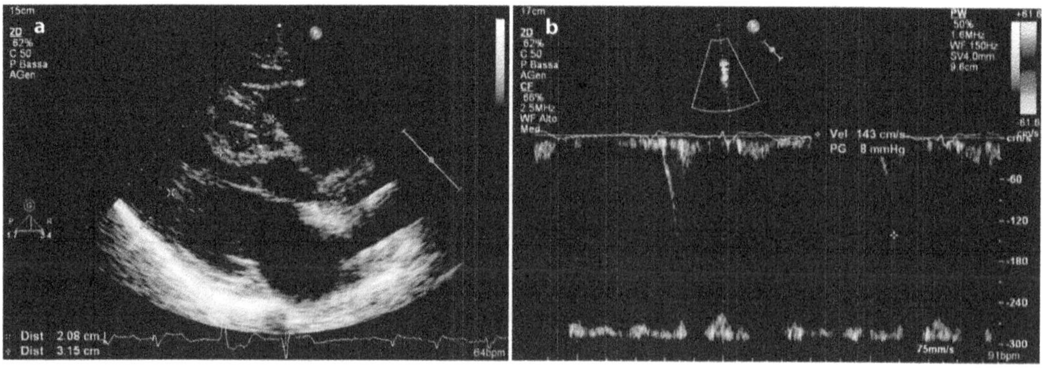

Fig. 19.1 Ecocardiographic images of a young volley-ball player during pre-participation screening. a (M-mode) thickness of SIV and posterior wall (31 and 20 mm respectively). b evidence of the lack of intraventricular pressure gradient. The diagnosis of HCM has been confirmed by genetic analysis

Table 19.2 Elements that suggest hypertrophic cardiomyopathy (HCM)

• Atypical LVH
• LV EDD < 45 mm
• Family history of HCM
• Female gender
• Abnormal transmitral flow

The differential diagnosis in this *gray zone* of overlap (about 2% of elite male athletes) can usually be resolved with some clinical and echocardiographic criteria (Table 19.2). An end-diastolic diameter (EDD) >55 mm and a reduction of the LV wall thickening after three months of detraining (<13 mm) are suggestive of the athlete's heart [3].

Magnetic resonance imaging (MRI) may be of diagnostic value when echocardio- graphic studies are technically inadequate or in identifying segmental LVH undetectable by echocardiography. Moreover late gadolinium enhancement may be helpful in identifying areas of intramyocardial fibrosis [4].

Also the *cardiopulmonary test* may contribute to the differential diagnosis between HCM and the athlete's heart: the athletes have usually a VO_2 peak value >50 ml/kg/min, in comparison with HCM patients that presents VO_2 peak value in the range of normality [4].

Actually genetic analyses are useful in distinguishing the benign consequences of systematic athletic training from pathological left ventricular hypertrophy with the potential for sudden cardiac death [2]. With regard to pedigree assessment, it is obligatory for the subject to be informed of the familial nature and autosomal dominant transmission of HCM. Screening of first-degree relatives, including medical history and physical examinations, and 2-dimensional echocardiography and ECG should be encouraged, particularly if adverse HCM-related events have occurred in the family. If a subject is positive for one of the 10 most common HCM-causing mutant genes tested in the panel, the test result is definitive. On the other hand, such genetic testing has potential limitations. For example, negative tests in subjects, while common, are non-diagnostic because they may frequently represent false negative results. In addition, commercial testing is costly (in the range of $5,000 for all 10 genes), and it is presently unpredictable whether that expense will always be covered by insurance carriers. However, if the gene defect responsible for HCM in the family becomes known, other family members can easily be tested definitively and inexpensively.

19.1.2 Risk Stratification and Sport Eligibility

The importance of correct risk stratification and the eventual disqualification from sport of HCM affected patients are based on the evidence that sudden death is often the first clinical manifestation of the disease, in particular in young people (<30 years).

The vast majority of athletes who die suddenly with HCM are free of symptoms or the suspicion of cardiovascular disease [1]. Sudden collapse usually occurs with physical exertion, predominantly in the late afternoon and early evening hours, corresponding to the peak periods of competition and training, and particularly in organized team sports, such as football and basketball [5]. In addition, underlying genetic heart diseases are more likely to cause sudden unexpected death in trained athletes than in their sedentary counterparts. These observations substantiate that, in the presence of cardiovascular disease, physical activity represents a trigger and important precipitating factor for sudden death in athletes.

The vast majority of athletic field deaths occur in men (about 90%). This relative infrequency in women probably reflects lower participation rates, sometimes less intense levels of training, and the fact that women do not engage in some of the higher-risk sports (e.g., football). Most athletes are involved in high-school sports at the time of death (about 75%), and less commonly in college or professional competitions.

Although the majority of sudden deaths in competitive athletes have been reported in white males, a substantial proportion (more than 40%) are African-Americans [5] (including the majority of HCM-related athletic field deaths). The substantial number of HCM sudden deaths in young black

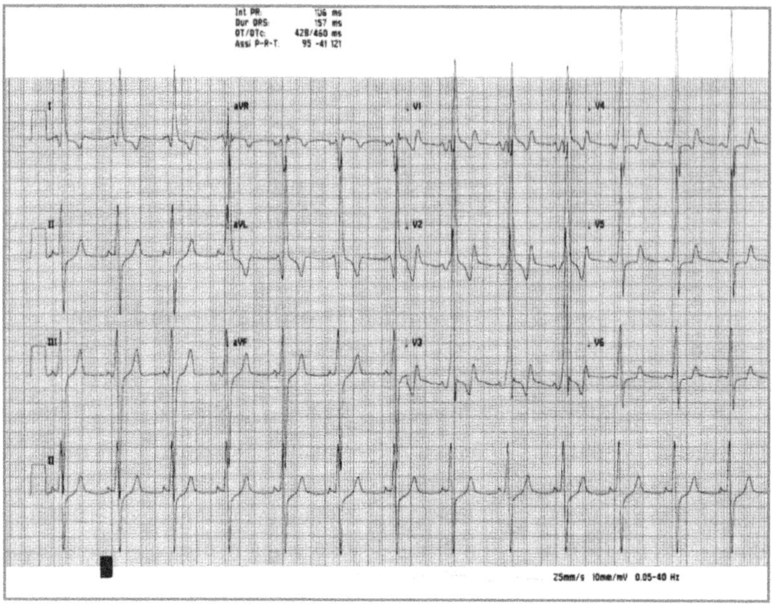

Fig. 19.2 ECG at rest of a non-agonistic athlete with a suspicion of Wolf-Parkinson-White Syndrome. ECG suggests the diagnosis of HCM, later confirmed by imaging

male athletes contrasts sharply with the infrequent identification of black patients with HCM in hospital-based populations. These observations emphasize the disproportionately lesser access to subspecialty medical care between the African-American and white communities in the United States, which makes it less likely that young black males will receive the diagnosis of HCM. Consequently, African-American athletes with HCM are also less likely to be disqualified from competition to reduce their risk for sudden death, in accordance with the recommendations of Bethesda Conference [6].

In Italy, unlike the USA, the introduction in the last 25 years of a systematic preparticipation screening program, which routinely includes a 12-lead ECG has enabled the identification of many athletes previously undiagnosed with HCM, as the electrocardiogram is abnormal in up to 95% of HCM patients [7,8].

In particular, Italian investigators have reported an almost 90% decline in the annual incidence of sudden cardiovascular death in competitive athletes (a result largely due to reduced mortality from cardiomyopathy) for the Veneto region of northeastern Italy. This change in the death rate occurred in parallel with progressive implementation of nationwide mass screening and the increasing identification of affected athletes who were then disqualified from competitive sports to lower their risk (Fig. 19.2).

The 12-lead ECG pattern is abnormal in 75% to 95% of HCM patients and typically demonstrates a wide variety of patterns, including elevated QRS voltages, intra-atrial or left intraventricular conduction abnormalities, pathological Q waves (depth > 2 mm) and significant repolarization abnormalities (ST depression, negative T waves).

However these ECG patterns, some of which may be observed in well trained athletes, raise the suspicion of HCM, but have a poor diagnostic value in the absence of evidence of structural abnormalities.

When a cardiovascular abnormality is identified in a competitive athlete, several considerations arise:

1. the level of risk for sudden death if participation in organized sports continues;
2. the likelihood that risk would be reduced if systematic training and competition were terminated;
3. the criteria used to formulate appropriate eligibility or disqualification decisions.

Unfortunately, on occasion the medical disqualification decision-making process can become polarized, given the personal aspirations of the athlete versus the mandate of the physician to protect patients from circumstances which could provoke unacceptable risks.

It should be underlined that the risk associated with intense physical exertion for sports participants with cardiovascular abnormalities is difficult to quantify with any precision, given the extreme and unpredictable physiological circumstances to which individual athletes may be exposed. Indeed, only some HCM-related sudden deaths are associated with intense physical activity and not all trained athletes with this disease die suddenly during their competitive phase.

In this regard, the American College of Cardiology's (ACC) 36th Bethesda Conference and the European Society of Cardiology (ESC) offer expert consensus panel recommendations and clear benchmarks for clinical practice. In line with these recommendations, young athletes with a confirmed diagnosis of HCM are discouraged from competitive athletic participation, with the exception of low-intensity sports (e.g., golf and bowling).

If individual risk stratification is difficult, the identification of low-risk patients is nevertheless easier.

In relation to medical decisions, it is possible to define HCM patients with the following characteristics as low risk in terms of sudden death:

1. absence of symptoms, in particular syncope or prolonged, recurrent and effort palpitations;
2. mild hypertrophy (<18 mm);
3. absence of atrial enlargement;
4. absence of dynamic LVOT obstruction or mitral regurgitation at rest and during exercise;
5. absence of effort hypotension (blood pressure reduction >20 mmHg during exercise;
6. normal transmitral flow patter and normal TDI of the right ventricle;
7. absence of significant supraventricular and ventricular arrhythmias:
8. absence of *late enhancement* in MRI.

These low-risk patients are eligible, under periodic controls, for low-intensity sports (e.g., golf, sailing, riding and bowling).

It should be emphasized that the customary practice in the USA is limited to patients' medical history and physical examinations [6,9].

19.2 Arrhythmogenic Right Ventricular Cardiomyopathy/Dysplasia

19.2.1 Definition

Arrhythmogenic right ventricular cardiomyopathy/dysplasia (ARVC/D) is an inherited heart muscle disease that predominantly affects the right ventricle and is characterized pathologically by progressive replacement of the right ventricular myocardium with fibrofatty tissue [10]. Clinically, the disease presents with myocardial electrical instability leading to ventricular tachycardia or ventricular fibrillation, which may precipitate cardiac arrest, particularly during physical exercise.

19.2.2 Epidemiology in Athletes

Systematic monitoring and pathological investigation of sudden death in young people and athletes in the Veneto region of Italy has shown that ARVC/D is the most common pathological substrate, accounting for nearly one-fourth of fatal events on the athletic field [11,12]. The incidence of sudden death from ARVC/D in athletes is estimated to be 0.5 cases per 100,000 persons per year. Adolescents and young adults involved in sports activity have a 2.8 times greater risk of sudden cardiovascular death than their non-athletic counterparts [13]. In particular, the risk of sudden death in ARVC/D is 5.4 times higher during competitive sports than during sedentary activity.

The introduction of a prevention strategy based on systematic cardiovascular screening (including 12-lead ECG) of all subjects embarking upon sports activity has the potential to identify athletes who are at risk and to reduce mortality

Moreover, this preparticipation screening of young competitive athletes, which has been practiced in Italy for more than 20 years, has changed the prevalence of the pathological substrates of sports-related sudden death. For example, sudden death from hypertrophic cardiomyopathy in athletic fields can be successfully prevented by the identification and disqualification of affected athletes As a consequence of this process, other cardiovascular conditions, such as ARVC/D, now account for a greater proportion of all sudden deaths in Italian athletes. In particular, ARVC/D has been demonstrated to be the leading cause of sudden death in athletes in the Veneto region of Italy.

19.2.3 History

The first historical description of the condition was in the book *De Motu Cordis et Aneurysmatibus*, published in 1736 by Giovanni Maria Lancisi, the Pope's physician and Professor of Anatomy in Rome. He reported a family with disease recurrence over four generations. Symptoms included palpitations, heart failure, dilatation and aneurysms of the right ventricle, and sudden death. However, the first comprehensive clinical description of the disease was reported in 1982 in adults with ventricular tachyarrhythmias of left bundle branch block morphology. The electrocardiographic features of the disease, including the characteristic epsilon wave, were first described in 1984. Since then, the disease has been recorded an important cause of sudden death in young people and particularly in athletes.

19.2.4 Genetics

ARVC is a familial disease in at least 50% of cases and is typically transmitted as an autosomal dominant trait with variable penetration. On the basis of clinical studies and data obtained from preparticipation screening for sport activity, the estimated prevalence of the disease in the general population ranges from 1 in 1,000 to 1 in 5,000.

19.2.5 Clinical History

ARVC/D, although genetically determined, is an acquired and progressive disease which shows an age-related penetrance. Clinical manifestations of ARVC/D usually occur during adolescence and young adulthood. Syncope, palpitations, and ventricular arrhythmias are also the usual presenting symptoms in pediatric patients.

Four clinical phases of the disorder have been described:

- *subclinical phase* with concealed structural abnormalities and no symptoms, even though sudden death might be the first manifestation;
- *an overt right ventricular electrical disorder*, with palpitations, syncope, and ventricular arrhythmias of left bundle branch block morphology, ranging from isolated premature ventricular complexes to sustained VT and VF (either spontaneous or triggered by intracavitary electrophysiological testing);
- *right ventricular failure* due to progressive loss of myocardium with severe dilatation and systolic dysfunction, in the presence of preserved left ventricular function;
- *late-stage biventricular failure* with left ventricular involvement, that can mimic dilated cardiomyopathy severe enough to require cardiac trans- plantation. By this stage, patients could have endocardial mural thrombosis, and be at risk of pulmonary and systemic thromboembolism.

Three distinct patterns of ARVC have been identified by the clinicogenetic characterization of families:

1. a right ventricular phenotype (either isolated or associated with some left ventricular involvement;
2. a left dominant phenotype, with early and prominent left ventricular manifestations;
3. a biventricular phenotype, characterized by equal involvement of both ventricles.

Arrhythmias of right ventricular or left ventricular origin, or both, and inferolateral ECG abnormalities are seen in the last two patterns, which might be misdiagnosed as dilated cardiomyopathy, although ECG abnormalities and arrhythmic symptoms predominate. Genotype–phenotype correlations have shown a higher occurrence of left ventricular involvement in carriers of desmoplakin mutations. These findings question the view that left ventricular involvement occurs only in the late stages of the disease, and support the adoption of the broader term arrhythmogenic cardiomyopathy.

Cardiac arrest due to VF can occur at any time during the disease course, and the incidence of sudden death varies from 0.1% to 3.0% per year in adults with ARVC/D.

However, this rate might be higher in young people, when sudden death can be the first sign of the disease.

19.2.6 Pathogenesis

The replacement of the right ventricular myocardium by fibrofatty tissue is progressive, starting from the epicardium or mid-myocardium and then extending to become transmural. Progression then leads to wall thinning and aneurysms, typically located at the inferior, apical, and infundibular walls (so-called triangle of dysplasia), the hallmark of ARVC/D [10].

19.2.6.1 Triangle of Dysplasia

These typical morphological characteristics of the right ventricle may be useful in the differential diagnosis with training-induced right ventricular adaptation (*athlete's heart*), usually consisting of global right ventricular enlargement without regional dilatation or deformities. Moreover, in about 50% of cases, the posterior sub-epicardial segment of the left ventricle is also interested.

Histologically, fibrofatty infiltration is usually associated with focal myocardial necrosis and patchy inflammatory infiltrates. Fibro-fatty scars and aneurysms are potential sources of life-threatening ventricular arrhythmias. The histopathological arrangement of the surviving myocardium embedded in the replaced fibro-fatty tissue may lead to inhomogeneous intraventricular conduction predisposing to re-entrant mechanisms [10]. Impaired mechanical coupling might account for abnormal electrical coupling by gap junction remodeling.

The correlation between the acute arrhythmic events and the exercise is of not univocal interpretation:

1. Physical exercise acutely increases right ventricular afterload and cavity enlargement which, in turn, may elicit ventricular arrhythmias by stretching the diseased right ventricular myocardium, in particular the areas more susceptible to sheer stress, favoring cellular death and ventricular arrhythmias, in the presence of genetic disorders;
2. wall mechanical stress, such as that induced by right ventricular volume overload during exercise, and increased heart rate may contribute to the cardiac ryanodine channel dysfunction.
3. the progressive fibro-fatty replacement of the right ventricle may damage the sympathetic nerve trunks, which would be hypersensitive to the free catecholamines and responsible for re-entrant mechanisms and arrhythmias (*denervation supersensitivity*);
4. a potential arrhythmogenic mechanism of sport-related cardiac arrest in patients with ARVC/D is triggered activity due to late after-depolarizations, which are provoked by intracellular calcium overload and enhanced by adrenergic stimulation.

19.2.7 Diagnosis

The disease affects men more frequently than women and becomes clinically overt usually from the second to the fourth decade of life. Symptoms and signs do not usually appear before puberty or beyond the age of 60 years. However, occasionally the first clinical manifestations arise even in patients older than 70 years of age.

The practising physician should be aware of the possibility of ARVC/D when presented with adolescents or young individuals with palpitations, syncope, or aborted sudden death. Ventricular tachycardia (VT) of left bundle branch block morphology is the primary reason to suspect ARVC/D, and idiopathic right ventricular outflow tachycardia is the main differential diagnosis. ECG changes such as T wave inversion in V1–V3 or premature ventricular complexes of left bundle branch block morphology should also raise suspicion of ARVC/D, even in asymptomatic individuals (Fig. 19.3).

The diagnosis of ARVD/C is currently based on the presence of major and minor standardized Task Force Criteria [14], including ECG, ventricular arrhythmias, right ventricular function and morphology, histopathology and family history (Table 19.3).

Diagnosis is established when two major, one major plus two minor, or four minor criteria from different groups are fulfilled.

These criteria have been a guide to ARVC/D diagnosis over the past 15 years and have been partic-

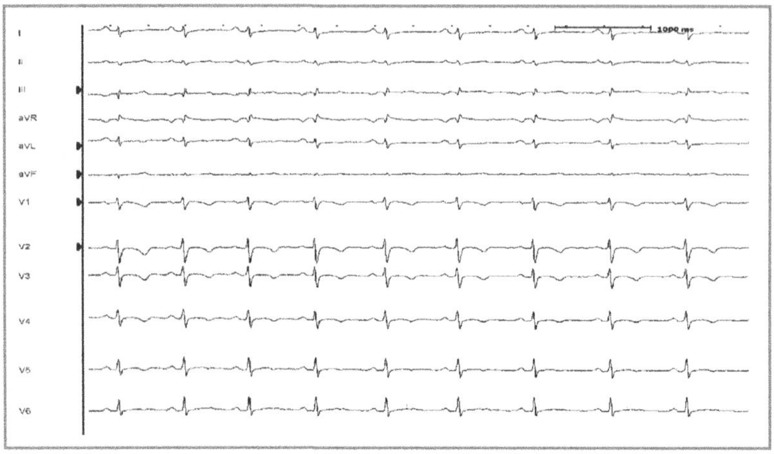

Fig. 19.3 Man, 32 years old, with sporadic palpitations. At pre-participation screening T wave abnormalities in V1-V4. The subsequent medical evaluation will make diagnosis of ARVC/D

Tabella 19.3 Task Force Criteria [modified from 14]

Global or regional dysfunction and structural abnormalities	Major	2D Eco	Akinesia, regional dyskinesia or RV aneurysm 1 of the following (tele-diastole) - PLAX RVOT >32 mm (PLAX/BSA >19 mm/m^2) - PSAX RVOT>36 mm (PSAX/BSA >21 mm/m^2) - or fractional area change <33%
		MRI	Akinesia, regional dyskinesia or dyssynchrony 1 of the following - ratio EDV/BSA >110 mL/m2 (male) or >100 mL/m^2 (female) - or EF VDx <40%
		RV angiography	Akinesia, regional dyskinesia or RV aneurysm
	Minor	2D Eco	Akinesia, regional dyskinesia of the RV 1 of the following (tele-diastole) - PLAX RVOT >29 and <32 mm (PLAX/BSA >16 and <19 mm/m^2) - PSAX RVOT >32 and <36 mm (PLAX/BSA >18 and <21 mm/m^2) - or fractional area change >33% e <40%
		MRI	Akinesia, regional dyskinesia or dyssynchrony 1 of the following - ratio EDV/BSA >100 and <110 mL/m^2 (male) or >90 mL/m^2 and <100 (female) - or EF VDx >40% and <45%
Tissue characteristics	Major		Residual myocites <60% to the morphometric analysis (or <50% estimated),fatty replacement of the free-wall RV >1 sample, with or without fatty replacement at endomyocardial biopsy
	Minor		Residual myocites >60% and <75% to the morphometric analysis (or <50%-75% estimated),fatty replacement of the free-wall RV >1 sample, with or without fatty replacement at endomyocardial biopsy
Repolarization abnormalities	Major		Negative T wave in right precordial leads and over in subjects >14 years older (without RBBB)
	Minor		Negative T wave in V1-V2 in subjects >14 years old (without RBBB) or in V4-V6 Negative T wave in V1-V2 in subjects >14 years old with RBBB

(cont. →)

Tabella 19.3 *(continued)*

Depolarization /conduction abnormalities	Major	ε wave in right precordial leads (V1-V3)
	Minor	Late potentials (SAECG) in >1of 3 parameters in absence of QRS>110 msec at 12 lead EKG Filtered QRS> 114 ms Terminal (last 40 msec) QRS duration >38 ms Root mean square < 20mV Terminal QRS duration >55 ms without RBBB
Arrhythmia	Major	sVT or nsVT with LBBB morphology and superior axis (positive QRS in aVL)
	Minor	nsVT or sVT LBBB morphology and inferior/undetermined axis PVCs>500 in 24 hours
Familial history	Major	1 I-degree relative affected by ARVD (current definition) Autoptic diagnosis of ARVD in a I-degree relative (current definition) Genetic abnormality associated with ARVD
	Minor	History of ARVD/C in a I-degree relative Sudden death (<35 years) in a I-degree relative suspected for ARVC/D ARVC/D diagnosis in a II-degree relative

ARVD/C arrhythmogenic right ventricular dysplasia/cardiomyopathy, *RBBB* right bundle branch block, *BSA* body surface area, *EDV* end diastolic volume, *EF* ejection fraction, *nsVT* non sustained ventricular tachycardia, *sVT* sustained ventricular tachycardia, *PLAX* parasternal long axis, *PSAX* parasternal short axis, *SAECG* signal averaging ECG, *RVOT* right ventricle outflow tract

ularly useful for differential diagnosis with dilated cardiomyopathy and idiopathic right ventricular outflow tract tachycardia, despite the lack of quantification of the various degrees of morpho-functional right ventricular abnormalities.

A modification of Task Force Criteria [15] has been proposed to allow detection of ARVD/C in first degree relatives with early or incomplete phenotyping during family screening of subjects with clinically or pathologically proven ARVC/D (Table 19.4).

The presence of any criteria such as inverted T waves (V1–V3) in individuals older than 14 years, late potentials on signal-averaged ECG, more than 200 premature ventricular complexes in 24 h, VT of left bundle branch block morphology, or mild right ventricular structure or function abnormalities can be diagnostic without the requirement to fulfill traditional Task Force Criteria.

Moreover, *echocardiography* is the first-line imaging method for both diagnosis and follow-up, for the assessment of typical structural changes in the right ventricle, i.e. wall motion abnormalities, trabecular derangement, and sacculations. Recently, quantitative criteria for defining abnormal size and function have been proposed, and diastolic dilatation of the right ventricular outflow tract has been a consistent feature in ARVC/D subjects (100%), with sizes of more than 30 mm in 89% of cases.

Magnetic Resonance Imaging (MRI) is a promising imaging method due to its ability for tissue characterization, but has limited diagnostic

Table 19.4 EKG criteria for diagnosis of ARVD (italics, criteria introduced later from the Task Force)

Depolarization abnormalities	QRS >110 msec in V1-V3 ε wave *TAD >55 msec in V1-V3*
Repolarization abnormalities	Onde T neg. in V1-V3 SA-ECG patologici
VT	LBB VT *LBB TV and superior axis* *Polimorhic VT*

TAD terminal activation delay of QRS; *VT* ventricular tachicardia; *LBB* left brunch block; *SA-EKG* signal averaged ECG specificity in the absence of concomitant wall motion abnormalities, because fatty tissue in the right ventricular free wall is common in normal hearts, particularly in obese and elderly people.

Thus, cine-MRI can be useful for estimating wall motion abnormalities, in association with right ventricular volume or structure.

Moreover, MRI with gadolinium enhancement can detect intra-myocardial fibrosis, a finding that can precede functional abnormalities, thus allowing disease detection at an earlier stage than the Task Force Criteria.

The angiography has a sensitivity >90% to assess akinetic and dyskinetic bulging at the level of the triangle of dysplasia.

Three-dimensional electroanatomical mapping can reveal low voltage areas that correspond to fibro-fatty myocardial replacement and could assist in the differential diagnosis with diseases that mimic ARVC/D, such as inflammatory cardiomyopathy and idiopathic right ventricular outflow tract tachycardia.

In some cases, *transvenous endomyocardial biopsy* can assist diagnosis by indicating fibro-fatty replacement and allowing exclusion of phenocopies, such as myocarditis and sarcoidosis. Actually, on morphometric analysis of endomyocardial biopsy specimens, myocardial atrophy due to fibro-fatty replacement, with a residual amount of the myocardium of less than 60%, should be regarded as a major diagnostic criterion, whereas an amount of 60–75% is a minor diagnostic criterion. Moreover the possibility to detect changes in the various intercalated disk proteins with immunohistochemical staining suggests a potential role of endomyocardial biopsy even for early diagnosis of ARVC/D.

Follow-up assessment is based on serial non-invasive tests, such as ECG (at rest and during exercise), ECG Holter monitoring and echocardiography. In case of ventricular arrhythmias, an invasive electrophysiological study needs to be planned.

19.2.8 Differential Diagnosis with Athlete's Heart

The ARVC/D diagnosis may be difficult in young athletes, in particular in the presence of training-induced right ventricular adaptation (*athlete's heart*), usually consisting of global right ventricular enlargement without regional dilatation or deformities.

Morphological criteria suggesting true ARVC/D rather than physiological ventricular enlargement include global right ventricular systolic dysfunction and regional wall motion abnormalities, such as bulging or aneurysm. In the absence of obvious structural changes of the right ventricle, frequent premature ventricular complexes or inverted T-waves in precordial leads can be benign. However, caution is justified before considering these features as part of the athlete's heart syndrome, and further non-invasive investigations are advised to avoid the catastrophic consequences of a missed diagnosis. The advent of molecular genetics will provide new insights into the definite diagnosis of ARVC/D [16].

19.2.9 Pre-participation Screening

A systematic pre-participation screening program has been developed by the Center for Sports Medicine in Padua [6,17].

When compared with the pre-screening period (1979–1981), the relative risk of sudden cardiovascular death has been 44% lower in the early screening period (1982–1992) and 79% lower in the late screening period (1993–2004).

Most of the reduced death rate has been due to fewer cases of sudden death from cardiomyopathy, mostly from ARVC/D. Time-trend analysis has showed that the incidence of sudden death from this latter condition fell by 84% over the 24-year span (from 3.8/100,000 person-years to 0.4/100,000 person-years).

This decline of mortality from cardiomyopathy paralleled the concomitant increase in the number of athletes with cardiomyopathy (both hypertrophic cardiomyopathy and ARVC/D) who were identified and disqualified from competitive sports.

Thus, the early identification of the athletes affected by ARVC/D has a crucial role in the prevention of the sudden death. Most of the young athletes who die suddenly of ARVC/D show ECG abnormalities that could raise the suspicion of underlying cardiovascular disease at preparticipation evaluation and lead to further testing for a definitive diagnosis. Right precordial T-wave inversion (beyond V1) appears to be the most useful clinical marker for the presence of potentially fatal ARVC/D in apparently healthy young competitive athletes, considering that T-wave inversion in V1-V3 occurs in less than 1% of men with apparently normal hearts who are aged 19-45 years [18]. More than 80% of the athletes who died from ARVC/D in the Veneto region had a history of syncope, ECG changes, or ventricular arrhythmias [12].

In a retrospective analysis by Turrini et al. [19], a QRS dispersion greater than or equal to 40 milliseconds represents the strongest independent predictor of sudden death with a sensitivity and specificity of 90% and 77%, respectively.

A life saving screening in the athletes has to start with an accurate clinical and family history, physical examination and with a basal 12-lead ECG, which represents a sensitive and powerful tool in the identification, risk stratification and treatment of patients affected by ARVC/D [20]. In fact, also in asymptomatic subjects, depolarization and repolarization abnormalities in the right precordial leads have to be considered with caution. Finally, selected patients in whom a non-invasive assessment is inconclusive may require further examination by MRI, contrast angiography and endomyocardial biopsy to confirm diagnosis.

Comprehensive mutation screening of known ARVC/D genes can detect genetic abnormalities in at least 40–50% of subjects [10]. Candidates for genetic screening include both index cases with borderline diagnostic findings and family members of gene-positive subjects. A significant proportion of family members carry the genetic mutation but do not present with clinical signs (*healthy carriers*). As the disease is progressive and can appear late in life, these asymptomatic subjects must be considered potentially at risk and should undergo serial and frequent cardiac follow-up, including medical history, basal 12-lead ECG, 24-h Holter monitoring, exercise testing and echocardiography. Thus, physical activity/competitive sports should be always forbidden considering the legal implications. Non-competitive sports may be allowed, provided there are regular check-ups in the follow-up period.

On the other hand, about 50% of the family members have negative results for the disease gene mutation (*non-carrier*). These subjects can be considered healthy, do not need further check-ups, and can be assured that they will not transmit the disease to offspring.

Only one-third of family members with positive genetic tests fulfill the diagnostic criteria, while 15% share some ECG abnormalities (e.g., premature ventricular beats, positive late potentials), although they are not enough to achieve the diagnosis.

19.2.10 Recommendations for Sport Activity in Athletes Affected by ARVC/D

The prevention of the sudden death is the most important strategy in the management of ARVC/D [6,7,20].

Retrospective analyses have identified several risk factors, such as previous cardiac arrest, syncope, young age, malignant family history, participation in competitive sports, VT, severe right ventricular dysfunction, left ventricular involvement and QRS dispersion of 40 ms or more. However, the prognostic value of these single or combined risk factors has not been prospectively assessed.

In summary:

1. *Asymptomatic patients and healthy carriers* do not require prophylactic treatment. They should instead undergo cardiac follow-up, including medical history, basal 12-lead ECG, 24-h Holter monitoring, exercise testing, and echocardiography on a regular basis for the early identification of warning symptoms, new onset or worsening of morphofunctional right ventricular abnormalities and ventricular arrhythmias.
2. In patients affected by ARVC/D with hemodynamically stable arrhythmias, such as non-sustained or sustained VT, either β-blockers or class III antiarrhythmic drugs (sotalol and amiodarone), used alone or in combination, are the most effective agents, with a low proarrhythmic risk. Catheter ablation of VT is suc-

cessful in 60-90% of cases, but the recurrence rate is considerable, because of the progressive nature of the disease

3. Treatment with ICD is indicated *in patients with cardiac arrest, syncope, or hemodynamically poorly-tolerated VT despite antiarrhythmic therapy*. On the other hand, ICD implantation for the primary prevention of sudden death in patients with multiple risk factors, family history of sudden death, or VT/VF inducibility with programmed ventricular stimulation is controversial and needs individual clinical decisions.

According to US and European recommendations for sports eligibility, athletes with a clinical diagnosis of ARVC/D should be excluded from all competitive sports. This recommendation is independent of age, gender, and phenotypic appearance and does not differ for those athletes without symptoms, or for those treated with drugs, surgery, catheter ablation, or an implantable defibrillator. The presence of a free-standing automated external defibrillator at sporting events should not be considered absolute protection against sudden death, nor should it be considered a justification for participation in competitive sports in athletes with previously diagnosed ARVC/D.

In fact, the definitive cure for the disease is still elusive. All of the previously mentioned therapeutic and preventive measures are palliative and not curative. Cardiac transplantation is used to treat end-stage cardiac failure or refractory electrical instability.

References

1. Maron BJ (2002) Hypertrophic cardiomyopathy: a systematic review. JAMA 287:1308-1320
2. Maron BJ, McKenna WJ, Danielson GK et al (2003) American College of Cardiology/European Society of Cardiology clinical expert consensus document on hypertrophic cardiomyopathy. A report of the American College of Cardiology Task Force on clinical expert society of cardiology committee for practice guidelines committee to develop an expert consensus document on hypertrophic cardiomyopathy. J Am Coll Cardiol 42:1687-1713
3. Maron BJ (2009) Distinguishing hypertrophic cardiomyopathy from athletes heart physiological remodeling: clinical significance, diagnostic strategies and implications for preparticipation screening. Br J Sports Med 43:649-656
4. Medicina dello Sport (2010) Rivista trimestrale della Federazione Medico-Sportiva Italiana. Protocolli cardiologici per il giudizio di idoneità allo sport agonistico 2009. Marzo 2010, vol 63
5. Maron BJ (2007) Hypertrophic cardiomyopathy and other causes of sudden cardiac death in young competitive athletes, with considerations for preparticipation screening and criteria for disqualification. Cardiol Clin 25:399-414
6. Maron BJ, Zipes DP (2005) 36th Bethesda Conference: eligibility recommendations for competitive athletes with cardiovascular abnormalities. J Am Coll Cardiol 45:1312-1375
7. Corrado D, Pelliccia A, Bjørnstad HH et al (2005) Cardiovascular preparticipation screening of young competitive athletes for prevention of sudden death: proposal for a common European protocol Consensus Statement of the Study Group of Sport Cardiology of the Working Group of Cardiac Rehabilitation and Exercise Physiology and the Working Group of Myocardial and Pericardial Diseases of the European Society of Cardiology. Eur Heart J 26:516-524
8. Pelliccia A, Maron BJ (1995) Preparticipation cardiovascular evaluation of the competitive athlete: Perspectives from the 30-year Italian experience. Am J Cardiol 75:827-828
9. Maron BJ, Thompson PD, Ackerman MJ et al (2007) Recommendations and considerations related to preparticipation screening for cardiovascular abnormalities in competitive athletes. 2007 Update: A scientific statement from the American Heart Association Council on Nutrition, Physical Activity, and Metabolism: Endorsed by the American College of Cardiology Foundation. Circulation 115;1643-1655
10. Basso C, Corrado D, Marcus FI et al (2009) Arrhythmogenic right ventricular cardiomyopathy. Lancet 373:1289-1300
11. Corrado D, Thiene G, Nava A et al (1990) Sudden death in young competitive athletes: clinico-pathologic correlations in 22 cases. Am J Med 89:588-596
12. Corrado D, Basso C, Schiavon M et al (1998) Screening for hypertrophic cardiomyopathy in young athletes. N Engl J Med 339:364-369
13. Corrado D, Basso C, Rizzoli G et al (2003) Does sports activity enhance the risk of sudden death in adolescents and young adults? J Am Coll Cardiol 42:1959-1963
14. McKenna WJ, Thiene G, Nava A et al. (1994) Diagnosis of arrhythmogenic right ventricular dysplasia/cardiomyopathy. Task Force of the Working Group Myocardial and Pericardial Disease of the European Society of Cardiology and of the Scientific Council on Cardiomyopathies of the International Society and Federation of Cardiology. Br Heart J 71:215-218
15. Hamid MS, Norman M, Quraishi A et al (2002) Prospective evaluation of relatives for familial arrhythmo-

genic right ventricular cardiomyopathy/dysplasia reveals a need to broaden diagnostic criteria. J Am Coll Cardiol 40:1445-1450
16. Maron BJ, Pelliccia A, Spirito P (1995) Cardiac disease in young trained athletes: insights into methods for distinguishing athletès heart from structural heart disease, with particular emphasis on hypertrophic cardiomyopathy. Circulation 91:1596-1601
17. Corrado D, Basso C, Pavei A et al (2006) Trends in sudden cardiovascular death in young competitive athletes after implementation of a preparticipation screening program. JAMA 296:1593-1601
18. Marcus FI (2005) Prevalence of T-wave inversion beyond V1 in young normal individuals and usefulness for the diagnosis of arrhythmogenic right ventricular cardiomyo-pathy/dysplasia. Am J Cardiol 95:1070-1071
19. Turrini P, Corrado D, Basso C et al (2001) Dispersion of ventricular depolarization-repolarization: a noninvasive marker for risk stratification in arrhythmogenic right ventricular cardiomyopathy. Circulation 103:3075-3080
20. Basso C, Corrado D, Thiene G et al (2007) Arrhythmogenic right ventricular cardiomyopathy in athletes: diagnosis, management, and recommendations for sport activity. Cardiol Clin 25:415-422

Myocarditis and Pericarditis in Young Athletes

20

Enrica Mariano, Maria Bianchi, Antonio Lucifero and Fiorella Caranci

20.1 Introduction

Electrocardiographic and echocardiographic alterations in young athletes are usually the expression of physiological heart adaptation to physical training (athlete's heart) [1-2]. This thesis may generate confusion about the interpretation of all EKG anomalies detected in young athletes, including arrhythmias and repolarization disorders.

On the other hand, the high percentage of histopathological findings documented in subjects sampled by endomyocardial biopsy that are typical of acute or subacute myocarditis, such as fibrosis, increased interstitial adipose tissue, is seen in subjects affected by arrhythmias in the absence of cardiopathies at the onset of symptoms [3].

Myocarditis has been suggested as the cause of ventricular repolarization disorders [4] and arrhythmias clinically documented [5-6] in apparently healthy athletes even if the presence of a direct correlation is not clearly demonstrated *in vivo* [7]. Moreover, the same disease in suspected as the pathophysiological substrate of some cases of sudden death in young athletes, probably triggering an episode of fatal ventricular fibrillation [8-10].

Zeppilli et al. [11] documented in 1994 unequivocal diagnosis of myocarditis in four young athletes (two subjects with fibrosis and two without fibrosis) of a group of six patients subjected to endomyocardial biopsy for minor heart rhythm disturbances and aspecific echocardiographic anomalies (Fig. 20.1); in the other two athletes morphological and functional anomalies are associated with aspecific fibrosis findings in histological samples and clinical data suggestive of myocarditis.

The experience of these authors underlines the fact that echocardiographic assessment of these patients is to be careful, especially in the presence

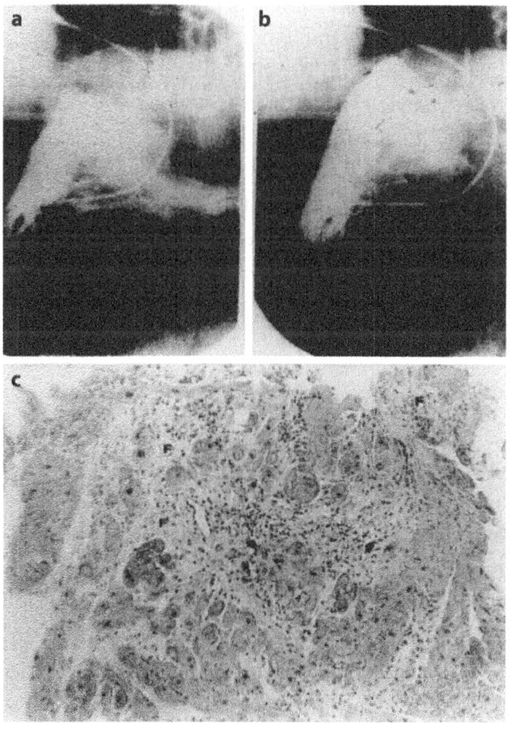

Fig. 20.1 a Right ventriculography (*left diastole, right systole*) that shows mild right ventricle dilatation and apical hypokinesia. b Endomyocardial biopsy findings suggestive of myocarditis with fibrosis and some cell necrosis (hematoxylin-eosin coloration, magnification x 1000)

E. Mariano (✉)
Interventional Cardiology Unit
"Tor Vergata" University, Rome, Italy

M. Fioranelli and G. Frajese (eds.), *Sports Cardiology*,
DOI: 10.1007/978-88-470-2775-6_20, © Springer-Verlag Italia 2012

of non-significant anomalies such as slight depression of the ejection fraction and the presence of minor segmental dyssynergia, and in such cases, to be repeated after an adequate period of physical *detraining*, in order to rule out the confusing factor of the *athlete's heart* phenomenon in the clinical interpretation of the data collected.

Dilated cardiomyopathy, at the onset of symptoms, for example, when the ejection fraction is still conserved, may mimic all echocardiographic alterations typical of *athlete's heart.*

Stress echocardiography has a key role in the diagnostic stratification of subjects with altered contractility only after strenuous exercise.

Arrhythmogenic right ventricle dysplasia (ARVD) has been recognized as the principle cause of sudden death in young athletes for years, even leading to false diagnosis, because ventricular arrhythmias with the appearance of left bundle branch block are not always due to the same substrate. These alterations are, sometimes, the consequence of the action of some pathogen agents, which provokes transitory alterations in the acute phase of myocarditis like dilatation and apical right ventricle hypokinesia, which progressively regress during follow-up [12].

Early detection of myocarditis in young athletes dictates the prescription of a period of physical training abstention, because strenuous exercise may negatively influence immunological process correlated to myocardial inflammation [13].

20.2 Myocarditis in Young Athletes

20.2.1 Diagnostic Procedure

Myocarditis is defined as an inflammatory process of the cardiac tissues. Infective forms, which normally have a viral etiology, are of great interest in the field of sports.

Common symptoms in acute forms are characterized by chest pain, palpitations and effort dyspnea associated with an increase in inflammation markers, while many cases have an asymptomatic clinical presentation (asthenia, transitory fever and rare palpitations) and are, therefore, underestimated by athletes. Physical examination in the acute phase normally documents an apex sound corresponding to mitral insufficiency and the presence of a third or fourth tone.

ECG tracings show low QRS voltages in precordial leads, arrhythmias, ventricular repolarization and atrioventricular conduction disturbances.

Doppler echocardiography shows, especially in extensive cases, overall left ventricular depression of systolic function associated with left chamber dilatation. The seriousness of these anomalies may be slight and segmentary and may regress after myocarditis recovery. MRI too may integrate Doppler data, detecting *delayed enhancement,* which is a typical radiological finding of the myocarditis process.

Endomyocardial biopsy plays a key role in the diagnostic confirmation of myocarditis, especially as it is crucial for therapeutic purposes. Young athletes with confirmed diagnosis of myocarditis are ineligible for any fitness competition until complete disease resolution, and in any case, within six months of the onset of symptoms. After this period, a careful re-evaluation of the case, in the absence of clinical and biological signs of the disease, is necessary in order to rule out morphological and functional heart sequelae and arrhythmias and to enable agonistic activity. Nevertheless, periodical check-ups are provided for this kind of patient.

20.2.2 Myocarditis as a Cause of Sudden Death

Myocarditis, especially in its acute and subacute forms, is a frequent cause of sudden death [14] in young athletes. A large amount of data from the literature correlates myocarditis with up 11-20% of cases of sudden death during sport [15]. *Sudden death* is defined as every case of death that happens out of the hospital within one hour from the onset of symptoms and correlated with any cardiac disease [16]. This problematic issue is exacerbated by the fact that these subjects are normally considered at low risk for developing this fatal event, making it difficult to prevent sudden death in this cohort of patients.

Fortunately, sudden death occurs in only 1-2%

of all cardiac deaths in young athletes (< 35 years). An Australian study demonstrated that in up to 29% of cases the heart is completely healthy, suggesting a genetic syndrome as the most common background followed by myocardial infarction (25%), myocarditis (12%) and hypertrophic cardiomyopathy in only 6% of all cardiac deaths in young athletes. On the other hand, in the USA hypertrophic cardiomyopathy is considered the principal cause of sudden cardiac death while in northern Italy arrhythmogenic right ventricle dysplasia is ascertained as the most important etiology of *sudden death*. Early detection of myocarditis is crucial in young athletes because of the controversial role of strenuous physical activity in causing sudden death.

20.2.3 Diagnosis

The clinical diagnosis of myocarditis is usually difficult. Many international and national task forces have defined clinical and ECG criteria for confirmed diagnosis of myocarditis [17], while laboratory diagnosis is based on inflammation parameters and specific bacteria or virus antibody serology.

Myocarditis is an inflammatory process of the myocardial tissue, usually secondary to respiratory or gastrointestinal infections. Histological findings in biopsy specimens are usually characterized by lymphomonocytic foci associated with non-ischemic necrosis of myocytes [18].

The incidence of myocarditis is probably higher in young athletes because of the variability in the clinical presentation and the uncertainty of non-invasive diagnostic criteria.

The most common pathogenic noxae are represented by adenovirus, citomegalovirus, enterovirus, herpes virus and parvovirus B 19. Bacterial forms include *Chlamydia*, *Pneumoniae*, *Borrelia* e *Bartonella*. Viral myocarditis diagnosis requires genomic confirmation of endomyocardial or epicardial biopsies. Animal studies have demonstrated that a murine infection is exacerbated by physical exercise, malnutrition and sex hormones, etc. [48]. Infected mice show three phases of the disease, which may probably be applied to human model.

The acute phase (days 0-3) is characterized by direct cardiomyocyte toxicity due to cytokines like TNFα, IFNγ and IL-1b in the absence of inflammatory cells. The subacute phase (days 4-14) is characterized by inflammatory infiltrates associated with the secretion of many cytokines like IL-1, IL-2, IL-6, IL-8 and adhesion molecules stimulated by NF-κB transcription markers. The third phase (days 15-90) may lead to the development of dilated cardiomyopathy with an increase in fibrosis and viral replication.

It is known that the treatment of heart failure prevention is based on the use of beta-blockers, ACE inhibitors and aldosterone antagonists. These drugs associated with physical activity suspension for at least six months, reduce mortality, according to observations by Burch and McDonald and Burch and Giles, which clearly showed the normal appearance of the cardiac silhouette in 60% of patients affected, after one year of rest [49-50].

20.2.4 Rule of Conduct

National and international guidelines have been proposed for the diagnosis, treatment and follow-up of patients affected by myocarditis [1-10]. These guidelines clearly underline the fact that subjects with confirmed or very probable diagnosis of myocarditis are ineligible for any competitive sport until complete disease recovery and in any case within six months from the onset of symptoms [8,11]. After this period an adequate re-evaluation of the case is necessary in order to rule out any morphological and functional heart sequelae.

A resumption of physical training is reconsidered in the absence of contractile function depression and significant arrhythmias upon Holter monitoring or a maximal ergometric test. Young athletes are in any case to be periodically checked by expert cardiological centres.

Felicani et al. [18] prepared some *screening protocols* as shown by Naccarella's experience at the Bologna Main Hospital. This study collected two sets of prospective case records: the first from 1990 to 2005, with 119 athletes and the second from 2006 that documented 11 consecutive cases of myocarditis in young athletes. Screening is pro-

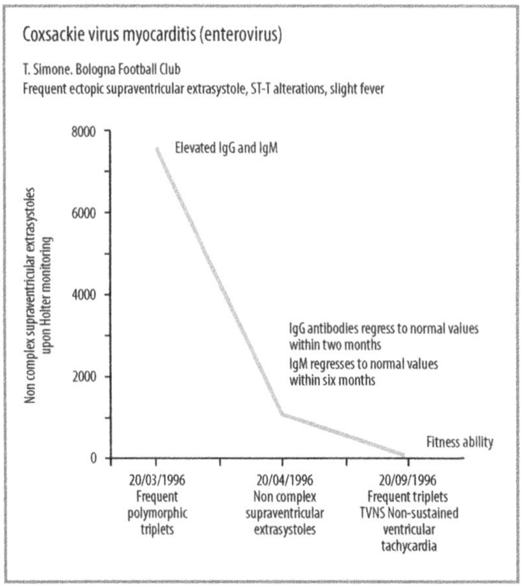

Fig. 20.2 Correlation between arrhythmia and serology evolution in a patient affected by enterovirus infection

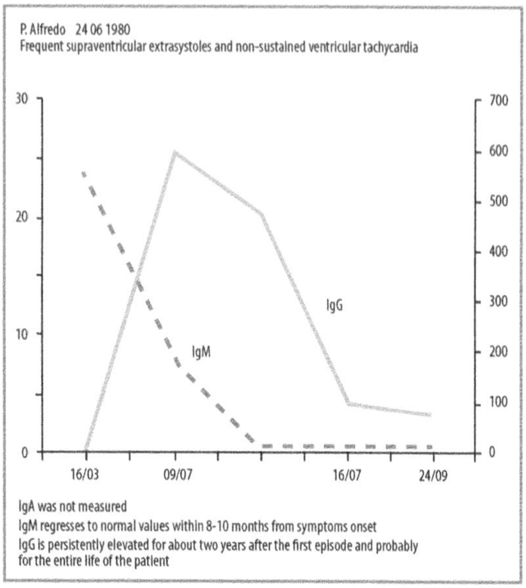

Fig. 20.3 Correlation between arrhythmia and serology evolution in a patient affected by toxoplasmosis

posed for subjects with weak signs of systemic infection, the onset of ventricular arrhythmias and ST-T EKG anomalies [18]. 56 (47%) of the 119 screened patients showed positive serology for viral or bacterial myocarditis, as reported in table 20.1. Serological verifications are performed at the initial check-up and three and six months before physical activity resumption. Only 28 (50%)of these 56 patients presented clinical signs of myocarditis associated with systemic infection. All patients presented fever, signs of recent respiratory or gastrointestinal infection. In 5 cases signs, heart failure or cardiomegaly were present. In two cases, congestive heart failure, with pericardial or pleural effusion, was detected. In one case myocarditis simulated acute myocardial infarction, with various forms of atrio-ventricular and bunch block, dilated cardiomyopathy and acute cardiac failure. Arrhythmic complications were usually ventricular (27 of 28 cases, 96%) and in 6 cases intraventricular block and transitory or permanent atrioventricular block. In 26 cases of 28 patients physical training was interrupted for 6-12 months, according to COCIS protocols [19].

Table 20.1 Aetiologies of atypical viral myocarditis

- 12 cases of echo-coxsackie B, enterovirus (one fatal case of giant-cell viral myocarditis)
- 4 cases of toxoplasmosis (one fatal case)
- 4 cases of infective mononucleosis
- 2 cases of *Mycoplasma pneumoniae*, two cases in association with *herpes virus* and *herpes zoster* infections
- 1 case of borelliosis or Lyme syndrome
- 1 case of legionellosis

Concerning the *etiology*, in 56 subjects who were positive for serological screening, 28 patients with clinical signs of myocarditis were particularly analysed (Table 20.1). In Figures 20.2 e 20.3, correlations between ventricular arrhythmias and serology evolution in subjects affected by enterovirus, toxoplasmosis and legionellosis are graphically represented.

Right ventricle endomyocardial biopsy was performed only in two cases according to criteria proposed by literature [17].

In seven cases, endocavitary electrophysiological mapping was performed after clinical recovery, in order to verify major arrhythmias inducibility, with a protocol similar to the protocol used for other arrhythmic syndromes [14].

This protocol has been integrated with other invasive or non-invasive diagnostic tools, for ruling out other pathologies associated with myocarditis, like Brugada syndrome [14] or arrhythmogenic right ventricle dysplasia [18].

Lymphocytic typing provided in the protocol enabled the detection of two cases: one of congenital immunodeficiency characterized by recurrent infections and another of acquired immunodeficiency in a patient with HIV syndrome, in a young subject with pulmonary, pleuropericardial and endocardial recurrent infections associated with septic emboli [17]. Autoantigen and autoantibody serology made it possible to diagnose a case of perimyocarditis during a systemic connective tissue infection like LES.

Disease evolution is generally favourable after specific drug treatment, physical activity withdrawal and rest for 6-12 months. Physical training was resumed in 18 cases of 28 (64%). No serious or fatal sequelae are described in this first group, except for the three deaths ascertained. Relapse of myocarditis occurs in 4 cases out of 18 (22%).

Ablations for ventricular or supraventricular arrhythmias were performed in 6 cases out of 28 (21%) while competition-level fitness was allowed only in 3 out of six cases (50%) after an ablation procedure.

Fitness competition ability was generally denied in 10 cases out of 28 (35.7%) because of serious sequelae on ejection fraction or persistence of major ventricular arrhythmias.

20.2.5 Incidence and Prevalence

It is probable that the incidence of myocarditis is lower in the general young population in comparison with young athletes, as clearly documented by international case records of young soldiers or college students [5,8-9]

Concerning prevalence, it is strictly correlated with the type of case record and method of selecting patients [14,20].

A key role is played by the periodical measurement of antibodies against specific viruses or bacteria, IgM and IgA typologies in the acute phase and IGg typologies in the chronic phase that represents an immunological memory of the previous infection.

Sometimes antibody serology is altered only for few days in the acute phase and is thus difficult to document. In the chronic phase, elevated IgG levels against specific bacterial infections are usually documented while antibodies against viral infections are more difficult to detect.

20.2.6 Systemic and/or Myocardial Infection?

It is therefore clear that the aspects discussed above are indicative of systemic infection with tropism of the myocardial tissue.

The only examination that is suitable for confirming myocarditis is right ventricle endomyocardial biopsy, which is represented by an invasive procedure that consists of sampling a specimen from the interventricular septum during heart catheterization. Nevertheless, endomyocardial biopsy results are frequently negative and holds a limited diagnostic value if the disease is not largely diffused in myocardial tissues.

Right ventricle free-wall endomyocardial biopsy is more specific and sensitive even if associated with more hemopericardium and cardiac tamponade complications. Left ventricle endomyocardial biopsy may alternatively be performed [15-17].

20.2.7 Clinical Presentation

Normalization of inflammation markers and antiviral or antibacterial serology is typically correlated with complete regression of major ventricular arrhythmias (Figs. 20.1-20.2).

Echocardiographic assessment plays a key role in following disease evolution according to the evaluation of regional contractile anomalies, pericardial effusion, fibrosis or pericardial surface thickening.

20.2.8 Prognosis

The course is generally favourable, allowing for good prognosis after specific treatment [17-18]. Physical activity withdrawal and strict rest for 6-12 months is fundamental for patient recovery. In the Bologna group's experience, sport activity was resumed in a high percentage of cases (18 out of 28 cases, 64%).

It is important to recall that pericardiomyocarditis, once erroneously called *benign*, has a tendency to recur.

4 out of 18 cases (22%) relapsed even many years after the initial episode. In 6 cases out of 28 (21%) ablation procedures were performed for ventricular or supraventricular arrhythmias. Eligibility for competition was allowed only in 3 out of 6 cases (50%). In a large cohort of patients (10 out of 28) resumption of physical activity was denied because of serious sequelae on myocardial contractility and persistence of complex and frequent ventricular arrhythmias. Two acute and one follow-up case and two cases of dilated cardiomyopathies (only one severe) are described.

Rare cases of post ventricular arrhythmias ablation procedures deaths and even more rare cases after supraventricular ablation procedures are sometimes documented [9].

Young athletes subjected to transcatheter ablation may resume physical activity after adequate re-evaluation that includes an echocardiographic assessment, Holter monitoring, and sometimes an electrophysiological study, provided that:

1. there is another heart disease;
2. a period of 3-6 months from intervention has passed;
3. there are no ECG preexcitation signs in cases of Wolff-Parkinson-White syndrome or ventricular and supraventricular anomalies;
4. they are asymptomatic, without supraventricular tachycardia or atrial fibrillation relapse.

20.3 Pericarditis in Young Athletes

Pericarditis is defined as pericardial inflammation, which normally involves cardiac tissue on subepicardial surfaces and is caused by a viral infection. It is normally rapid and clinical recovery occurs within two weeks, even if complete biological resolution may require a longer period. Moreover, relapses are described, especially for 6-12 months after the onset.

In some cases of pericarditis, such as the tubercular form, the biological evolution of inflammatory process may induce pathological thickening of pericardial surfaces, leading to chronic constrictive pericarditis, even if this event is very rare in young athletes.

Typical symptoms are represented by acute chest pain that changes with respiratory movements and position, and fever that is usually associated with increased inflammatory markers such as VES and PCR; sometimes, evolution may be insidious with asthenia, transitory fever and stubbing chest pain. Physical examination documented the presence of pericardial or pleuropericardial rubbings associated with paraphonic heart tones and pericardial effusion. ECG normally showed diffuse ST elevation while echocardiography documented, in acute phase, pericardial effusion accompanied by pericardial surface thickening and augmented echo-reflection.

Diagnosis is mostly clinical because echocardiographic findings of pericardial effusion or thickening are not constantly detected [20]. On the other hand, pericardial effusion is present in up to 20-30% of cases and is correlated with the prognosis. Subjects with confirmed diagnosis of pericarditis are ineligible to participate in any fitness competition until complete recovery and in any case for a six-month period from the onset of symptoms.

Athletes may resume competitive activity only after adequate demonstration of a completely normal pericardium by clinical-instrumental evaluation. In cases of myocarditis-pericarditis with considerable myocardium involvement, the same clinical and therapeutic criteria for myocarditis are to be followed.

References

1. Maron BJ (1986) Structural features of the athlete's heart as defined by echocardiography. J Am Coll Cardiol 7:190-203
2. Zeppilli P (1988) The athlete's heart. Practical Cardiol 14:61-84
3. Pelliccia A, Maron BJ, Spataro A et al (1991) The upper limit of physiologic cardiac hypertrophy in highly trained elite athlete. N Engl J Med 324:295-301
4. Hosenpud JD, McAnulty JH, Niles NR (1986) Unexpected myocardial disease in patients with life threatening arrhythmias. Br Heart J 56:55-61

5. Strauzemberg Se, Olsen G (1980) The occurrence of electrocardiographical abnormalities in athletes: an expression of cardiovascular adaptation or a sign of a myocardial lesion? In: Lubich T, Venerando A (eds) Sports Cardiology. Bologna: Aulo Gaggi, pp 415-432
6. Palileo EV, Ashley WW, Swirin S et al (1982) Exercise provocable right ventricular out flow tract tachycardia. Am Heart J 104:185-193
7. Arbustini E, Grasso M, Diegli ML et al (1989) Utilità della biopsia endomiocardica nell'individuare i substrati aritmogeni nelle aritmie ventricolari dell'atleta apparentemente sano. Atti IV Congresso della Società Italiana dello Sport, Venezia, pp 332-336
8. Maron JB, Roberts WC, Mc Allister MA et al (1980) Sudden death in young athletes. Circulation 62: 218-229
9. Corrado D, Thiene G, Nava A et al. Sudden death in young competitive athletes: clinicopathologic correlation in 22 cases. Am J Med 89:588-596
10. Burke AP, Farb A, Virmani R et al (1991) Sports-related and non-sport-related sudden cardiac death in young adults. Am Heart J 121:568-575
11. Zeppilli P, Santini C, Palmieri V et al (1994) Role of myocarditis in athletes with minor arrhythmias and/or echocardiographic abnormalities. Chest 196:373-380
12. Scognamiglio R, Fasoli G, Nava A et al (1987) Two dimensional echocardiographic features in patients with spontaneous right ventricular tachycardia without apparent heart disease. J Cardiovasc Ultrasonography 6:113-118
13. Hosenpud JD, Campbell SM, Niles RN et al (1987) Exercise induced augmentation of cellular and humoral autoimmunity associated with increased cardiac dilatation in experimental autoimmune myocarditis. Cardiovasc Res 21:217-22
14. Naccarella F, Bracchetti D, Quadrelli S et al (1996) Un protocollo per la diagnosi e il follow-up della sospetta miocardite in atleti. Int J Sport Cardiol 5:2-12
15. Maron BJ, Zipes DP (2005) 36th Bethesda Conference: eligibility recommendations for competitive athletes with cardiovascular abnormalities. J Am Coll Cardiol 45:1313-1375
16. Goldberger JJ, Cain ME, Hohnloser SH et al (2008) AHA/ACC scientific statement on noninvasive risk stratification techniques for identifying patients at risk for sudden cardiac death. A scientific statement from the American Heart Association council on clinical cardiology committee on eletrocardiography and arrhythmias and council on epidemiology and prevention . Circulation 118:1497-1518
17. Bowles NE, Ni J, Kearney DL et al (2003) Detection of viruses in myocardial tissues by polymerase chain reaction. Evidence of adenovirus as a common cause of myocarditis in children and adults. J Am Coll Cardiol 42:466-472
18. Rampazzo A, Nava A, Danieli GA et al (1994) The gene for arrhythmogenic right ventricular cardiomyopathy maps to chromosome 14q23-q24. Hum Mol Genet 3:959-962
19. Bachl N, Benazzo F, Biffi A et al (2010) Protocolli cardiologici per il giudizio di idoneità allo sport agonistico. Medicina dello Sport 63:1
20. Luft FC, Gilman JK, Weyman AE (1980). Pericarditis in the patient with uremia: clinical and echocardiographic evaluation. Nephron 25:160

Non-Structural Causes of Sudden Death

21

Giuseppe Picciolo

21.1 Introduction

Sudden cardiac death is always a dramatic event and, besides raising issues and questions, makes it doubtful whether it is possible to predict it somehow; its impact is even greater when it confirms that competitive athletes, by definition, should be the healthiest and most controlled population. Behind these deaths there is, in most cases, a structural disease, often on a genetic basis and previously unidentified, such as hypertrophic cardiomyopathy or arrhythmogenic right ventricular cardiomyopathy [1-2]. Nevertheless there are a series of diseases that could lead to arrhythmic sudden cardiac death without evident macroscopic or histopathological cardiac alterations; the current classification includes these along with *genetic primary cardiomyopathies* under the name of *ion channel disorders* [3]: long QT syndrome (LQTS), Brugada syndrome (BS), short QT syndrome (SQTS), catecholaminergic polymorphic ventricular tachycardia (CPVT). The common feature is the presence of mutations that, at different levels, alter membrane ion channels features and consequently the action of potential myocells, generating electrical instability that could lead to malignant ventricular arrhythmias and thus sudden cardiac death. Although the post-mortem diagnosis is not simple and can be made only through molecular analysis, thc *pre-event* diagnosis can be done on the basis of a simple 12-lead electrocardiogram (ECG) or at most with a stress test (CPTV), hence the importance of knowing the clinical and electrocardiographic features to suspect them, so that patients could be directed to further investigations to confirm diagnosis.

G. Picciolo (✉)
Cardiac Intensive Care
AOU Policlinico S. Martino, Messina, Italy

21.2 Long QT Syndrome

Long QT syndrome is a group of genetic diseases sharing the phenotypic manifestation of elongation of the QT interval, syncope and sudden cardiac death due to the risk of ventricular fibrillation. The first described hereditary variants were Jervell and Lange-Nielsen syndrome and Romano-Ward syndrome. Over the years the molecular basis of these two variants had been understood and mutations of about 10 genes had progressively been identified as responsible for LQTS (Table 21.1). Mutations involve mainly potassium channels (LQT1-2-5-6-7),

Table 21.1 Genetic basis of LQTS

Form	Gene	Function	Frequency
LQT1	KCN	$\downarrow I_{ks}$	30-35%
LQT2	KCN	$\downarrow I_{kr}$	25-30%
LQT3	SCN5A	$\uparrow I_{Na}$	5-10%
LQT4	ANK2	$\downarrow I_{Na,K}$	1-2%
LQT5	KCN	$\downarrow I_{ks}$	1%
LQT6	KCN	$\downarrow I_{kr}$	Rare
LQT7	KCN	$\downarrow I_{k1}$	Rare
LQT8	CACNA1C	$\uparrow I_{Ca,L}$	Rare
LQT9	CAV3	$\uparrow I_{Na}$	Rare
LQT10	SCN4B	$\uparrow I_{Na}$	Rare

M. Fioranelli and G. Frajese (eds.), *Sports Cardiology*,
DOI: 10.1007/978-88-470-2775-6_21,

sodium channels (LQT3-10), or proteins that can indirectly alter membrane ion conductance, such as ankyrin (LQT4) or caveolin (LQT9). Although the number of proposed or confirmed LQTS forms is increasingly growing, it is important to figure out that currently a mutation could be identified in only 70% of affected patients and in 90% of them it involves genes responsible for the first three variants (LQT1, LQT2, LQT3). In the LQTS ion channels alterations imply alterations in trans-membrane ion currents with a subsequent prolongation of repolarization phase, refractory periods dispersion, and genesis of early post-depolarization (EAD) that can trigger torsades de pointes (TdP) [4], syndrome-characteristic arrhythmia; TdP may end on its own, causing brief symptoms as palpitations and/or syncope, or degenerate into ventricular fibrillation with consecutive sudden cardiac death of the subject.

21.2.1 Electrocardiographic Features and Clinical Presentation

The main electrocardiographic feature is *heart rate corrected QT interval (QTc) prolongation*. Correction could easily and accurately be achieved using Bazett's formula, which divides the QT interval by the square root of the preceding RR interval:

$$QTc = \frac{QT}{\sqrt{RR}}$$

The QT interval should be measured in the lead where it is longest; however a U-wave could be present at times, making measurements difficult: in these cases a lead in which the U-wave is absent or smaller, or assuming as T-wave end the crossing point between the tangent of the descending branch of the T-wave and the virtual line continuing in the TP tract, representing the isoelectric line [5]. Abnormal values are usually considered QTc >440ms in men and QTc >460ms in women, keeping in mind that the longer the QTc interval, the higher the arrhythmic risk, and it is very high over >500ms. Some patients affected by LQTS have a QTc interval within normal limits because of possible low penetration of the mutation. *ST-T tract* gene-specific features have been described: in LQT1 patients, the T-wave has a normal morphology with a wide base; in LQT2 the T-wave has a lower voltage with a *notch*; in LQT3 the T-wave has a very late onset [6]. A beat to beat T-wave alternans could be present at times, often before the onset of TdP: this is an important marker of electrical instability. Finally the presence of low sinus frequencies or sinus pauses that are not correlated with sinus respiratory arrhythmia have been described: the latter could can play a role in causing, particularly in LQT3 patients.

LQTS clinical manifestations are represented by syncope and sudden cardiac death. Both exercise and emotional stress can trigger clinical events, basically by increasing serum catecholamine level; usually catecholamines shorten the QT interval by acting on a slow potassium current (IKs); in LQTS patients, particularly in LQT1, this current is altered resulting in a failed QT shortening with a consequent change in repolarization, EAD appearance and the major likelihood of arrhythmic events; this current is normal in LQT2 and LQT3 patients, in which events are rarely related to exercise (LQT2) or occur even during sleep (LQT3). Specific arrhythmic triggers exist in fact for each LQTS variant: in LQT1 events are triggered mainly by exercise (swimming), in LQT2 by emotional stress (sudden high intensity sounds such as a telephone ringing or alarms), though they can occur during exercise or rarely at rest, and during post-partum; in LQT3, in which mutation is in sodium channels, arrhythmias occur mainly during sleep [7]. In Jervell and Lange-Nielsen syndrome patients, congenital deafness is present.

Many drugs could prolong QT interval both in normal subjects and affected patients without electrocardiographic alterations, unmasking the syndrome phenotype and potentially increasing the risk of arrhythmic events. Other conditions such as electrolyte disturbances, autoimmune diseases or pathologies provoking marked autonomic imbalance can be involved in the genesis of arrhythmic events in these patients.

21.2.2 Diagnosis

Clinical diagnosis is based on electrocardiographic features, personal medical history, and

Table 21.2 Diagnostic criteria of LQTS

	Score
Electrocardiographic criteria	
QTc interval (ms):	
≥480	3
460-480	2
450 (in me)	1
Torsades de pointes	2
T-wave alternans	1
Notched T-wave in 3 leads	1
Low heart rate for age	0.5
Clinical History	
Stress syncope	2
Syncope at rest	1
Congenital deafness	0.5
Family medical history	
Relatives with diagnosed LQTS	2
Unexplained sudden death in a relative <30 years old	1

family medical history; Schwartz and colleagues have given a score to each clinical and electrocardiographic feature (Table 21.2); if the total score is >3.5 there is a high likelihood of LQTS, an intermediate likelihood if the total score is between 1 and 3, and low if it is <1 [8]. Currently a *genetic diagnosis* is also available, which makes it possible to identify the mutation that is responsible for the disease in 70% of subjects. *Arrhythmic risk stratification*, which is particularly challenging in this population, is paramount; in this respect, besides clinical parameters, an increasingly deep knowledge of molecular mechanisms that underlie each mutation makes it possible to obtain prognostic information even by molecular genetics. Patients with *previous cardiac arrest* or documented spontaneous TdP are considered to have a very high risk. Also patients with a QTc >500 ms are at very high risk. Subjects with LQT1 and LQT2 seem to have more events than those with LQT3, but in this last group events have a higher lethality; patients with LQT1 seem to have less lethal events because of a higher percentage of silent mutation carriers. Regarding sex, female LQT2 and male LQT3 patients seem to be at higher risk [9-10]. Syncope is a very important characteristic for risk stratification, and it is important to know not only the presence in the medical history but also the frequency and time distribution: it assumes a different significance depending on the age of presentation; hence the need not to *crystallise* the patient in a risk zone, but to evaluate him or her periodically [11]. To these parameters must be added, if possible, molecular information to further refine the risk stratification: for example, the mutation in carboxyl-terminus of gene KCNQ1 seems to be related to a more mitigated phenotype, while mutations in the pore region in patients with LQT2 seem to be related to a higher risk of major cardiac events.

21.2.3 Therapy

Therapy is first based on beta-blockers. For their widespread and well-established use propranolol and nadolol are preferred. Beta-blockers have been shown to reduce the risk of major events significantly in patients affected by LQTS, although there are great benefits in LQT1, fewer benefits in LQT2, and controversial benefits in LQT3 [12]. In the latter, in fact, sodium channel mutation leads to a gain in function of the channel with a subsequent prolongation of repolarization time, the mechanism that beta-blockers have difficulty influencing; in LQT3, therefore, the use of sodium channel blockers such as mexiletine or flecainide has been proposed on an individual basis, and in some cases ranolazine, a late sodium current inhibitor, has been used. Despite beta-blocker therapy, a high percentage of subjects have syncope recurrence: 10%, 23%, 32% respectively in LQT1, LQT2, and LQT3. For this reason, in these patients an ICD implantation is recommended. For patients experiencing arrhythmic disorders despite beta-blocker therapy, *left stellectomy* is possible. Cardiac pacing, finally, may be used in patients in whom sinus pauses triggering TdP are present, although in these patients an excessive high incidence of sudden death had been reported in follow-up.

Currently, international guidelines recommend the use of class I beta-blockers in patients presenting a prolonged QTc and class beta-blockers IIa in those with molecular diagnosis of LQTS and normal QTc. Class I ICD implantation is recommended instead in patients who have survived cardiac arrest and class IIa in those with recurrent syncope despite beta-blocker therapy. Moreover, class IIb ICD implantations are suggested for primary prevention in patients with an elevated theoretical risk profile, such as patients with QTc > 500 ms and patients with LQT2 and LQT3.

Concerning athletic eligibility, LQTS contraindicates every kind of sport even in the absence of documented ventricular arrhythmias.

21.3 Brugada Syndrome

Brugada syndrome (BS) is a recently identified arrhythmogenic disease [13-14], characterized by a particular electrocardiographic aspect associated with malignant ventricular arrhythmias and sudden cardiac death in the presence of an apparently morphologically healthy heart.

It seems to have an incidence of 5 per 10,000 subjects and it is responsible for about 4% of all sudden cardiac deaths and 20% of cases in patients with apparently healthy hearts [15]. The disease has a genetic basis with a dominant autosomal transmission and variable phenotypic expression. It was initially associated with SCN5A gene mutation by encoding the sodium channel alpha subunit, which is fundamental for cardiac depolarization, determining a reduction of inward sodium current during phase 0 of the action potential; this mutation is present in no more than 25% of patients affected. Subsequently mutations of the GPD1-L gene were later detected, encoding for glycerol-3-phosphate dehydrogenase (a glycoprotein essential for proper function of the sodium channel, the mutation of which leads to reduced sodium conductance) [16], and of genes CACNA1C and CACNA2B encoding for L-type calcium channels [17].

21.3.1 Electrocardiographic Characteristics and Clinical Picture

Electrocardiographically there are three Brugada ECG patterns:

- type 1 is characterized by an elevation of the J point ≥ 2 mm in one or more of the right precordial leads (V1-V3), followed by a ST tract rapidly descending and a negative T wave without an interposed isoelectric line (*coved ST*) (Fig. 21.1a);
- type 2 has an elevation of the J point in V1-V3 ≥ 2 mm as well but followed by the ST tract slowly descending with a positive or biphasic T wave (*saddleback ST*) (Fig.21.1b);
- type 3 is characterized by an elevation of the J

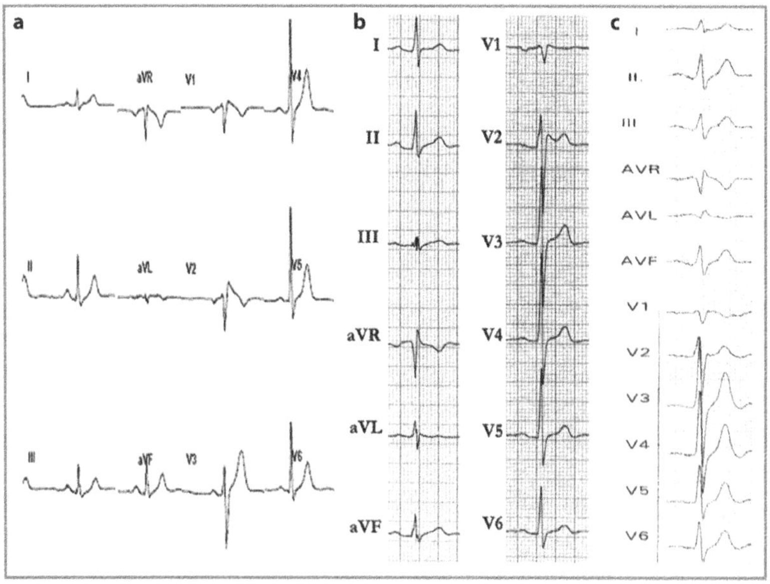

Fig. 21.1 The three ECG Brugada syndrome patterns: (a) type 1, (b) type 2, (c) type 3. Tracings b and c were recorded in the same patient at different times

point < 1 mm and may be followed by a coved or saddleback pattern (Fig.21.1c).

Only the coved type 1 pattern among the three is considered diagnostic [18]. The hallmark is the dynamicity of repolarization alterations: in the same patient, at different times, it is possible to record types 1, 2 and 3, and even a completely normal ECG; this ECG pattern dynamicity makes diagnosis more complex, and in doubtful cases (e.g. type 2 or 3 ECG) further diagnostic tests are required, such as shifting V1 and V2 leads at the III or II intercostal space or a pharmacological test that contemplates the use of a sodium channel blocker (ajmaline 1mg/kg over 5 minutes or flecainide 2mg/kg over 10 minutes). Furthermore, surface ECG can point to other alterations such as long PQ interval, right bundle branch block or left anterior fascicular block (expression of intra- and infra-hisian conduction disorders) and a long QT interval, but may sometimes also be shorter than expected as in calcium channel gene mutations. Clinical features are characterized by syncope and sudden cardiac death. Events occur during the third and fourth decade of life in males and mostly during sleep, particularly in the early hours of the morning. Fever may unmask a ECG type 1 pattern and be combined with arrhythmic events. In patients affected by supraventricular arrhythmias as atrial fibrillation, atrioventricular nodal re-entrant tachycardia and atrioventricular re-entrant tachycardia, sinoatrial conduction disorders are frequent.

21.3.2 Diagnosis

Diagnosis of the syndrome is confirmed when a spontaneous or drug-induced type 1 ECG pattern (only this one!) is associated with one of six of the following elements: documented ventricular fibrillation (VF), polymorphic ventricular tachycardia (VT), family history of sudden cardiac death < 45 years, type 1 ECG in one of the family members, inducibility of VT/VF at the electrophysiological testing, syncope or functional equivalent of syncope (convulsion or nocturnal agonal respiration).

Before confirming diagnosis, it is paramount to rule out pathologies that may mimic ECG characteristics of the syndrome (arrhythmogenic right ventricular dysplasia, myocarditis, acute ischemia and extrinsic compression of the right ventricular outflow tract, variant angina, use of antiarrhythmic, antianginal, psychiatric drugs, alcohol or cocaine intoxication, early repolarization etc.); in particular, arrhythmogenic right ventricular dysplasia and myocarditis must be carefully investigated and ruled out with tests such as echocardiography and magnetic resonance imaging with contrast, which are normal in BS; in this respect, however, there is no general agreement in the scientific community: some doctors, in fact, suggest an exclusive functional genesis, others think that the ECG pattern typical of the syndrome is a *container* of heterogeneous pathologies with genetic, inflammatory, infective or degenerative genesis. Beyond this controversy it is important to underline that BS diagnosis should be of exclusion which arrive after a careful and complete clinical and instrumental study of the patient. Genetic analysis, though available, currently does not play a central role as it is positive in no more than 30% of patients and, although positive, has a low predictive value of events. A significant issue is arrhythmic risk stratification; many studies have attempted to identify reliable predictors of events, with often discordant results. Currently identified predictors are: type 1 ECG, previous cardiac arrest, syncope, family history of sudden cardiac death, and inducibility of VT/VF at the electrophysiological testing; however there are uncertain topics to discuss. Most of the authors agree that the risk is highest in patients with type 1 ECG patterns and previous cardiac arrest and it reduces progressively in patients with syncope and in those who are asymptomatic. There is agreement that patients presenting spontaneous type 1 ECGs are more at risk than those in whom the pattern is drug-induced. Males seem to be more at risk than females.

There is controversy surrounding the role of electrophysiological testing: some authors give an important predictive value that should be crucial in the indication for ICD implantation, while others consider it to be an unreliable and non-predictive test and therefore to be excluded from risk stratification methods; in a recent Italian prospective study carried out by Delise et al. in patients with type 1 ECG patterns without previous cardiac arrest, three risk factors (syncope, family history of sudden cardiac death, and ventricular arrhythmias inducibility at electrophysiological testing) were identified, none of which could alone predict future events, as predictability would be high in the presence of two or more risk factors. Clearly, much work is still necessary to clarify the uncertainty regarding risk stratification in patients with BS.

21.3.3 Therapy

Currently there is no effective drug therapy to prevent arrhythmic events and sudden death; quinidine has been proven to normalize the ST tract and seems to reduce arrhythmic events, but its efficacy has not been demonstrated clearly; isoproterenol has been used to control arrhythmic storms that can be present in these patients, particularly in those with an ICDs, but obviously cannot be used chronically; moreover, most of the antiarrhythmic drugs and cardiac and psychiatric drugs are contraindicated in BS patients because they are believed to unmask electrocardiographic alterations and thus increase the risk of events. The only therapy currently able to prevent sudden death is ICD implantation. Given current data in international guidelines, ICD implantation is recommended in patients with type 1 ECG patterns (spontaneous or induced) and previous cardiac arrest (class I), in patients with spontaneous type 1 ECG patterns and syncope (class IIa) and in asymptomatic patients with type 1 ECG patterns with ventricular arrhythmias inducible under electrophysiological testing (class IIb).

In such a complex and uncertain scenario, it seems appropriate to deny athletic eligibility in symptomatic and asymptomatic patients presenting spontaneous or induced type 1 ECG patterns.

21.4 Short QT Syndrome

Short QT syndrome (SQTS) is a rare genetic ion channel disease described in 2003 by an Italian group that associated the presence of a short QT and sudden death [19]. It is characterized by a QTc interval <360 ms (typically <300 ms) with minimal variability in heart rate variation. Almost a quarter of patients have atrial fibrillation. In patients affected by the syndrome three genes encoding different potassium channels have been identified, resulting in a gain of function (opposite behaviour from LQTS): KCNH2, responsible for I_{Kr}, in SQT1; KCNQ1, responsible for I_{Ks}, in SQT2; KCNJ2, responsible for I_{K1}, in SQT3. Electrocardiograms show, besides a short QT interval, an almost non-existent ST tract and narrow and high symmetric T-waves, except in SQT3 in which the T wave is highly asymmetric with a steep downslope. In some patients the QTc interval further shortens during bradycardia. No structural alterations are present during echocardiography. The intra-cardiac electrophysiological testing shows very short atrial and ventricular effective refractory periods and easy inducibility of atrial and ventricular fibrillation. The role of ventricular arrhythmia inducibility in electrophysiological testing is unclear in risk stratification.

21.4.1 Diagnosis

Currently there are no certain diagnostic criteria for this syndrome, but diagnosis should be based on a set of information: a short QT interval (≤360 ms in males and ≤370 ms in females, typically ≤320 in both sexes), syncope, polymorphic VT or VF documentation, family history of syncope, SQTS or VF, presence of atrial fibrillation, in the absence of structural cardiopathy or external conditions that may shorten QTc (e.g. hypocalcemia).

21.4.2 Therapy

The only available therapy that is effective in preventing sudden death is ICD implantation. There are no guidelines on implantation indications, although it is clear that patients in secondary prevention should receive an ICD. Unfortunately, after implantation, these patients are frequently inclined to receive inappropriate shocks because of a double count of the T-wave, which is morphologically narrow and high, and because of the presence of atrial fibrillation. Pharmacologically, quinidine has proved to be effective in prolonging the Qtc interval, in normalising the response to RR interval variations, and in preventing arrhythmic events in some patients. More data, however, are required to validate the use. Sport is strongly not recommended in both symptomatic and asymptomatic patients.

21.5 Catecholaminergic Polymorphic Ventricular Tachycardia

Catecholaminergic polymorphic ventricular tachycardia (CPVT) is a rare arrhythmogenic disease on a genetic basis characterized by the presence of specific ventricular arrhythmias (bidirectional ventricular tachycardia) induced by exercise and a high risk of sudden death [20]. It has a genetic origin; the genes currently known to be involved are:

- RyR2 gene encoding ryanodine receptor, which is paramount for the homeostasis of intra-cellular calcium, and responsible for the autosomal dominant form, CPVT1, identified in 50-65% of cases;
- the CASQ2 gene encoding calsequestrin, which is also paramount for the homeostasis of intracellular calcium, is autosomal recessive and responsible for the rare CPVT2.

There is a third form of this disease, CPVT3, an autosomal recessive form detected on the chromosome 7 short arm, whose responsible gene is not yet known; finally in 45% of subjects it is impossible to identify the mutation responsible for the disease.

21.5.1 Clinical Presentation and Diagnosis

Clinical manifestations of the disease occur during infancy or in the first stages of adolescence with repeated syncopal episodes triggered by exercise or emotions. The electrocardiogram is almost normal; at times a prominent U-wave is present and the heart rate is lower than normal at rest. Echocardiography is normal too. Paramount for the diagnosis, therapeutic management and follow-up is a stress test, thanks to which it is possible to record CPVT-related arrhythmias. They usually begin at a heart rate of 100-110 beats per minute as isolated premature supraventricular and ventricular beats; with increasing exercise we see the organization first in bigeminism, and subsequently in couples and brief supraventricular and ventricular tachycardias until the appearance of ventricular tachycardia that gradually becomes more rapid and eventually, if exercise is not stopped, may degenerate into ventricular fibrillation. Normally arrhythmias disappear during recovery, when at times a beat to beat U-wave alternans may be noticed.

CPVT hallmark ventricular tachycardia is a bidirectional ventricular tachycardia characterized by beat to beat inversion of 180 degrees on the QRS axis; in rare cases it is possible to observe polymorphic tachycardia. It has been observed that the beat triggering the tachycardia has often the same morphology and that in 90% it origins from right ventricular outflow tract, or secondly from left ventricular outflow tract. Moreover, increasing heart rate has been noticed with the shortening of the ectopic beat from the preceding beat coupling, suggesting delayed post-depolarizations or triggered activity such as the basic mechanism of arrhythmia. During the stress test atrial fibrillation can also be observed.

The stress test is paramount not only for diagnosis but also for drug therapy titration: the arrhythmogenic threshold, in fact, seems stable enough and repeatable individually, so it is possible to evaluate therapy effects with repeated stress tests.

Holter monitoring is useful in recording the real-life burden of arrhythmia and monitoring the response to emotive stimuli, another important trigger in this these patients.

Once the disease is clinically diagnosed, it is important to suggest that the patient and his/her relatives undergo genetic diagnosis. CPVT is a potentially lethal disease with a high mortality rate in those not receiving drug therapy. The initial event, which can be arrhythmic syncope but also sudden death, occurs at an average age of 8 years, although an initial presentation in adulthood has been reported.

Few data are available for risk stratification: arrhythmic events seem to be more likely at a younger age in patients with CPVT1 than in those with other forms and the male sex seems to be a risk factor for syncope in CPVT1 patients. Intracardiac electrophysiological testing does not seem to play any role neither for diagnosis nor for risk stratification.

21.5.2 Therapy

Therapy is mainly with beta-blockers: some authors reported nearly a 100% success rate in preventing arrhythmic events; others, instead, describe arrhythmic event recurrences near 40% with beta-blocker therapy. Some other drugs have been proposed in association with beta-blockers in patients who are not well controlled by the latter, such as sodium channel blockers, amiodarone, and calcium channel blockers, but their use is not well defined. In patients who have experienced cardiac arrest or who keep having syncope or arrhythmias on beta-blockers, ICD implantation is indicated.

Current international guidelines suggest the use of beta-blockers in patients with is indicated clinical diagnosis of CPVT in the presence of spontaneous or stress-induced ventricular arrhythmias (class I), in patients with genetic diagnosis during infancy even in the absence of clinical manifestations (class IIa) and in adult patients with genetic diagnosis in the absence of symptoms (class IIb); ICD implantation in association, with beta-blockers, is recommended in patients who have survived cardiac arrest (class I) and in those in whom syncope and ventricular arrhythmias persist despite beta-blocker therapy.

Because of the very nature of the disease, athletic eligibility cannot be granted.

References

1. Maron BJ (2003) Sudden death in young athletes N Engl J Med 349:1064-1075
2. Corrado D, Basso C, Schiavon M et al (1998) Screening for hypertrophic cardiomyopathy in young athletes. N Engl J Med 339: 364-369
3. Maron BJ, Towbin JA, Thiene G et al (2006) Contemporary definitions and classification of the cardiomyopathies: an American Heart Association Scientific Statement from the Council on Clinical Cardiology, Heart Failure and Transplantation Committee; Quality of Care and Outcomes Research and Functional Genomics and Translational Biology Interdisciplinary Working Groups; and Council on Epidemiology and Prevention. Circulation 113:1807-1816
4. Morita H, Wu J, Zipes DP (2008) The QT syndromes: long and short. Lancet 372:750-763
5. Rautaharju PM, Surawicz B, Gettes LS (2009) AHA/ACCF/HRS Recommendations for the Standardization and Interpretation of the Electrocardiogram: Part IV: The ST Segment, T and U Waves, and the QT Interval A Scientific Statement From the American Heart Association Electrocardiography and Arrhythmias Committee, Council on Clinical Cardiology; the American College of Cardiology Foundation; and the Heart Rhythm Society Endorsed by the International Society for Computerized Electrocardiology. J Am Coll Cardiol 53: 982-991
6. Moss AJ, Zareba W, Benhorin J et al (1995) ECG T-wave patterns in genetically distinct forms of the hereditary long QT syndrome. Circulation 92:2929-2934
7. Schwartz PJ, Priori SG, Spazzolini C et al (2001) Genotype-phenotype correlation in the long-QT syndrome: gene-specific triggers for life-threatening arrhythmias. Circulation 103:89-95
8. Schwartz PJ, Moss AJ, Vincent GM et al (1993) Diagnostic criteria for the long QT syndrome. An update. Circulation 88:782-784
9. Priori SG, Schwartz PJ, Napolitano C et al (2003) Risk stratification in the long-QT syndrome. N Engl J Med 348: 1866-1874
10. Priori SG, Napolitano C, Schwartz PJ (2008) Genetics of cardiac arrhythmas. In: Libby P, Bonow RO, Mann DL, Zipes DP (eds) Braunwald's Heart Disease, 8th. Philadelphia: Saunders; pp 101-109
11. Goldenberg I, Moss AJ (2008) Long QT syndrome. J Am Coll Cardiol 51:2291-2300
12. Priori SG, Napolitano C, Schwartz PJ et al (2004) Association of long QT syndrome loci and cardiac events among patients treated with beta-blockers. JAMA 292:1341-1344
13. Martini B, Nava A, Thiene G et al (1989) Ventricular fibrillation without apparent heart disease: description of six cases. Am Heart J 118:1203-1209
14. Brugada P, Brugada J (1992) Right bundle branch block, persistent ST segment elevation and sudden cardiac death: a distinct clinical and electrocardiographic syndrome. A multicenter report. J Am Coll Cardiol 20:1391-1396
15. Antzelevitch C, Brugada P, Borggrefe M et al (2005) Brugada syndrome: report of the second consensus conference. Heart Rhythm 2:429-440
16. London B, Michalec MS, Mehdi H et al (2007) A mutation in glycerol-3-phosphate dehydrogenase 1 like gene (GPD1-L) decreases cardiac Na+ current and causes inherited arrhythmias. Circulation 116:2260-2268
17. Antzelevitch C, Pollevick GD, Cordeiro JM et al

(2007) Loss-offunction mutations in the cardiac calcium channel underlie a new clinical entity characterized by ST-segment elevation, short QT intervals, and sudden cardiac death. Circulation 115:442-449
18. Wilde AA, Antzelevitch C, Borggrefe M et al (2002) Proposed diagnostic criteria for the Brugada syndrome: consensus report. Circulation. 106:2514-2519
19. Giustetto C, Di Monte F, Wolpert C et al (2006) Short QT syndrome: clinical findings and diagnostic-therapeutic implications. Eur Heart J 27:2440-2447
20. Priori SG, Napolitano C, Memmi M, et al. Clinical and molecular characterization of patients with catecholaminergic polymorphic ventricular tachycardia. Circulation 2002 106: 69-74

The Paradox of Sudden Cardiac Death in the Young: The Main Mission of a Sports Cardiologist

22

Paolo Angelini

22.1 The Issue

Rare, unexpected – and usually unexplainable – sudden cardiac death (SCD) in young student athletes appears to be occurring more frequently, especially with the prevalent reporting of such events via the Internet and other mass media. The literature presently contains contradictory reports as to the incidence of SCD in young persons [1-5]. The Minneapolis Heart Foundation released a survey spanning a 27-year period and conservatively quantified the phenomenon as occurring about 60 to 70 times per year in the United States; however, only *athletes* were considered and mainly Internet-based records were consulted [4]. In a similar study, the National Collegiate Athletic Association (NCAA) reported an incidence of 1 in 43,770/year in collegiate-level athletes in the United States. Some commentators added that the Internet method of obtaining data for similar investigations is likely to identify only 25% of all real cases occurring in a certain community [6]. However, we must realise that the reason for continuing to use such an unreliable approach, beyond its expediency, is that SCD, especially in the young, is likely not observed in hospital. Most SCD events occur on athletic fields, which leads to the cause rarely being known before death. In fact, mortality from sudden cardiac arrest (SCA) occurring outside the hospital environment is more than 90% [7-12].

P. Angelini (✉)
Medical Director, Center for Coronary Artery Anomalies
Texas Heart Institute at St. Luke's Episcopal Hospital
Houston, USA

This chapter reviews the current understanding of what amounts to an apparent failure in healtcare delivery and the opportunities for improving outcomes in these young patients.

22.2 The Incidence of Sudden Death in the Young

Many factors are at play in the continuing inconsistencies in the data. Recently, three critical age groups in the general population were recognized as featuring different peaks in the incidence of SCD and related to different causes: the newborn and infantile period (0–1 year), the young period (12–35 years), and the adult period (older than 35 years) [10-12]. Each group appears to have differences in the most frequent and specific causative factors, such as complex congenital heart conditions in the early age group, congenital coronary anomalies and congenital cardiomyopathies in the young age group, and acquired coronary atherosclerotic disease in the adult age group.

What is clinically important to recognize is the multiplicity of the ultimate causative factors and that, simultaneously, various precipitating factors must also be involved ahead of a crisis. For example, a child born with a potentially serious coronary artery anomaly (e.g. originating from the wrong side of the aorta) could become a highly trained runner, until one day, that person experiences SCD while participating in an athletic competition (cardiac output may increase 4–5 times baseline, heart rate 3–4 times baseline, and significant dehydration may be present). Such cases should indeed be labelled sudden *cardiac* death because the ultimate

M. Fioranelli and G. Frajese (eds.), *Sports Cardiology*,
DOI: 10.1007/978-88-470-2775-6_22, © Springer-Verlag Italia 2012

cause was cardiac, despite extreme exertion being a necessary contributing factor [13]. Effective prevention of SCD demands recognition and aggressive treatment of pre-existing cardiac anomalies (such as by surgical intervention) if simple avoidance of extreme competitive exercise in at-risk patients is not an acceptable and effective alternative.

Worldwide, the incidence of SCD in the young has been variably reported as between 0.1 to 0.5 per 100,000 *normal* individuals per year [11] but up to 5 to 10 per 100,000 in some athletic specialties [5,14-15]. The most relevant issues affecting the incidence reporting of SCD relate to the presence of a clear definition of a cardiac cause – currently, autopsy is the gold standard for determining the cause [14-16]. Unfortunately, most autopsy series have not been diligent in clarifying the number and prevalence of risk factors in the population being studied (the denominator of the fraction in which autopsy cases are the numerator). The term SCD should be applied only to cases with reliably proven, predominant cardiac causes; however, it has been loosely used in studies reported in the literature and applied also to cases where there was an absence of autopsy-proven causes, resulting in a varying reported incidence of *autopsy-negative SCD* of 5% to 35%.

The American Heart Association and American College of Cardiology [2-4] state that 90-95% of cases of sudden death in the young have known cardiac causes and other investigators state that up to 35% do not [16]; thus, we must conclude that the science is still unreliable in both the methods and quality of data. The most disciplined and documented study currently available on the subject was performed by the US Army Pathology Institute, which, in 2004, reported results from 6.3 million military recruits surveyed over a 27-year period [14]. The mean age of the recruits was 19±2 years and the setting an 8-week period of strenuous boot camp training. Routine autopsy was performed in all fatalities. Even in such a large number of recruits, only 64 deaths were attributed to cardiac causes. One-third of the deaths comprized 1 (and only 1) type of congenital coronary anomaly—anomalous origin of the left coronary artery from the right sinus of Valsalva. Interestingly, the incidence of SCD varied in different subgroups: of 6.6/100,000 recruits/year in total, it was only 3.8/100,000 in women versus 7.1/100,000 in men and 12.0/100,000 in African American men. Unfortunately, the investigators did not include a clear description of the preparticipation screening policy, but it was likely similar to the one used before sports participation in the United States. The study showed that 86% of the SCDs were reported as occurring during exercise.

22.3 The Challenge

The most delicate and urgent questions surrounding health policy for this issue are "Do we accept the relatively *low risk* of sudden cardiac death in the young as unavoidable?", "Do we limit our policy to treat events only when they occur?", and "Do we strive to prevent such tragedies through accurate and prospective screening?" The answers will only come when we acknowledge the overwhelmingly poor prognosis of cases of SCA that occur outside the hospital environment. Surely, the human cost (emotional and medical-legal) and the direct and indirect health care costs associated with SCD in the young, occurring in the absence of effective prevention, at least warrant its more careful study.

An acceptable novel prevention programme should include affordable costs, effective prevention, and minimally invasive screening acceptable to the candidates, all the while using accurate and reproducible protocols. In addition, the decrease in the incidence of SCD should be documented after such screening and follow-up intervention programme are implemented. It is possible (but still requires a prospective study) that any screening protocol could introduce excessive diagnostic uncertainty and inappropriate exclusion from sporting activities in addition to exorbitant follow-up costs for cardiac evaluation. Definitive and comprehensive studies are necessary to address these concerns.

22.4 The Mechanisms of Sudden Cardiac Death

Cardiac dysfunction can lead to sudden death through several factors or mechanisms, but, essentially, the final mode of SCD from any cause is an abnormal rhythm: either too slow (resulting in asystole) or too rapid (ventricular fibrillation). Usually after a prolonged episode of SCA, irreversible brain damage occurs, and, thus, death could be related to issues with the brain more than with the heart if there is prolonged survival after an SCA episode. However, SCD in the young generally differs from that in older patients, for whom coronary artery disease is most frequently the cause of death, usually shortly after the onset of coronary thrombosis. With SCD in the young, there is usually no clear evidence at autopsy of sudden onset changes in the heart anatomy, even if pre-existing congenital abnormalities may have been present.

The most frequent conditions causing sudden death in the young are:

1) hypertrophic cardiomyopathy (HCM), in which primary hypertrophy generally occurs because of congenital defects and/or genetic disorders, which may lead to scarring and heart rhythm irregularities. The typical mode of death is ventricular fibrillation;
2) dilated cardiomyopathy (DCM), in which the cardiac chambers are enlarged and the heart muscle is usually intrinsically diseased or scarred because of genetic disorders or acquired disease (myocarditis). Again, this may lead to ventricular fibrillation as the most likely cause of SCD [2-4,15];
3) congenital coronary artery anomalies (CAAs), which have recently come to be recognized as a cause of SCD due to coronary dysfunction, typically coronary ischemia. Although only a few CAAs can intrinsically cause critical ischemia by clear mechanisms, variable severity in each case may be present. They are typically identified as an anomalous origin of a coronary artery from the opposite sinus of Valsalva (recently named ACAOS), with a necessary intramural course (the cause of ischemia only in some cases) inside the aortic wall [17-21];
4) congenital anomalies of critical myocardial structural proteins that control electrical activity of the cardiac muscle (typically, channelopathies). Dysfunction of the ion flow in the cardiac muscle may lead to occasional arrhythmias and, most importantly, ventricular fibrillation [16]. Such conditions only occasionally lead to clinical manifestations in the form of an unfortunate and dramatic episode of SCA.

The introduction of automated cardiac defibrillators (AEDs) to venues where sports activities are conducted has had a definite though inadequate impact on out-of-hospital outcomes for SCA. Although AEDs are capable of automatically ascertaining the clinical impairment mechanism and selecting the appropriate electrical shock treatment, the devices, in most cases, cannot ascertain the cause. Ultimately, the general expert opinion is that SCA prevention is better than secondary treatment and should be the preferred option.

22.5 Current Approaches

Despite such an urgent call for action, the American Heart Association Council on Nutrition, Physical Activity, and Metabolism, as endorsed by the American College of Cardiology, has only come to agree to a call for voluntary screening of candidates performed by primary care physicians or their assistants [2]. Such policy is often reluctantly carried out by those with neither a clear mandate nor specialization in the field. It is likely that less than 5% of the possible causes of SCD can be identified by such screening methods.

Conversely, the Italian Public Health System, which has had a mandate for preventing SCD in athletes since 1976, recently suggested that general electrocardiographic screening for all athletes or all candidates for school sports activities could decrease mortality in athletes by 90% [22-25] (Fig. 22.1). The claim is based on a finding of an unusually high prevalence of a rare degenerative disease of the right ventricle (arrhythmogenic right ventricular dysplasia or myopathy [ARVD] or [ARVM]) in a specific region of Italy (Veneto) (Table 22.1). The elaboration on specific diagnostic protocols for electrocardiogram (ECG) interpretation pursued by the same investigators [24] has resulted in unexpected improvements in the incidence of SCD in the Veneto region. Indeed, such an entity likely has a genetic cause that is more prevalent in this region, but electrocardiographic screening is inadequate for other high-risk cardiovascular conditions related to the occurrence of SCD in the young, in-

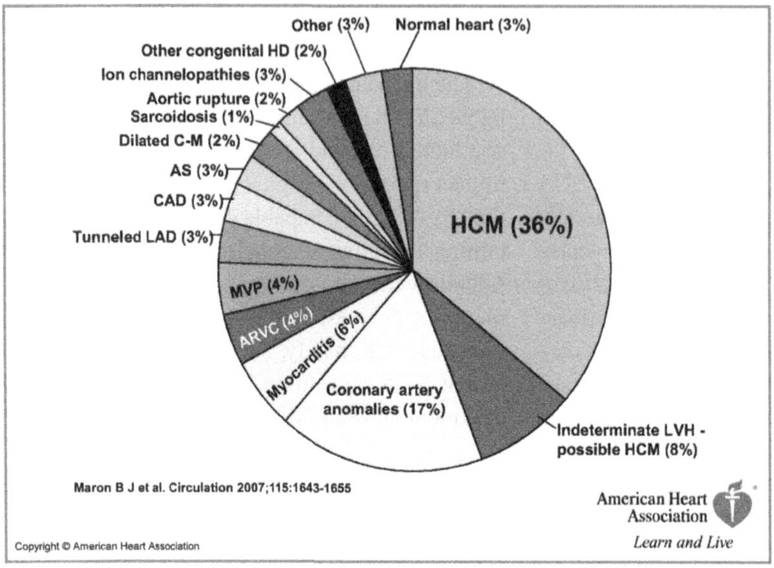

Fig. 22.1 Distribution of cardiovascular causes of sudden cardiac death in 1435 young competitive athletes. Reprinted with permission [2]

cluding mild to moderate hypertrophic or dilated cardiomyopathies and coronary anomalies where persons usually have a *normal* resting ECG.

International discussion has ensued since the original Italian series and has led to serious challenges to electrocardiographic screening programs for young athletes [26-27]. At present, in the United States, electrocardiographic screening alone is considered as having too limited accuracy. The relatively high incidence of false-positive results may lead to increased preventive care costs and an unacceptable exclusion rate for persons with an *abnormal ECG* without accurate justification. Any extensive prevention programme will need to em-

Table 22.1 Causes of sudden deaths in athletes and non-athletes (aged ≤35 years) in the Veneto region of Italy from 1979 to 1996

	Athletes (n=49) n (%)	Non-athletes (n=220) n (%)	Total (n=269) n (%)
Arrhythmogenic RV cardiomyopathy	11 (22.4)	18 (8.2)*	29 (10.8)
Atherosclerotic coronary artery disease	9 (18.5)	36 (16.4)	45 (16.7)
Anomalous origin of coronary artery	6 (12.2)	1 (0.4)**	7 (2.6)
Conduction system pathology	4 (8.2)	20 (9)	24 (8.9)
Mitral valve prolapse	5 (10.2)	21 (9.5)	26 (9.7)
HCM	1 (2)	16 (7.3)	17 (6.3)
Myocarditis	3 (6.1)	19 (8.6)	22 (8.2)
Myocardial bridge	2 (4)	5 (2.3)	7 (2.6)
Pulmonary thromboembolism	1 (2)	3 (1.4)	4 (1.5)
Dissecting aortic aneurysm	1 (2)	11 (5)	12 (4.5)
Dilated cardiomyopathy	1 (2)	9 (4.1)	10 (3.7)
Other	5 (10.2)	61 (27.7)	66 (24.5)

*P=0.008 for the comparison with the athletes.
**P<0.001 for the comparison with the athletes.
Modified from Corrado et al. [24], with permission.

ploy more reliable and accurate diagnostic modalities, while answering the obvious and legitimate questions of affordability.

22.6 What Lies Ahead?

Current assumptions are first, that most cases of SCD in the young are indeed cardiac related and that a cardiac cause usually can be identified at autopsy. Second, most causes of SCD are potentially curable or treatable with currently available interventions. Third, exercise, especially extreme or competitive exercise, is the main precipitating cause of SCD (at least 80% of cases) in individuals with *high-risk* cardiac defects [5,19].

Currently, what are still missing are reliable, population-based data about the following critical points. A) The prevalence of high-risk cardiovascular conditions in the general population. B) The quantification of the risk of SCD related to each of the claimed risk factors. C) The quantification of the individual severity for each individual risk factor (e.g. in cases of CAAs, the severity of coronary stenosis in individual candidates). Preliminary data seem to indicate that the risks of SCD can be anywhere from baseline to more than 300 times higher (as seen in individuals with anomalous origin of the left coronary artery from the right sinus of Valsalva, and a more than 50-55% area of cross-sectional stenosis). We need to determine why only a few individuals may die and more precisely relate the likelihood of SCD to the specific severity of the pre-existing condition versus the critical precipitating circumstances versus a combination of the 2. D) The cost of accurately and safely diagnosing large, at-risk groups. (Additionally, are sedentary people with the same conditions free from the risk of SCD?) E) An effective, accurate, and reproducible screening strategy could indeed significantly reduce the incidence of SCD [28].

22.7 The Mission of the Center for Coronary Artery Anomalies

The Center for Coronary Artery Anomalies (CCAA) at the Texas Heart Institute was created in 2008 to programmatically address the above-mentioned issues and provide a better outcome for young athletes. Initially, the programme's mandate is to establish definitive documentation of the problem and causes of SCD in the young through a screening program of a large sample of the *normal population* and a survey of a large, continuous series of autopsy studies of people who died suddenly, likely from cardiac causes.

The first study, the *MRI-based screening study*, includes 3 sources of data from a large Houston-area population of children aged 11–15 years: clinical information obtained from a self-completed questionnaire, a resting ECG, and cardiac magnetic resonance imaging (MRI) to obtain a screening-quality cardiac image to identify coronary anomalies and hypertrophic and dilated cardiomyopathies. The objective is to gather prospective information about not only the prevalence of typical symptoms of interest in the context of SCD prevention (e.g. shortness of breath, chest pain, and fainting spells) but also the prevalence of abnormalities on ECG and MRI that are said to be associated with SCD in the young.

Simultaneously, in collaboration with the Harris County Institute for Forensic Studies, the CCAA is organising and carrying out the *necropsy-based study*, a large, prospective survey of the causes of SCD in the young versus those in other groups, including older individuals or non-SCD cases, based on forensic cases from the Houston area. About 6,500 cases are being screened over 2 years using a prospective protocol and working with the forensic pathologists at the centre.

We believe that our innovative and comprehensive approach to the multiple issues involved in SCD in the young will help in finally establishing a solid discipline in this emerging field of cardiology. Clinicians at the CCAA are motivated by the belief that diagnosing curable, potentially lethal conditions is an urgent and promising call that is now a realistic option because of the accurate diagnostic technology available for a general screening programme.

Because sporting activities are both popular and widely encouraged for promoting and maintaining health and well-being among the general public, screening programmes by sports cardiologists are clearly needed for establishing a solid foundation for protecting the health of the younger generation – and this realization is half of the solution [29].

The results of the CCAA studies will start to become available in 2012, and the studies are expected to be completed in 2015.

References

1. Harrell E (2009) Sudden cardiac death: should young athletes be screened? Time Magazine
2. Maron BJ, Thompson PD, Ackerman MJ, et al (2007) Recommendations and considerations related to preparticipation screening for cardiovascular abnormalities in competitive athletes: 2007 update: a scientific statement from the American Heart Association Council on Nutrition, Physical Activity, and Metabolism: endorsed by the American College of Cardiology Foundation. Circulation 115:1643-455
3. Corrado D, Pelliccia A, Bjørnstad HH, Vanhees L, Biffi A, Borjesson M, Panhuyzen-Goedkoop N, Deligiannis A, Solberg E, Dugmore D, et al (2005) Cardiovascular pre-participation screening of young competitive athletes for prevention of sudden death: proposal for a common European protocol. Consensus Statement of the Study Group of Sport Cardiology of the Working Group of Cardiac Rehabilitation and Exercise Physiology and the Working Group of Myocardial and Pericardial Diseases of the European Society of Cardiology. Eur Heart J 26:516-24
4. Maron BJ, Doerer JJ, Haas TS, Tierney DM, Mueller FO (2009) Sudden deaths in young competitive athletes: analysis of 1866 deaths in the United States, 1980-2006. Circulation 119:1085-92
5. Harmon KG, Asif IM, Klossner D, Drezner JA (2011) Incidence of sudden cardiac death in national collegiate athletic association athletes. Circulation 123:1594-600
6. Steinvil A, Chundadze T, Zeltser D, et al (2011) Mandatory electrocardiographic screening of athletes to reduce their risk for sudden death: proven fact or wishful thinking? J Am Coll Cardiol 57:1291-6
7. Atkins DL, Everson-Stewart S, Sears GK, et al (2009) Epidemiology and outcomes from out-of-hospital cardiac arrest in children: the Resuscitation Outcomes Consortium Epistry-Cardiac Arrest. Circulation 119:1484-91
8. Donoghue AJ, Nadkarni V, Berg RA, et al (2005) Out-of-hospital pediatric cardiac arrest: an epidemiologic review and assessment of current knowledge. Ann Emerg Med 46:512-22
9. SOS-KANTO (2007) Cardiopulmonary resuscitation by bystanders with chest compression only (SOS-KANTO): an observational study. Lancet 369:920-6
10. Young KD, Gausche-Hill M, McClung CD, et al (2004) A prospective, population-based study of the epidemiology and outcome of out-of-hospital pediatric cardiopulmonary arrest. Pediatrics 114:157-64
11. Winkel BG, Holst AG, Theilade J, et al (2011) Nationwide study of sudden cardiac death in persons aged 1-35 years. Eur Heart J 32:983-90
12. Weeke P, Folke F, Gislason GH, Lippert FK, Olesen JB, Andersson C, Wissenberg M, Poulsen HE, Nielsen SL, Køber L, Torp-Pedersen C (2011) Hospital admissions and pharmacotherapy before out-of-hospital cardiac arrest according to age. Resuscitation
13. Corrado D, Basso C, Rizzoli G, et al (2003) Does sports activity enhance the risk of sudden death in adolescents and young adults? J Am Coll Cardiol 42:1959-63
14. Maron BJ (2003) Sudden death in young athletes. N Engl J Med 349:1064-75
15. Eckart RE, Scoville SL, Campbell CL, et al (2004) Sudden death in young adults: a 25-year review of autopsies in military recruits. Ann Intern Med 141:829-34
16. Ackerman MJ (2009) State of postmortem genetic testing known as the cardiac channel molecular autopsy in the forensic evaluation of unexplained sudden cardiac death in the young. Pacing Clin Electrophysiol 32 Suppl 2:S86-9
17. Taylor AJ, Rogan KM, Virmani R (1992) Sudden cardiac death associated with isolated congenital coronary artery anomalies. J Am Coll Cardiol 20:640-7
18. Frescura C, Basso C, Thiene G, et al (1998) Anomalous origin of coronary arteries and risk of sudden death: a study based on an autopsy population of congenital heart disease. Hum Pathol 29:689-95
19. Basso C, Maron BJ, Corrado D, et al (2000) Clinical profile of congenital coronary artery anomalies with origin from the wrong aortic sinus leading to sudden death in young competitive athletes. J Am Coll Cardiol 35:1493-501
20. Angelini P (2007) Coronary artery anomalies: an entity in search of an identity. Circulation 115:1296-305
21. Angelini P, Flamm SD (2007) Newer concepts for imaging anomalous aortic origin of the coronary arteries in adults. Catheter Cardiovasc Interv 69:942-54
22. Corrado D, Basso C, Pavei A, et al (2006) Trends in sudden cardiovascular death in young competitive athletes after implementation of a preparticipation screening program. JAMA 296:1593-601
23. Maron BJ, Haas TS, Doerer JJ, et al (2009) Comparison of U.S. and Italian experiences with sudden cardiac deaths in young competitive athletes and implications for preparticipation screening strategies. Am J Cardiol 104:276-80
24. Corrado D, Pelliccia A, Heidbuchel H, et al (2010) Recommendations for interpretation of 12-lead electrocardiogram in the athlete. Eur Heart J 31:243-59
25. Corrado D, Pelliccia A, Bjørnstad HH, Vanhees L, Biffi A, Borjesson M, Panhuyzen-Goedkoop N, Deligiannis A, Solberg E, Dugmore D, et al (2005) Cardiovascular pre-participation screening of young competitive athletes for prevention of sudden death: proposal for a common European protocol. Consensus Statement of the Study Group of Sport Cardiology of the

Working Group of Cardiac Rehabilitation and Exercise Physiology and the Working Group of Myocardial and Pericardial Diseases of the European Society of Cardiology. Eur Heart J 26:516-24
26. Glover DW, Maron BJ (2007) Evolution in the process of screening United States high school student-athletes for cardiovascular disease. Am J Cardiol 100:1709-12
27. Chaitman BR (2007) An electrocardiogram should not be included in routine preparticipation screening of young athletes. Circulation 116:2610-4
28. Thompson PD, Levine BD (2006) Protecting athletes from sudden cardiac death. JAMA 296:1648-50
29. Anderson L, Exeter D, Bowyer L (2011) Sudden cardiac death: mandatory exclusion of athletes at risk is a step too far. Br J Sports Med

Peripheral Vascular Disease in Athletes

23

Ombretta Martinelli, Luigi Irace and Paolo Gozzo

23.1 Introduction

Athletes who carry out competitive sporting activities often complain of symptoms, especially pain, which in most cases are related to musculoskeletal injuries. However, when the sporting activity involves frequent and repetitive movement of the upper or lower limbs, the same clinical manifestations may be a result of an arterial disease, causing ischemia which is induced by muscular exercise [1].

Although this can be corrected using surgical revascularization or intravenous procedures, sport-related arterial disease is often undetected during routine physical examination. Using experience of vascular complications in competitive athletes over a six-year period, Arko et al. [2] observed arterial lesions affecting the subclavian-axillary axis due to thoracic outlet syndrome (TOS) in 50% of cases, entrapment of the popliteal artery in 43% and external iliac artery stenosis in 7%, while subclavian thrombosis vein was the only venous complication found. The possible reasons for the lack of recognition of vascular disease in athletes are attributed to the similarity of symptoms of vascular disease with those more commonly found in musculoskeletal diseases and the difficulty in confirming vascular clinical changes, which often can only be identified using provocative tests and not in basic conditions.

Precise anatomical identification of vascular damage is extremely important in terms of prognosis and treatment and, when combined with the identification and definition of pathophysiological mechanisms of arterial disease, enables prompt selection of more suitable treatment strategies for the remission of symptoms and for adequate functional recovery that, when possible, also allows athletes to return to competitive activities. Many pathophysiological factors and mechanisms may be involved in the onset of vascular disease in young athletes, especially those who take part in competitions. These involve direct vascular compression of muscles and/or tendons that cause insults of repeated demands on a segment of the vascular wall as in the case of TOS in baseball players [3], but it is also possible that vascular disease is the result of an abnormal autoimmune or inflammatory response to mechanical stimuli of vascular strain or compression following specific movements made during certain types of sporting activity, such as iliac endofibrosis in endurance athletes [4].

In subjects who practise sporting activities, particularly at competitive level, peripheral vascular disease in the upper or lower limbs is often suspected based on the clinical picture, which in reality is common to various possible pathological conditions; this results in the need for a diagnostic procedure that is sometimes long and complicated and takes into consideration all possible causes of such clinical manifestations. This justifies the potential delay in diagnosing vascular changes, which often is more than 6-12 months from the onset of clinical symptoms, and can reasonably be explained by the difficulty in managing such patients using conventional epidemiological criteria that are taken into account for

O. Martinelli (✉)
Department of General Surgery
"La Sapienza" University of Rome

M. Fioranelli and G. Frajese (eds.), *Sports Cardiology*,
DOI: 10.1007/978-88-470-2775-6_23, © Springer-Verlag Italia 2012

screening and diagnostic evaluation of arterial and venous diseases in young athletes who regularly undergo medical visits and instrumental control tests to rule out pathological conditions, particularly cardiovascular conditions, that contraindicate physical activity.

It is also the case that minor peripheral arterial lesions often remain asymptomatic in conditions of rest and moderate physical activity and become manifest only when physical force increases. This explains the corresponding delay in identifying the vascular etiology of symptoms in young subjects and, above all, in athletes of all ages. It is also difficult to establish a causal relationship between instrumentally confirmed vascular lesions and the clinical picture when the force test during instrumental analysis does not reproduce the symptoms felt during sporting activity and/or when instrumental findings normal during rest. This problem may be avoided by including non-invasive instrumental tests aimed at ruling out abnormalities or anatomical variants and/or vascular changes that may cause symptomatic vascular damage or be clinically silent in the lower limbs and, more rarely, the upper limbs in diagnoses carried out at the start of sporting activity, particularly at competitive level, and during subsequent routine controls.

In terms of the *lower limb* vessels, the most common diseases in athletes, for which clinical and instrumental evaluation is required, are: popliteal artery entrapment, iliac endofibrosis, primary varicose veins and, more frequently, secondary varicose veins. TOS, on the other hand, is the main condition affecting the *upper limbs*.

23.2 Iliac Endofibrosis

This is a pathological condition mainly located in the iliac arteries, occurring in association with intermittent claudication due to intense physical exercise and hemodynamically significant stenosis (> 70% of the vascular lumen) of the iliac axis. It was first described twenty-five years ago by Mosimann et al. [5] and is a rare and little known disease caused by non-atherosclerotic, lesions affecting the iliac arterial axis; the etiology is still not fully known. It involves gradual thickening of the endothelium of the vascular wall due to the accumulation of fibrous material; this process of endofibrosis is typically found in the proximal segment of the left external iliac artery, but may be bilateral or also involve other arterial segments (e.g., the common femoral artery).

It mainly affects young athletes, especially cyclists, who undergo intense training, with none of the classic risk factors for atherosclerosis in the medical history. The main finding in professional cyclists has led to the view that the main pathogenic factor may be repeated straining of the walls of the external iliac artery in correspondence along with articulation of the hip while pedalling. However, similar iliac lesions have been found in rugby players, long-distance runners, body builders and football players, supporting the hypothesis of a multifactorial etiopathogenesis, which is still not completely understood, of this disease. The possible causes of iliac endofibrosis include arterial compression by a segment of the hypertrophic psoas muscle, hyperdynamic blood flow due to muscular force, prolongation of the external iliac artery, or straining of the arterial wall where the vessel is attached to its collateral branches proximally and to the inguinal ligament distally.

Unlike atherosclerotic arterial wall lesions, endofibrotic parietal damage is often difficult to identify during diagnosis, not only based on its clinical importance but also using ultrasound instruments and/or radiological imaging, including color-Doppler ultrasound, MR angiography and spiral CT angiography with 3D reconstruction, as well as endoluminal ultrasound (EUS) and digital subtraction angiography (DSA).

Endofibrosis may be asymptomatic for a long time at rest and only has clinical manifestations when maximum force is exerted; arterial lesions are not easy to see at first and are therefore often unrecognized and associated with normal instrumental findings in basic conditions; this justifies the frequent significant delay in diagnosing iliac endofibrosis, which on average happens 16 months after the start of the first symptoms in professional athletes and 12 months in amateurs. In more advanced stages of the disease patients may complain of various other factors: intermittent claudication, edema, pain leading to functional impotence or paresthesia of the gluteal muscles, thigh or calf of the homolateral limb in cases of iliac stenosis.

Upon objective examination, the absence of a femoral arterial pulse is a pathognomonic sign of hemodynamically significant obstruction or stenosis of the upstream iliac axis and may therefore lead to the suspicion of endofibrosis in this area in subjects who practise intense physical training, if there is no possible vascular damage resulting from hypercoagulability, the use or drugs of anabolic steroids, and orthopedic or neurological changes. However, the absence or hyposphygmia of the femoral pulse downstream from iliac stenosis is recognisable in a limited number of cases: Alimi et al. [6], in a case study involving 14 patients, recorded a normal sphygmic arterial pulse in 12 cases, a slow femoral pulse in 1 patient and no pulse in another. The limited significance of objective findings means that any suspicion of iliac endofibrosis must be checked using instrumental data that, at least in preliminary phases, should be gathered with non-invasive echocardiographic methods [7]. Among the forms of echocardiography, Doppler arterial tensiometry has a specific, elective indication in measuring the pressure index in the ankle and arm (ankle-brachial index, ABI) with continuous wave Doppler. This index should be measured in both rest conditions and after maximum physical exercise (treadmill test). After the treadmill test an ABI that has fallen below 0.66 enables reliable diagnosis of iliac stenosis. Chevalier [30] maintains that measuring ABI after the force test can be considered the analysis of first choice. It is also currently believed that the ABI sensitivity of Doppler arterial tensiometry is closely linked to the effectiveness of the force test, and some authors (including Alimi) have therefore decided to reduce the ABI cut-off point to 0.56 in order to increase sensitivity to this parameter. It is also important to consider that ABI measurements do not provide any information on the place and type of arterial lesion that decreases this index, and that prompt, detailed identification of the site, extent and possibly the characteristics of the arterial lesion is essential for correct and effective planning of the most appropriate therapeutic approach to diseases such as iliac endofibrosis, which is an isolated arterial lesion that can be treatment successfully with surgery or intravenous procedures.

Analysis of data collected during a review of the literature suggest that endofibrotic iliac stenosis should be suspected in athletes when one or more of the following instrumental factors occurs:

- stenosis affecting the external iliac artery, but sometimes the common or internal iliac artery too;
- external iliac dolichoartery;
- one or more collateral arteries of the iliac axis and tributaries of the psoas muscle.

These data are currently obtainable with various diagnostic techniques such as color-Doppler ultrasound, spiral CT angiography with 3D reconstruction, MR angiography, and possibly DSA, which, alone or in combination, provide reliable information for the diagnosis of such diseases. Color-Doppler ultrasound performed by expert examiners with high-definition equipment enables identification of external iliac artery stenosis with a sensitivity rate of 84% even if specificity is only 66%. Color-Doppler ultrasound also has satisfactory reliability in measuring the length of external iliac artery stenosis, while the accuracy of this diagnostic method decreases significantly in determining common iliac artery stenosis and visualising the psoas muscle artery. Abraham et al. [8] report a higher rate of sensitivity and specificity for color-Doppler ultrasound in identifying changes along the iliac vessels (kinking), even if the pelvic bone structures often make it difficult to see the internal iliac artery with greater diagnostic accuracy when the examination is performed by bending of the hip joint to 90°.

Radiological imaging techniques (CT angiography or MR angiography) enable diagnostic confirmation of segmental stenosis and possible tortuosity of the iliac vessels that have already been identified with color-Doppler ultrasound, and also enable visualization of the tributary arteries of the psoas muscle. The diagnostic reliability of such methods is currently high enough to represent a valid alternative to DSA, the use of which can be limited to cases in which data gathered using other less invasive techniques are insufficient. Preoperative diagnosis can later be confirmed with EUS during treatment of endofibrotic stenosis. Whatever the method of diagnosis, instrumental evaluation must be dynamic since moderate stenosis cannot adequately be identified in static conditions even in consideration of the possibility that eccentric stenosis cannot be seen in any static views. This allows iliac endofibrosis to be diagnosed promptly and treated early and full functional recovery to be achieved in athletes who can return to sporting activity at the highest level.

23.3 Varicose Veins

Mean or maximum cardiac force during any sporting activity involves significant hemodynamic changes, particular in relation to peripheral vasodilation with consequent repercussions on venous circulation. This is especially true in the superficial venous circulation of the upper and lower limbs.

Approximately 5% of athletes are affected with varicose veins in the lower limbs; this is more common in wrestlers and weigh-lifters and is associated with static force together with sudden and intense increases in intra-abdominal pressure with subsequent obstruction of venous return that is characteristic of these sports. Sudden changing the position of the body and adopting certain postures can lead to mechanical obstruction of venous flow and a sudden rise in peripheral venous pressure. These conditions are also confirmed during other sporting activities such as football, high jump, long jump, rowing, and martial arts such as judo and karate.

The development of varicose veins in the lower limbs of athletes who practise these sports competitively is, however, linked to congenital miopragia of the venous walls and, in particular, vulnerability of the venous valve system; these are conditions that predispose subjects to the onset of chronic superficial venous insufficiency. The diagnosis of this pathological condition is based on objective reports of ecstatic and tortuous veins in one or both of the upper or lower limbs. In particular, in the legs, diagnosis is made using color-Doppler ultrasound, which allows the site, extent and presence of venous reflux to be identified, which is to be considered pathological if it lasts longer than 0.5 seconds. Ultrasound findings also enable true varicose veins to be identified and distinguished from those considered *false*. The former are characterized by ecstatic and tortuous veins and are associated with hemodynamic changes that can be identified instrumentally, while in the latter case the superficial veins are predominant and there are no significant hemodynamic changes, due to marked hypertrophy of the muscular mass.

The choice of treatment for varicose veins during conventional surgical intervention (stripping, crossectomy, phlebectomy and ligation of incontinent perforant veins) or with ablative procedures using lasers or radiofrequencies depends on the location and seriousness of the varicose disease. These operations enable full patient recovery and a return to sporting activity, but the subject remains predisposed to possible relapse.

23.4 Entrapment Syndromes

The best known and most studied of these syndromes is the result of popliteal artery entrapment. Entrapment of popliteal vessels – arteries and possibly veins – may be due to developmental changes to the gastrocnemius muscle and, more rarely, the deep popliteus muscle or other muscles, or may lead to the formation a fibrous band or abnormalities along the course of the artery itself; these anatomical changes may be the cause of intermittent compression of the vessels that lead from the popliteal cavity and adductor canal, with resulting histopathological changes to the arterial and/or venous walls and compression of the distal vascular bed.

Popliteal artery entrapment is much more common in males aged under 30 years and is often bilateral; it is characterized by intermittent claudication in the calves and feet, sometimes associated with paresthesia, pallor and subjective hypothermia in the feet. Exceptionally, patients may feel pain when resting or trophic ischemic lesions.

Clinical manifestations of popliteal entrapment are often difficult to diagnose with routine physical and instrumental examinations, even in young patients because intermittent claudication often occurs only during intense physical activity involving the lower limbs, such as walking or running.

It is now known that popliteal artery entrapment

should be taken into consideration in the differential diagnosis of intermittent claudication in young adults, particularly in those who practise sporting activities. Levien et al. [9] report a popliteal artery entrapment rate of 60% in young athletes in whom, where there is no muscular or tendon-related anatomical abnormalities, it is linked to extrinsic compression of the popliteal artery as part of the medial head of the hypertrophic gastrocnemius muscle following physical exercise. Entrapment of the entire vasculonervous bundle in the popliteal cavity can also be confirmed by compression against the rigid band of the bundle that forms the posterior margin of the soleus canal. The exclusively functional variant of popliteal artery entrapment due to muscular hypertrophy with no anatomical abnormalities is less common and more difficult to diagnose than entrapment resulting from structural damage of vascular walls due to anatomical changes affecting the popliteal cavity [10].

Popliteal artery entrapment mainly involves intermittent cramp-like pain in the soleus muscle and plantar paresthesia after physical exercise and only causes distal ischemic lesions in very rare cases; these symptoms tend to occur after repeated muscular activity or orthopedic injuries that are more likely in athletes [11]. Venous compression may be a cause of perimalleolar edema, albeit rarely, cutaneous cyanosis and turgor of the superficial veins of the legs, which is more evident after walking or running.

Objective pathological findings such as the absence of a subgeniculate arterial pulse and/or signs of venous stasis in the leg can be completely absent at rest; this leads to the need for provocative tests that enable identification of popliteal vessel compression in relation to various knee articulation positions. In fact, contraction of the calf muscles as a result of dorsiflexion and extension movements with the foot or rising on the ball of the foot can cause the pulse to disappear in the posterior tibial artery and homolateral foot upon entrapment. These dynamic manoeuvres undeniably help with diagnosis even if their positivity has also been recorded in 50% of healthy volunteers [12].

Dynamic stress tests can also lead to false negative results in the presence of vascular compression when muscular contraction is not sufficient to cause vascular compression [13]. This results in different levels of popliteal entrapment and the need for maximum muscular force during tests [14].

The dynamic manoeuvres suggested as integral and unavoidable components of a physical examination are equally vital during instrumental evaluation of this disease. Regarding more appropriate instrumental analyses of popliteal artery entrapment, angiography has for many years been considered the reference examination for this disease; in fact, this allows recordings to be made of deviations along the popliteal artery, segmental obstruction of the medial part and/or post-stenotic dilatation, and the disappearance of flow during dynamic acquisitions [15].

The growing use and ever increasing reliability of ultrasound examinations (continuous wave Doppler and color-Doppler) have enabled the indication for angiography to be modified. Determining ABI with continuous wave Doppler in both basic conditions and in forced plantar positions, is highly sensitive and is indicated for screening and preliminary investigation of popliteal artery entrapment as well as the follow-up of patients undergoing surgical correction of entrapment. An ABI reduction of more than 0.20 during dynamic manoeuvres is considered to be indicative of popliteal artery entrapment. Doppler arterial tensiometry is currently combined with color-Doppler ultrasound to enable visualization of the popliteal artery and vein along the entire course, defining the relationship with adjacent structures; it also allows the reduction to be recorded until the blood flow, color and Doppler signals disappear, which is related to vascular compression during provocative tests (Fig. 23.1). Color-Doppler ultrasound also provides useful information on the distal arteries and is combined with the dynamic investigation of satellite popliteal veins.

Further ultrasound studies may be conducted with spiral CT angiography or MR angiography of the same area, thus enabling direct visualization of the muscles and tendons responsible for entrapment. Spiral CT angiography, in fact, provides accurate details on anatomical structures next to the vascular bundle, as well as excellent images of the vessels.

MR angiography is increasingly used to evaluate popliteal artery entrapment as it enables or-

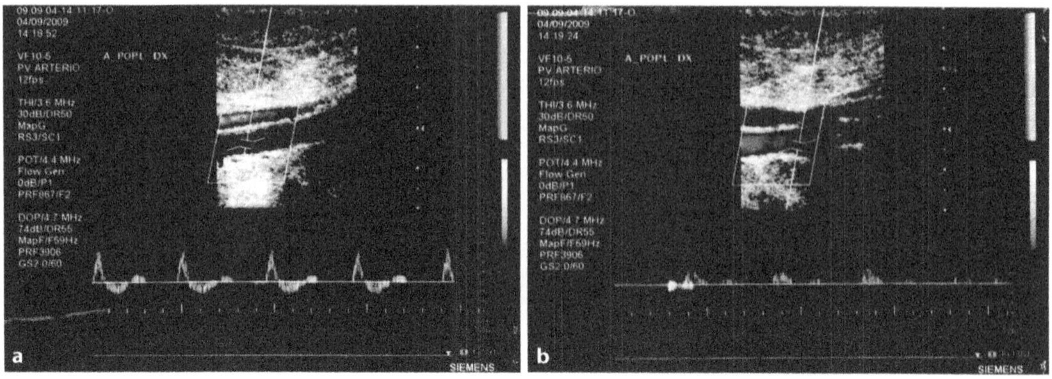

Fig. 23.1 Popliteal artery entrapment. a Color-Doppler evaluation in basic condition. b The same case during dynamic maneuvers showing a progressive decrease of the Doppler signal due to popliteal artery compression at the level of the adductor canal

ganic forms to be distinguished from functional forms, even if the diagnostic accuracy of this technique is restricted by the potential presence of movement-related artefacts during dynamic studies [16]. Regardless of the type of instrumental diagnosis, findings must always be matched with the clinical picture. In fact, there is currently no other clinical evidence that patients with functional entrapment are at greater risk of changes to the popliteal vessels than control subjects, at least those who do not complain of specific symptoms. Therefore, surgical treatment for popliteal arteries decompression by means of fasciotomy, myotomy or section of the aberrant fibrotendinous structures, with or without direct arterial reconstruction, is indicated only in cases where there are significant symptoms that restrict physical activity in patients [17].

23.5 Chronic Compartment Syndrome

Chronic compartment syndrome (CCS) is related to transient ischemia of a lower limb. This ischemia is the result of hypertension in the muscle compartments, surrounded by aponeurotic fascia that cannot be extended by increasing the volume of the hypertophic muscular mass during maximum physical exercise.

This pathological condition is responsible for about 75% of cases of chronic pain in the lower limbs, which can occur during any sport: marathons and even skiing, football, tennis and rugby, with a similar incidence rate in athletes of both sexes. In 80% of cases such pain is bilateral, typically occurring after a well defined and planned period of physical exercise, and recedes when exercise stops.

In cases in which CCS is related to hypertension of the anterior compartment of the leg, which is most often affected, and ischemic involvement of the external sciatic and popliteal nerves leads to a deficiency in the dorsiflexion movement and paresthesia.

Clinical suspicion of CCS may be the result of palpations of the small muscular hernias due to repeated stress of the fascia. However, it is based on an instrumental study of intra-compartimental pressure that may be > 15 mmHg at rest and rise by a further 30 mmHg after 1 minute of maximum physical exercise.

Post-exercise hypertension is clearly related with MRI findings and near-infrared spectroscopy findings, which show oxygen desaturation of the muscular mass following ischemic involvement due to an increase in compartmental pressure.

The treatment of first choice for this disease involves a reduction in training, the use of non-steroidal anti-inflammatory drugs and individualized elastocompressive protection for each athlete, as well as stretching exercises for the limb in question.

If the clinical picture persists despite conservative measures, fasciotomy may be necessary. This involves complete remission of compartment syndrome affecting the anterior and lateral components of the leg, but offers less of a guarantee of success for hypertension of the posterior compartment. Athletes considering a return to maximum sporting activity after fasciotomy should bear in mind the time required for full and adequate healing of tissues in order to avoid relapse.

23.6 Thoracic Outlet Syndrome

Vascular damage due to thoracic outlet syndrome (TOS) can have a debilitating effect or also lead to a serious risk for the strength of the homolateral upper limb. This syndrome is linked to compression of the vasculonervous fascia of the subclavian vein and artery and the brachial plexus in the upper chest region, at the level of:

- the triangle formed by the anterior and medial scalene muscles and the first rib;
- the costoclavicular space;
- the angle defined by the coracoid process and the pectoralis minor muscle.

Compression of the subclavian artery and/or the brachial plexus may also be a result of bone abnormalities such as a cervical rib, an abnormal first rib or the outcome of a clavicle fracture.

In athletes, compression occurs more often due to medial and anterior scalene muscle hypertrophy, resulting from particular movements of the homolateral upper limb, as in baseball pitchers. In particular, hypertrophy of the anterior and medial scalene muscles in athletes can cause extrinsic compression of the superclavicular segment of the subclavian artery with parietal damage that leads to thrombotic obstruction and possible distal embolism and makes it necessary, in addition to surgical decompression of TOS with scalenectomy, to resect the first rib and possibly carry out direct termino-terminal arterial reconstruction.

Damage to the axillary artery and/or its branches by the tendon of the pectoralis minor muscle against the head of the humerus is less known and harder to identify and, even if it is not correct anatomically, it can be included as a compressive disease of the thoracic outlet relating to similar vascular damage, clinical manifestations and the diagnostic and therapeutic approach. In fact, hypertrophy of the head of the humerus caused by intense exercise involving the upper limb can be an additional causal mechanism of axillary arterial compression; in fact, external extrarotational movements with hyperabduction of the upper limb can cause strain leading to intimal laceration or weakening of the axillary artery wall attached to its collateral branches by traction of the vessel against the head of the humerus. Similar parietal damage can affect the same axillary collateral branches, particularly the tributary circumflex arteries at the head of the humerus, as a result of repeated intense movements of the scapulohumeral joint [18].

Repeated compression of the arteries in relation with the thoracic outlet is a cause of changes to the vascular wall that may occur in patients with intraluminal thrombosis or with the development of an aneurysm with parietal thrombotic apposition and possible subsequent distal embolization.

Suspicion of TOS during diagnosis is the most common indication for physical and instrumental examination of upper limbs vessels in subjects who practise sport. In fact, the rate of neurovascular compression in the thoracic outlet is higher in athletes than in the general population, due to hypertrophy of the muscular mass following physical exercise.

Specific movements by the upper limbs in any type of sport, such as weight-lifting, baseball, shot put or javelin throwing, may cause marked muscular hypertrophy associated with the thoracic outlet and subsequent vasculonervous compression in the same area. Compression of part of the hypertrophic pectoralis minor muscle is the most common cause of TOS in athletes and is shown by the fact that the clinical picture for TOS is mainly a consequence of nervous or venous compression, while parietal damage to the arteries is less common.

In clinical terms, most patients are asymptomatic or have mild symptoms; when it occurs, pain is often dull and intermittent, attributable to claudication of the forearm, arm or hand, extending to the neck and shoulders and exacerbated abduction and raising of the upper limbs. In most cases vascular symptoms are associated with neurological symptoms and range from mild paresthesia of the fingers of the homolateral hand to obvious ischemia due to embolic occlusion of the digital arteries, especially as a consequence of post-stenotic aneurysmatic dilatation of the compressed artery associated with the formation of a parietal thrombus in the aneurysmatic sac. Raynaud's phenomenon is typically present in only 25% of cases.

TOS has been demonstrated in baseball players, particularly pitchers, and volleyball players who develop hypertrophy of the anterior and medial scalene muscles due to repeated throwing movements [19].

Based on data in the literature, when the subclavian vessels and brachial plexus are compressed due to a marked development of the scalene muscles and the pectoralis minor muscle, the axillary artery and the humeral circumflex arterial branches may also be compressed following abduction manoeuvres with the homolateral upper limb during throwing movements that can occur in any sporting activity [20].

Roher et al. [21] report radiological evidence of axillary artery compression with a consequent gradient of 20 mmHg between the two upper limbs in pitchers. This compression may cause complete obstruction of the artery while throwing the baseball and is mainly linked to hypertrophy of the pectoralis minor muscle, even if it cannot be ruled out that in such athletes the head of the humerus may contribute to repeated injury of the third segment of the axillary artery. The results of surgical decompression of the vasculonervous fascia in the thoracic and/or axillary outlet closely depend on the precise location of the injury and the identification of anatomical structures that cause compression [22].

Diagnosis of TOS requires adequate knowledge and wide-ranging experience of the disease in order to carry out color-Doppler echocardiography and/or targeted radiological imaging, angiographic imaging, CT angiography or MR angiography in basic conditions and during external abduction-rotation movements or hyperabduction of the upper arm (Fig. 23.2). These dynamic manoeuvres simulate repetitive shoulder movements in athletes that occur during any sporting activity. The fact that physical and instrumental evaluation of upper limb vessels can be negative in basic conditions is taken into account, unless complete thrombotic obstruction of the subclavian-axillary veins or arteries does not occur or if embolic obstruction is found in the arteries of the forearm or hand. The importance of dynamic manoeuvres is therefore evident: standing to attention, with deep breathing and rotation of the head (Adson's manoeuvre) and, above all, hyperabduction of the arm (Wright's manoeuvre) (Fig. 23.3).

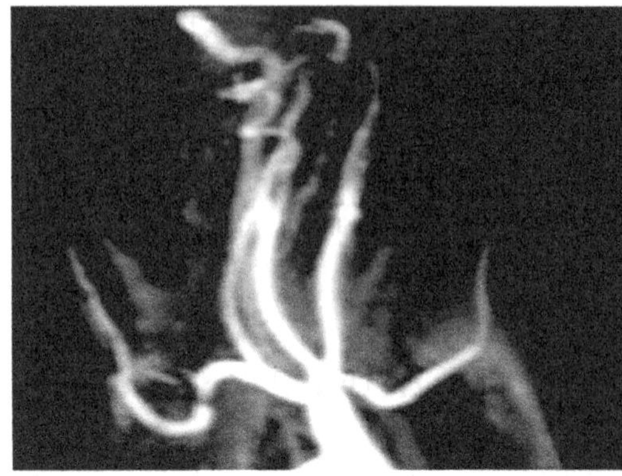

Fig. 23.2 Thoracic outlet syndrome: MR angiography evaluation showing right subclavian artery compression during hyperabduction of the homolateral upper limb

Accurate diagnosis of TOS is crucial because the efficacy and complexity of treatment relies on the early recognition and prompt removal of the mechanism of compression, possibly associated with direct arterial and venous revascularization surgery if there is irreversible parietal damage to the vessels of the thoracic outlet. In particular, there is sufficient standardization of the methods of treating subclavian artery compression that makes it necessary to perform decompressive surgery, which, in athletes, is often associated with direct arterial reconstruction. The treatment approach for lesions in the axillary artery is more controversial. In athletes who have no thromboembolic lesions in distal vessels, humeral compression on the axillary artery may be considered only as a warning sign for parietal stress affecting the artery. In this case an initial attempt at physiotherapy rehabilitation may be considered with a change to the throwing movements associated with close clinical and instrumental monitoring with a color-Doppler examination. The persistence or worsening of symptoms associated with the occurrence of steno-obstructive lesions affecting this vessel or downstream arteries makes surgery necessary.

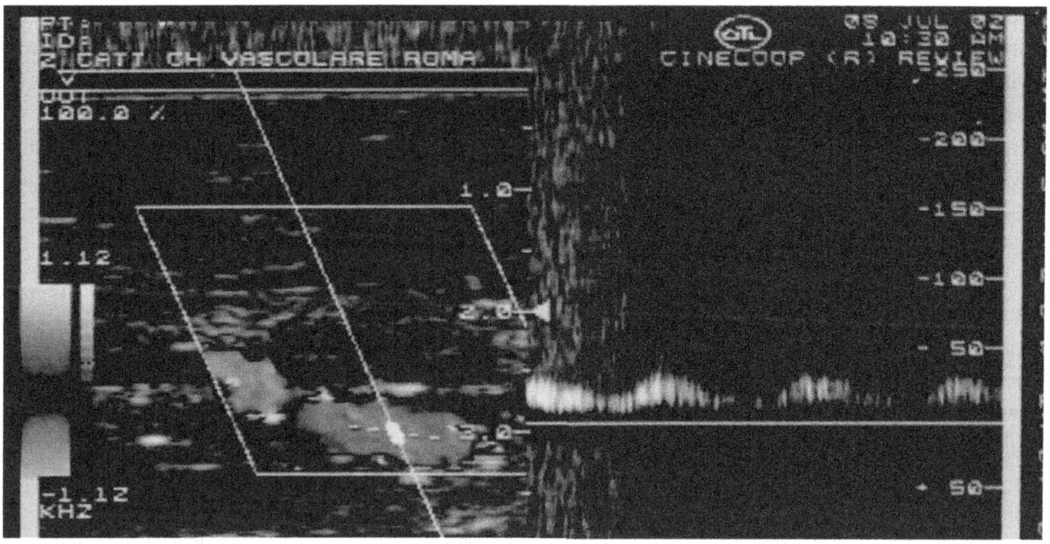

Fig. 23.3 Color-Doppler ultrasound: the hyperabduction manoeuvre of the homolateral upper limb shows left subclavian vessel compression at the level of the thoracic outlet due to scalene muscle hypertrophy

23.7 Paget-Schroetter Syndrome (Effort-induced Thrombosis)

Paget-Schroetter syndrome (PSS), or effort-induced thrombosis, often affects healthy young adults and is caused by repetitive arm movements that lead to repeated injury to the axillary-subclavian venous axis in the muscloskeletal structures of the thoracic outlet or the costoclavicular space and subsequent spontaneous venous thrombosis. In fact, prolonged and/or repeated extrinsic compression can cause micro-injuries and/or intimal lacerations of the venous wall with consequent activation of the blood coagulation cascade that triggers thrombotic events. The same pathogenetic mechanisms can cause fibrosis of the wall that stenotises the venous lumen and causes gradual deceleration of blood flow leading to thrombosis. This disease mainly occurs in males, more often involving the dominant upper arm, and representing 1-2% of cases of deep vein thrombosis (DVT) in the upper limbs, but it affects 15-24% of DVT cases in healthy young adults who practise sporting activities [23]. Sports such as tennis, swimming, gymnastics, rowing, baseball, weight-lifting and wrestling can cause effort-induced thrombosis; in athletes, due to their young age and good overall condition, thrombosis may go unrecognized with a subsequent delay in diagnosis and treatment, and may increase morbidity and affect quality of life [24]. The possible serious clinical and prognostic implications of delayed diagnosis of PSS make it necessary to carry out a suitable instrumental diagnostic procedure even if the clinical picture is of little significance, based on the patient's medical history of intense and repeated physical activity involving the upper limbs. Evaluation of the disease is initially based on data from blood chemistry and blood coagulation tests, even if effort-induced thrombosis is not necessarily associated with a state of hypercoagulability [25]. Radiological examination of the thoracic outlet may confirm bone abnormalities, but diagnosis of PSS must include instrumental identification of venous thrombosis and dynamic manoeuvres that provide evidence for venous compression as the causal agent.

Color-Doppler ultrasound is a non-invasive and readily available form of instrumental evaluation in clinical practice as well as in poorly equipped facilities. Its reliability is very satisfactory in the proximal segments of the subclavian and axillary veins, with specificity of between 88 and 100% and sensitivity of between 78 and 100% [26]. Diagnostic accuracy of this method, however, is affected by the difficulty in demonstrating thrombosis in the retroclavicular segment of the subclavian vein that is most often affected. In cases in which color-Doppler findings are not conclusive or contradict clinical findings, MR angiography may provide evidence of subclavicular DVT with, in addition to venous obstruction, as well as the presence of collateral circles and venous compression by the adjacent musculoskeletal structures. It cannot, however, be performed in claustrophobic patients or those with pacemakers or metallic prostheses; nor does allow for enable dynamic investigation of flow in the axillary-subclavicular axis. In cases in which color-Doppler is not reliable and MR angiography contraindicated, diagnostic confirmation of PSS may be achieved with CT angiography or phlebography, which should be carried out by changing the position of the upper limb to show extrinsic compression of the axillary or subclavian veins and/or their collateral branches. Phlebography is always performed during intravenous treatment of this condition. There is currently a general consensus for the indication of loco-regional thrombolysis as the most effective treatment of effort-induced thrombosis, even if patients undergoing this procedure and subsequent anticoagulation procedures remain at a high risk for relapse unless destruction of the thrombus is not associated with decompression of the venous axis and/or treatment of venous stenosis by angioplasty [27] (Fig. 24.1-24.3).

23.8 Conclusions

There are therefore a large number of vascular, arterial and venous diseases that can be associated with sporting activity; these diseases can be attributed to various causes and numerous pathophysiological mechanisms with a range of therapeutic implications [28].

It is therefore possible to identify a common facto in these pathological conditions: diagnosis must be made as early and accurately as possible, and this is closely connected with the choice of the most suitable treatment. Prompt diagnosis and treatment of vascular diseases in athletes is part of a multidiscipline approach based on the close cooperation of trainers, specialists in sports medicine, orthopedic surgeons, vascular surgeons and angiologists [29].

Bibliography

1. Mosley JG (2003) Arterial problems in athletes. Br J Surg 90:1461-1469
2. Arko FR, Harris EJ, Zarins CK, Olcott C (2001) Vascular complications in high performance athletes. J Vasc Surg 33:935-942
3. Dugas JR, Weiland AJ (2000) Vascular pathology in the throwing athletes. Hand Clin 16: 477-485
4. Ehsan O, Darwish A, Edmundson C et al (2004) Non-traumatic lower limb vascular complications in endurance athletes. Review of literature. Eur J Vasc Endovasc Surg 28:1-8
5. Mosimann R, Walder J, Van Melle G. (1985) Stenosis intimal thickening of the external iliac artery. Illness of competition cyclist. Vascular Surgery 19:258-263
6. Alimi YS, Accrocca F, Barthelemy P et al (2004) Comparison between duplex scanning and angiographic findings in the evaluation of functional iliac obstruction in top endurance athletes. Eur J Vasc Endovasc Surg 28:513-519
7. Doraiswamy VA, Giri J, Mohler E (2009) Premature peripheral arterial disease – difficult diagnosis in very early presentation. Int J Angiol 18:45-47
8. Abraham P, Saunet JL, Chevalier JM (1997) External iliac artery endofibrosis in athletes. Sports Med 24:221-226
9. Levien LJ, Veller MG (1999) Popliteal artery syndrome: more common than previously recognized. J Vasc Surg 30:587-598
10. Rignault DP, Pailler J, Lunel F (1985) The "functional" popliteal entrapment syndrome. Int J Angiol 4: 341-343
11. Turnipseed W (2002) Popliteal entrapment syndrome. J Vasc Surg 35:910-915
12. Erdoes LS, Devine JJ, Bernhard V et al (1994) Popliteal vascular compression in normal population. J Vasc Surg 20:978-986
13. Levien JM (2005) Non atheromatous causes of popliteal artery disease. In: Rutherford R Vascular surgery, 6th edn Saunders, Philadelphia
14. Edward PH, Wright MJAH (2005) A practical approach for the differential diagnosis of chronic leg pain in the athletes. Am J Sports Med 33:1241-1249
15. Andrish J, Lee JC, Drez DJ (1994) Orthopedic sports medicine: principles and practice. The Leg. Saunders, Philadelphia
16. Chernoff DM, Walker AT, Khorasani R et al (1995) Asymptomatic functional popliteal entrapment demonstration at MR imaging. Radiology 195:176-188
17. Symeonidis PD, Stavrou P, King D (2008) Bilateral functional popliteal artery entrapment in young athlete. The Knee 15:54-57
18. Nijhuis HHAM, Muller-Wiefel HM (1991) Occlusion

of the brachial artery by thrombus dislodged from traumatic aneurysm of the anterior humeral circumflex artery. J Vasc Surg 13:408-411
19. Nichols AW (1996) The thoracic outlet syndrome in athletes. J Am Bard Fam Pract 9:346-355
20. Durhan JR, Yao JS, Pearce WH et al (1995). Arterial injuries in the throracic outlet syndrome. J Vasc Surg 22:124-125
21. Roher MJ, Cardullo PA, Pappas AM et al (1990) Axillary artery compression and thrombosis in throwing athletes. J Vasc Surg 11:761-769
22. Yao JS (1998) Upper extremity ischemia in athletes. Semin Vasc Surg 11:96-105
23. Shebel ND, Marin A (2006) Effort thrombosis (Paget-Schroetter syndrome) in active young adults: current concepts in diagnosis and treatment. J Vasc Nurs 24:116-126
24. Lee MC, Grassi CJ, Belkin M (1998) Early operative intervention after throbolytic therapy for primary subclavian vein thrombosis: an effective treatment approach. J Vasc Surg 27:1101-1108
25. Martinelli I, Cattaneo M, Panzeri D (1997) Risk factors for deep venous thrombosis of the upper extremities. Ann Intern Med 126:707-711
26. Baarslag HJ, van Beek EJ, Koopman MM (2002) Prospective study of color duplex ultrasonography compared with contrast venography in patients suspected of having deep vein thrombosis of the upper extremities. Ann Intern Med 136:865-872
27. Molina JF, Hunter DW, Dietz CA (2007) Paget-Schroetter syndrome treated with thrombolytic and immediate surgery. J Vasc Surg 45:328-334
28. Takach TJ, Kane PN, Madjarov JM et al (2006) Arteriopathy in the high-performance athlete. Tex Heart Int 33:482-486
29. Melby SJ, Vedantham S, Narra VR (2008) Comprehensive surgical management of the competitive athlete with effort thrombosis of the subclavian vein (Paget-Schroetter syndrome). J Vasc Surg 47:809-821
30. Chevalier JM, Enon B, Walder J et al (1986) Endofibrosis of the external iliac artery in bicycle racer: an unrecognized pathological state. Ann Vasc Surg 1:297-303

24 Hypertension in Athletes

Mara Piccoli, Serafino Orazi and Massimo Fioranelli

24.1 Introduction

Systemic hypertension is the most frequent cardiovascular disease in athletes in spite of regular physical activity, and is associated with a reduction in normal blood pressure levels, with exercise itself representing an important therapeutic intervention for this condition. These conditions require special attention by the clinician both in the initial assessment of an athlete with hypertension, with special emphasis on gender and race, and in its proper therapeutic management.

The recent European Guidelines [1] define and classify hypertension in relation to blood pressure levels recorded in several separate measurements. In adolescents and children too (2), it is very important measure blood pressure values (Table 24.1).

In the general population, as with athletes, 95% of cases are of primary or essential hypertension, resulting from an interaction between genetic and acquired factors such as being overweight, excessive alcohol intake or high sodium intake. The main causes of secondary hypertension, which affects 20% of the general population, are renal, adrenal or renovascular dysfunction [3].

The severity of hypertension in athletes depends not only blood pressure but also on the presence of additional cardiovascular risk factors for organ damage. In particular, detection of left ventricular hypertrophy poses a serious problem for differential diagnosis because it is both a specific marker of organ damage and a physiological consequence of physical training.

Through correct evaluation of the electrocardiogram, echocardiography and cardiopulmonary exercise testing can provide a differential diagnosis between an athlete's heart and pathological forms of left ventricular hypertrophy. The use of detraining may improve the diagnostic definition, but if there is any doubt it is necessary to use more specific methods such as nuclear magnetic resonance and, in some cases, endomyocardial biopsy.

The importance of risk stratification for hypertensive athletes is derived from the need to deal quickly with those at high risk with medicinal treatment.

24.2 Effects of Exercise on Blood Pressure

The cardiovascular system is largely influenced by exercise, and hemodynamic changes are closely related to the different forms of training and specific activity levels. In particular, we recognize two basic categories of exercise: dynamic and static, which are classified according to the level of intensity: low, medium and high [3] (Table 24.2).

24.2.1 Dynamic Exercise

During dynamic exercise, along with an increase in oxygen consumption, stroke volume and peripheral oxygen extraction, blood pressure increases in relation to effort intensity [4], and this increase is greater for systolic pressure than diastolic, which

M. Piccoli (✉)
Cardiology Unit
Policlinico "Luigi di Liegro", Rome, Italy

M. Fioranelli and G. Frajese (eds.), *Sports Cardiology*,
DOI: 10.1007/978-88-470-2775-6_24, © Springer-Verlag Italia 2012

Table 24.1 Classification of hypertension

	Children – Adolescents SBP or DBP percentile	Adults SBP or DBP mmHg
Normal	<90th	<120/80
Prehypertension	90th or <95th or if BP exceeds 120/80 mmHg even if <90th percentile up to <95th percentile	120-139/80-89
Stage 1 hypertension	95th-99th percentile + 5 mmHg	140-159/90-99
Stage 2 hypertension	>99th percentile + 5 mmHg	>160/100

SBP systolic blood pressure; *DBP* diastolic blood pressure.

Increase in static component ↑ / Increase in dynamic component →	C. LOW (<40% max O_2)	B. MODERATE (40-70% maxO_2)	A. HIGH (>70% maxO_2)
III. HIGH (> 50% MVC)	Martial arts Weight lifting Windsurf Sailing Water skiing	Body building Snowboard Wrestling Skateboarding	Boxe Rowing Decathlon Triathlon
II. MODERATE (20-50% MVC)	Archery Equestrian sports Motorcycling	Rugby Running (sprinting) Surfing Synchronized swimming	Running Swimming Basketball Ice Hockey
I. LOW (<20% MVC)	Billiards Cricket Golf Bowling	Volleyball Baseball Table tennis	Skiing Running Soccer Tennis

Table 24.2 Classification of sports based on peak static and dynamic components achieved during competitions

remains normal or increases slightly. Exercise is usually followed by hypotension in the recovery phase, which can also be prolonged for several hours and is generally more pronounced in hypertensive subjects compared to normotensive patients [5]. Long and constant training can lead to a reduction systolic blood pressure at rest by about 10 mmHg [6].

Some longitudinal epidemiological studies suggest that physical inactivity as well as low-intensity training are associated with an increased incidence of hypertension in the general population [7]. Similarly, a recent meta-analysis of 72 randomized clinical trials has demonstrated that dynamic exercise produces a significant and ongoing reduction in blood pressure both at rest and during outpatient monitoring, and most significantly in hypertensive subjects [8]. Aerobic exercise produces important dynamic cardiovascular and hemodynamic changes with a substantial reduction in systolic and diastolic blood pressure at rest and mitigates the effects of the sympathetic nervous system and renin angiotensin system on vascular resistance.

24.2.2 Static Exercise

Static exercise, especially at high intensity, such as weightlifting, causes a marked and sudden increase in blood pressure, heart rate, peripheral vascular resistance and consequently left ventricular afterload. These hemodynamic changes cause concentric left ventricular hypertrophy and may be associated with reduction in stroke volume [9]. However, high blood pressure reached during exercise does not increase resting values, but is highlighted in a recent meta-analysis that moderate intensity resistance training can reduce levels of blood pressure at rest [10]. However, it remains an indication of the American College of Sports Medicine (ACSM) [6], which does not recommend endurance exercise, especially high-intensity exercise, as the first choice for hypertensive athletes.

24.3 Blood Pressure Patterns in Athletes

24.3.1 White Coat Hypertension

White coat hypertension is common in athletes, especially in the young population, and is often induced by anxiety related to the physical examination. It is very important to obtain blood pressure measurements in an out-of-office location (blood pressure at home in the morning and in the evening) or 24-hour outpatient blood pressure monitoring [11]. This hypertension pattern was defined as 24-hour systolic blood pressure < 140mmHg and 24-hour diastolic blood pressure < 90 mmHg. The prognostic significance is uncertain.

24.3.2 Spurious Systolic Hypertension

Spurious systolic hypertension is common in tall men who are active in sports and non-smokers. It may be explained by the first exaggerated systolic peak in the brachial artery pressure waveform [12], which is due to very high pulse pressure amplification and low arterial wave reflection due to elastic arteries. In these individuals, central systolic blood pressure is much lower (about 30-40 mmHg lower) than brachial systolic blood pressure. This condition may be represented as an intermediate form between normotensive patients and sustained hypertension, but further studies are necessary for its application in clinical practice.

24.3.3 Hypertension in Wheelchair Athletes

Wheelchair athletes with spinal cord injuries may present episodes of severe hypertension related to the presence of autonomic dysreflexia, a sympathetic spinal reflex, related to autonomic or bladder dysfunction. This special situation has an unpredictable cardiac risk, caused higher release of catecholamines during exercise with high blood pressure values [13]. These athletes should be evaluated and managed accurately. Some athletes with spinal cord injuries above T6 may participate in so-called *boosting* practice to increase performance by intentional and self induced bladder distension. This intentional autonomic dysreflexia is considered to be a prohibited form of manipulation according to the doping guidelines of the International Paralympics Committee and should strongly be discouraged.

24.4 Physical Evaluation

Physical evaluation of hypertensive athletes uses correct the physiology and family history to identify any secondary causes of hypertension. In this context it is also necessary to rule out the use of illegal drugs, anabolic steroids, alcohol, tobacco and non-steroidal anti-inflammatory drugs [14], which are widely used in such patients (Table 24.3). This first phase is crucial for the correct diagnosis of hypertension but also for risk profile stratification of athletes and the identification of potential comorbidities, such as early signs of organ damage. As previously documented, the diagnosis of hypertension is confirmed when pressure at rest is greater than 140/90 mmHg in further measurements. The presence of psychological and physical stress can mimic hypertensive states and may require outpatient blood pressure monitoring or self measurements at home with the aim of rul-

Table 24.3 Substances that may increase blood pressure

Sodium excess and saturated fat intake
Alcohol
Tobacco
Over-the-counter medicines - Cold remedies, decongestants - Diet pills
Ergogenic aides - Caffeine - Sudafed - Cocaine - Human growth hormone - Anabolic steroids and illicit drugs
Prescription medications - Non-steroidal anti-inflammatory drugs - Immunosupressants - Antidepressants - Oral contraceptives
Dietary and herbal supplements - Guarana - Ephedra - Ma huang

ing out forms of *white coat hypertension*. It requires a careful methodology for the evaluation of blood pressure devices validated according to criteria set by the European Society of Hypertension, with an appropriately sized cuff at the brachial artery (the bladder should encircle and cover at least 80% of the length of the arm) while the patient is seated and no caffeine or tobacco are consumed in the hour preceding the reading. Even when all the rules are observed, blood pressure measurements may not reflect the real values of the individual. Three options are therefore available: re-evaluating the athlete with serial visits at intervals established for a period of 3-6 months; addressing the athlete's own measurements and validated blood pressure devices with memory; and performing outpatient blood pressure monitoring.

In all cases of hypertension it is good practice to measure blood pressure in both the upper and lower limbs: a difference in BP > 20 mmHg in the upper limbs can be considered a diagnosis of aortic coarctation. Radial and femoral pulses should also be palpated simultaneously and if the femoral pulse is diminished or delayed in relation to radial pulse, further evaluation is needed to screen for coarctation of aorta.

The cardiac assessment should be performed in a quiet setting to facilitate heart auscultation. Good physical examination is important because it can reveal the presence of heart murmurs or added tones, which are characterized by their timing, location, character and intensity. Dynamic auscultation-squatting and Valsalva manoeuvres can clarify murmur types and bring out other murmurs that were not heard initially.

Routine laboratory tests should include assays for creatinine and uric acid, an estimation of

Table 24.4 Abnormal and exercise-induced left ventricular hypertrophy (LVH)

Cardiac test		Normal LVH	Abnormal LVH
ECG	LVH Sokolow-Lyon index	Present	Absent
	Presence of Q wave pathological, significant ST depression, T wave inversion in any derivations in Caucasian athletes, T wave inversion in inferior or lateral derivations in black athletes	Absent	Present
Echocardiogram	Kinetics of left ventricular wall	Normal	Abnormal
	Left ventricular dimension	Normal >55 mm	Reduced
	Left atrium diameter	<50 mm	>50 mm
	Systolic anterior movement of anterior mitral leaflet	Absent	Present
	Diastolic function	Normal	Abnormal
	Global longitudinal strain	Normal	Reduced
Cardio-pulmonary test	Maximal oxygen uptake	>50 ml/Kg/min or >120% of estimated value by age, gender and BMI	Altered

BMI Body Mass Index.

glomerular filtration rate, lipid profile and thyroid function; especially in young athletes with a negative family history for hypertension, controls of reninaemia, aldosterone and urinary electrolytes are recommended, as they are useful in identifying secondary hypertension. In all hypertensive athletes an electrocardiogram should be performed, which can reveal indirect signs of left ventricular hypertrophy or coronary artery disease. Often the ECG shows signs of vagal hypertonia (sinus bradycardia, first degree atrioventricular block, junctional rhythm), which normalizes upon standing. They can also be associated with high-amplitude R waves, a QRS semi-vertical axis, ST elevation or the presence of inverted T waves suggestive of ischemia. Although these changes are benign, physicians should be very cautious in assessing these athletes because 75% of cases of sudden death in young athletes occur during maximal exercise. However, in this situation, athletes must undergo second-level examinations such as echocardiography and exercise testing [10,14-15].

Echocardiograms show greater specificity than electrocardiograms in identifying left ventricular hypertrophy and in most cases in distinguishing between an athlete's physiological hypertrophy of and a pathological pattern. In athlete's hearts hypertrophy is a symmetrical distribution, ventricular normal volumes and normal diastolic function by Doppler flow (Table 24.4)

The exercise test is widely used to predict and identify different types of hypertension. Athletes with hypertension show during the test and during the recovery phase a rapid increase in systolic and diastolic pressure values. It should be considered abnormal if systolic blood pressure is > 240 mmHg during exercise. To some authors, an exaggerated increase in diastolic values during exercise may be considered a predictor of developing hypertension in normotensive subjects [16]. Further evidence also confirms that an excessive increase in systolic values during exercise tests may predict the onset of hypertension and left ventricular hypertrophy and may be indirectly related to a risk of death from cardiovascular causes [17].

24.5 Recommendations for Participation in Competitive Sport

The evaluation of competitive sport in secondary hypertension in athletes is conditioned by the abolition of secondary identified causes of hypertension itself.

Instead, essential arterial hypertension requires a comprehensive assessment in order to participate in competitive sports. Table 24.5 summarises recommendations for athletes with hypertension in relation to the cardiovascular profile and type of sport [3].

This classification has limitations because most sports involve various dynamic and static components. For example, it is not possible for an athlete with stage 2 hypertension to participate in sports classified as IIIA, IIIB and IIIC, but, if blood pressure is under control, it is possible to participate in IA sports. During the evaluation phase, it is reasonable to begin moderate-intensity exercise.

Asymptomatic athletes with controlled hypertension and no organ damage may participate in competitive athletics, but should be monitored accurately.

All athletes should be followed in terms of the severity of hypertension and the risk category, and should be educated about the appearance of sus-

Table 24.5 Recommendations for participation in competitive sport

	Type of sport
Normal	All sports
Prehypertension	Lifestyle changes
Stage 1 hypertension without organ damage	No limits, controlled pressure every 2 to 4 months
Stage 2 hypertension with organ damage (IIIA to IIIC)	Restriction sports especially with high static component
Hypertension and cardiovascular disease	Defined type and severity of the associated cardiovascular disease

pected symptoms such as dyspnea or chest pain that may need immediate counselling by qualified medical personnel.

24.6 Therapy

The therapeutic management of hypertensive athletes should reflect the proposals of recent international guidelines [1] for the treatment of systemic hypertension.

Regarding treatment lifestyle, modification measures (sodium intake reduction, increased fruit and vegetable consumption, alcohol reduction, avoidance of tobacco, relaxation techniques and weight control), should be routinely emphasized to athletes and active individuals with the same importance as for general population. Sodium intake recommendations for young people are 1.2 g/day for children aged 4 to 8 years, 1.5 g/day for children > 8 years and 2.4 g/day for adults.

Recently the DASH Diet (Dietary Approach to Stop Hypertension), with high levels of potassium, a low fat intake and a high intake of fruits and vegetables, had a positive effect on systolic and diastolic blood pressure [18] in the study population.

For athletes performing static sports, regular aerobic exercise is desirable.

Antihypertensive drug therapy should be initiated promptly in all patients who carry a high risk of cardiovascular complications. The therapeutic target is a reduction of blood pressure to below 140/90 mmHg in the general population and below 130/80 mmHg in diabetic patients and thosc with a high cardiovascular risk.

As suggested by the international literature [1], several classes of drugs may be considered when starting antihypertensive therapy: diuretics, beta-blockers, calcium channel blockers, angiotensin-converting enzyme (ACE) inhibitors and angiotensin receptor blockers (ARBs). In competitive athletes, diuretics and beta-blockers are not recommended [4] because diuretics are indicated in doping lists for all sports, because they can hide anabolic steroid use by diluting urine, and beta blockers are considered doping in high-precision sports as reported by the National Collegiate Athletic Association and World Anti-Doping Agency. ACE inhibitors, ARBs, dihydropyridine and calcium channel antagonists (especially in older and black athletes) are drugs of choice for athletes because they have no major adverse effects on energy metabolism, do not impair maximum oxygen intake, have reduced side effects and can be associated with insufficient control of blood pressure [19-20]. Older agents such as alpha-methyldopa and doxazosin, are rarely used, as they have a lower antihypertensive efficacy compared with ACE inhibitors and calcium antagonists.

References

1. Mancia G, Laurent S, Agabiti-Rosei E et al (2009) Reappraisal of European guidelines on hypertension management: a European Society of Hypertension (ESH) Task Force document. J Hypertension 27:2121–2158
2. American Academy of Pediatrics (2010) Policy statement – Athletic participation by children and adolescents who have systemic hypertension. Pediatrics 125:1287–1294
3. Kaplan NM, Gidding SS, Pickering TG, Wright JT (2005) 36th Bethesda Conference: recommendations for determining eligibility for competition in athletes with cardiovascular abnormalities: Task Force 5: systemic hypertension. J Am Coll Cardiol 45:1346-1348
4. Fagard R, Amery A (1995) Physical exercise in hypertension. In: Laragh J, Brenner B (eds) Hypertension: pathophysiology, diagnosis and management, 2nd edn. New York:Raven Press, pp 2669–2681
5. Pescatello LS, Franklin B, Fagard R et al (2004) American College of Sports Medicine Position Stand: exercise and hypertension. Med Sci Sports Exerc 36:533–553
6. Roitman JL, Herridge M (eds) (2000) American College of Sports Medicine Guidelines for Exercise Testing and Prescription, 6th edn. Philadelphia: Lippincott Williams & Wilkins
7. American College of Sports Medicine (1993) Position stand: Physical activity, physical fitness, and hypertension. Med Sci Sports Exerc 25:I–X
8. Cornelissen VA, Fagard RH (2005) Effect of resistance training on resting blood pressure: a meta-analysis of randomized controlled trials. J Hypertens 23:251–259
9. Deligiannis A, Björnstad HH, Carrè F et al (2006) ESC Study Group of Sports Cardiology position paper on adverse cardiovascular effects of doping in athletes. Eur J Cardiovasc Prev Rehabil 13:687–694
10. Pelliccia A, Fagard R, Björnstadt HH et al (2005) Recommendations for competitive sports participation in athletes with cardiovascular disease. A consensus document from the Study Group of Sports Cardiology of the Working Group of Cardiac Rehabilitation and Exercise Physiology, and the Working Group of Myocardial and Pericardial Diseases of the European Society of Cardiology. Eur Heart 26:1422–1445

11. Kouidi E, Fahadidou-Tsiligiroglou A, Tassoulas E et al (1999) White coat hypertension detected during screening of male adolescens athletes. Am J Hypertens 12:223–226
12. Mahmud A, Feely J (2003) Spurious systolic hypertension of youth: fit young men with elastic arteries. Am J Hypertens 16(3):229–232
13. Schmid A, Schmidt-Trucksäss A, Huonker M et al (2001) Catecholamines response of high performance wheelchair athletes at rest and during exercise with autonomic dysreflexia. Int J Sports Med 22(1):2–7
14. Fagard RH, Björnstad HH, Borjesson M et al (2005) ESC Study Group on Sports Cardiology recommendations for participation in leisure-time physical activities and competitive sports for patients with hypertension. Eur J Cardiovasc Prev Rehabil 12:326–331
15. Pelliccia A, Maron BJ, Culasso F, Spataro A, Caselli G (1996) Athlete's heart in women. Echocardiographic characterization of highly trained elite female atheltes. JAMA 276(3): 211–215
16. Singh JP, Larson MG, Manolio TA et al (1999) Blood pressure response during treadmill testing as a risk factor for new onset hypertension. The Framingham Heart Study. Circulation 99:1831–1836
17. Wilson NV, Meyer BM (1981) Early prediction of hypertension using exercise blood pressure. Preventive Medicine 10:62–68
18. Appel LJ, Moore TJ, Obarzanek E et al (1997) A clinical trial of the effects of dietary patterns on blood pressure. New Engl J Med 336:1117–1124
19. Vanhees L, Fagard R, Lijnen P, et al (1991) Effect of antihypertensive medication on endurance exercise capacity in hypertensive sportsmen. J Hypertens 9:1063–1068
20. Chick TW, Halperin AK, Gacek EM. (1988) The effects of antihypertensive medications on exercise performance: a review. Med Sci Sports Exerc 20:447–454

25 Sporting Activities for Patients with Chronic Ischemic Disease. Focus on Patients Treated with Angioplasty and Stent Implants

Chiara Leuzzi, Fabiana Rollini and Massimo Sangiorgi

25.1 Introduction

Ischemic heart disease is currently the main cause of death in industrialized countries, and in particular it is the main cause of sudden death during exercise in sedentary subjects aged over 35 years.

There are many mechanisms at the root of high mortality during exercise: sympathetic activation and release of catecholamine, platelet activation and consequent thrombotic activation, electrolyte disorders or stress-induced ischemia [1].

Despite high mortality rates due to physical activity, numerous data show how physical activity within determined parameters, as recommended by the national guidelines of the Italian Cardiology Society (SIC Sport) as well as international guidelines, has positive effects on patient health. In fact, regular sporting activity involving various muscle groups (e.g. walking or cycling), leads to adjustment of the cardiocirculatory system with a resulting increase in the capacity for and resistance to exercise. All this translates as a reduction in the risk of coronary events in healthy patients and an improvement in symptoms for subjects with cardiovascular diseases. The latter case involves the importance of secondary prevention and the overall issue of cardiac rehabilitation, especially after mechanical revascularization using angioplasty with stent implants, which is now the treatment of choice as well as the most common form of treatment in subjects with ischemic heart disease.

M. Sangiorgi (✉)
Interventional Cardiology
Policlinico Universitario, Modena, Italy

In this respect, various studies have shown how regular physical exercise improves the prognosis of patients with ischemic heart disease. Therefore, secondary prevention of a cardiovascular event includes not only adherence to medical therapy, but also the addition of a correct lifestyle (in terms of physical exercise). This involves regular sporting activity that enables the patient to restore his/her quality of life, but also to improve functional capacity, which is an important predictor of the subsequent clinical course.

Various randomized, controlled studies have been conducted in the past to study the effect of exercise-based cardiac rehabilitation in patients with heart disease, including those treated with angioplasty and possible stent implant. Unfortunately most of these studies were conducted before the current treatment planned for ischemic heart disease, before the arrival of primary angioplasty, and at a time when medical treatment had not yet been optimized (with beta blockers, ACE inhibitors and statins).

Data from one of the most recent meta-analyses on the subject show how sporting programmes reduce overall mortality by 27%, even if there is no effect on reducing the recurrence of heart attack. In this context, the lower mortality risk, even without a reduction in recurrent heart attack, may be explained by the ability of physical exercise to reduce the arrhythmogenic potential of the ischemic myocardium by decreasing the incidence of major ventricular arrhythmias associated with death [3].

There are, however, various types and various levels of physical activity; however, the recommended level of physical activity must take into account an assessment of the cardiovascular risk.

M. Fioranelli and G. Frajese (eds.), *Sports Cardiology*,
DOI: 10.1007/978-88-470-2775-6_25, © Springer-Verlag Italia 2012

Therefore, before prescribing physical activity to a patient with heart disease, it is necessary to evaluate certain parameters such as the level of cardiovascular risk and the level and type of physical activity in which the patient engages, and which he/she wants to practise depending on the type of revascularization.

This chapter will briefly review the various levels of cardiovascular risk in subjects with ischemic heart disease, taking into account the most recent guidelines and recommendations on the initiation and restoration of motor activity, in both sedentary patients and those who practized sport previously, as well as providing recommendations on how and how far to extend the regular physical exercise programme following mechanical revascularization surgery in the coronary network.

25.2 Cardiovascular Risk Level in Subjects with Heart Disease

Patients with chronic ischemic heart disease include those with a history of myocardial infarction, angina pectoris or instrumental signs of ischemia, as well as those who have undergone surgical revascularization (coronary artery bypass surgery) or percutaneous revascularization (coronary angioplasty with possible stent implant) [4].

When prescribing regular physical activity in these patients, age, sex, associated co-morbidities and medical treatment need to be taken into account. As well as these parameters, the daily physical activity prior to the cardiovascular event, the patient's preferences and the intended goals also need to be assessed. It is then necessary to identify the presence of conditions that present a high cardiovascular risk, identifying subjects with a severe prognosis among those who have:

- left ventricular dysfunction (ejection fraction <40%) with signs or symptoms of cardiac insufficiency;
- level, location and extent of coronary disease;
- complex ventricular arrhythmias induced by stress or at rest;
- possible residual inducible ischemia;
- previous complex revascularization surgery.

In clinically stable conditions, before prescribing physical activity to a patient with ischemic heart disease, it is always worthwhile – in accordance with international guidelines –to carry out a stress test. This examination will systematically be a guide for later prescription of physical activity, thanks to the ability to identify the presence of inducible ischemia and the inducibility threshold before the development of symptoms and/or ischemia, the patient's exercise capacity and individual response to stress, as well as possible complications caused by stress. Obviously the intensity of the stress must be considered for each individual: maximum stress is not required in all patients, but, for example, in those at high risk it is sufficient to carry out stratification with a sub-maximum test or the Six Minute Walk Test (Fig. 25.1).

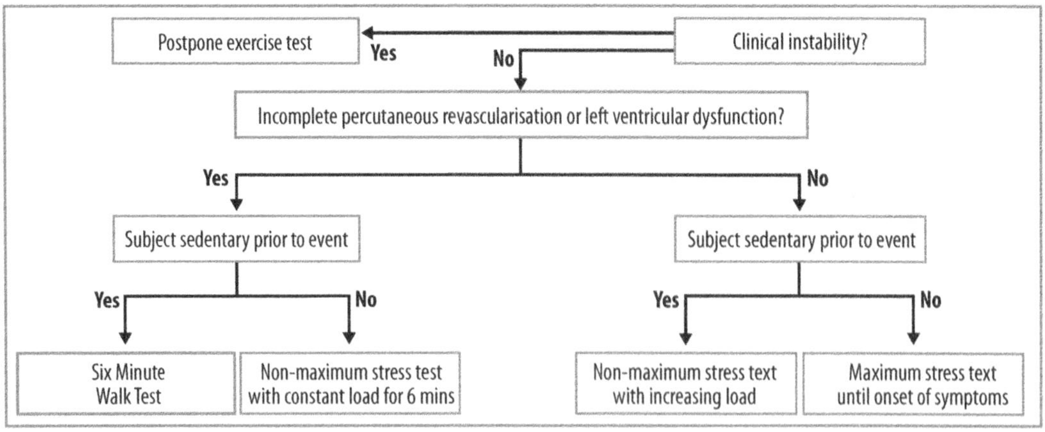

Fig. 25.1 Flow chart showing functional evaluation of the prescription of physical activity in patients with heart disease treated with percutaneous revascularization (amended from F. Piepoli et al. [2], with permission)

In subjects undergoing percutaneous revascularization (angioplasty and possible stent implant), it is important to be aware of the possible pre-operative and post-operative complications. If the procedure is not complicated, regular physical activity may be initiated the following day; if, however, the revascularization procedure was complex, introduction of physical activity must be postponed until the patient is clinically stable and exercise can be increased slowly, depending on the symptoms [2].

In the ETICA study in patients treated with angioplasty, trained patients had a significantly higher capacity for exercise and improved quality of life, even if the probability of angiographic restenosis was not affected. In subsequent months of follow-up, subjects who carried out physical activity had a reduction in cardiovascular events and rehospitalization that was statistically significant in comparison with those with no training [5].

Such positive effects are not only achieved in patients with coronary disease who undergo revascularization, but also in those who are not candidates for revascularization, with positive effects on the capacity for exercise and a reduction in the ischemic threshold. These effects are clearly mediated by less oxygen consumption and reduced heart rate and blood pressure in those who regularly carried out motor activity of any type.

25.3 Level and Type of Physical Activity

The level of physical activity should be chosen based on the clinical characteristics and as a result of instrumental examinations that the patient has undergone after the cardiovascular event and/or revascularization surgery. Even in this case, the recommended level of physical activity cannot disregard the patient's medical history (assessment of the usual level of physical activity before the cardiovascular event or before revascularization). Therefore, a sedentary subject will be advized to follow a different level of physical activity compared to those who usually practise sport. Generally speaking, in patients with chronic ischemic heart disease, after percutaneous revascularization, regular increasing aerobic physical activity is recommended.

It is also very important to consider various types of sport: numerous classifications have been introduced based on cardiovascular involvement. One of the most common is based on the response of some patients (heart rate (HR), arterial hypertension), and variations in peripheral resistance (PR) and cardiac output (CO). Based on these, four groups of sporting activities are distinguished:

1. Group A, i.e. sporting activity with *neurogenic* cardiocirculatory involvement, in which there is in particular a slight increase in HR following the emotive component, with no change to CO;
2. Group B, i.e. sporting activity with *neurogenic* cardiocirculatory involvement due to a moderate increase in HR, CO and PR;
3. Group C, i.e. sporting activity with pressure-related cardiocirculatory involvement, characterized by a sharp increase in HR and PR;
4. Group D, i.e. activity with a high level of cardiocirculatory involvement [6].

Generally speaking, physical activity is defined as each movement of the body produced by muscular energy, resulting in energy expenditure that is higher than at baseline, and is an integral part of intervention in terms of the subject's lifestyle. A cardiac rehabilitation programme should therefore include:

- an assessment of the subject's level of physical ability at home, at work and during recreational activities; activities related to age, sex and the subject's daily routine; the wish of the patient to change his/her sedentary behaviour; the conviction for starting an activity programme and possible obstacles or barriers to this; support from family and friends to positively change the level of physical exercise;
- suggestions for individualized physical activity, taking into account age, previous habits, comorbidities, preferences and the subject's desired objectives;
- recommendation of a minimum of 30-minute sessions of intense aerobic activity, at least 3-4 times a week, with gradual increase in daily exercise until a constant weekly activity programme is achieved;
- reassuring the subject about the safety and benefits of a daily exercise programme;
- encouragement of physical activity and group

programmes to avoid a return to sedentary behaviour over time;
- teaching the patient about the need to continue with physical activity throughout his/her life to reduce the risk of recurrence of cardiovascular events.

After acute coronary syndrome with a primary or selected uncomplicated angioplasty operation, physical activity may only be restored the following day. If myocardial injuries were significant or the procedure complicated, it is best to wait until the patient is clinically stable so that the level of activity can be increased slowly and gradually depending on symptoms.

If the capacity for exercise is preserved and there are no symptoms, physical activity (such as fast walking, gardening, climbing the stairs or cycling) is possible for at least 30 minutes and up to 60 minutes; if symptoms exist it is best to halve the maximum capacity for physical exercise and gradually to increase physical involvement [7-12].

On the other hand, a training programme for physical exercise is defined as a subcategory of physical activity in which planned, structured and repeated body movements are carried out to maintain or increase exercise capacity in a programmed way over a defined period. A training programme must therefore involve continued physical exercise with a gradual increase in the duration of exercise and regular controls (every 3-6 weeks) to change and correct the duration and level of stress once the tolerance level has been reached. Running, cycling, rowing, aerobic dance and gymnastics are considered to be the only forms of exercise that a patient with heart disease can practise under strict medical control.

The duration of training sessions should not be less than 20-30 minutes (preferably 45-60 minutes), at least four times per week (preferably 6-7 days) and with an intensity of 50-80% of oxygen consumption at the peak of exercise (close to the anaerobic threshold) or a frequency peak of 40-60% of the maximum frequency reserve (10/20-14/20 on the Borg rating of perceived exertion scale) [2].

A training programme for exercise should therefore include:
- assessment of the subject's physical capacity by comparing symptoms with the stress test (both cycloergometric and treadmill stress tests). In clinical practice it is not always possible to carry out this assessment, especially in patients with left cardiac dysfunction (ejection fraction < 40%), or after recent surgery. In such cases a sub-maximum stress test or a Six Minute Walk Test are required [13];
- suggesting individualized physical exercise, taking into account clinical conditions and risk factors;
- recommending reaching the maximum aerobic threshold for exercise;
- teaching patients to recognize symptoms caused by effort and adapting to anginal pain with a subsequent change in the exercise programme;
- during initial phases of the training programme, this should be performed in a hospital setting under strict medical control, especially in high-risk patients, such as those with reduced EF, severe comorbidities and recent clinical destabilization (< 1 week). In this way both the response and individual tolerance in a protected and secure area can be tested, and signs and symptoms can be identified that lead to immediate suspension of exercise. Supervision should include a visit with a physical examination, determination of possible arrhythmia, monitoring of heart rate and blood pressure before, during and after exercise. This monitoring period should be longer in patients with new episodes of symptoms, clinical signs of decompenzation, poor pressure control and supraventricular or ventricular arrhythmia during exercise [2].

25.4 Ischemic Heart Disease in Athletes

Another chapter covers the suitability of competitive sporting activity in athletes with ischemic heart disease.

These subjects must systematically be assessed using:
1. medical history: presence of symptoms or fewer symptoms, and type of sport practized;
2. ECG at rest and stress test: evaluation of inducible ischemia, symptoms, changes to the

STT tract, chronotope response to stress, arrhythmia;
3. echocardiogram: assessment of overall contractile function and possible existence of associated structural abnormalities;
4. Holter ECG monitoring: to assess possible arrhythmia or silent myocardial ischemia.

These instruments enable identification of subjects at high cardiovascular risk, a group to which competitive sporting activity cannot be allowed according to current guidelines.

In subjects, however, who are at low risk, competitive suitability for some sports may be allowed, with periodical reassessment of the cardiovascular risk profile [4].

Furthermore, following percutaneous revascularization there are no clear indications on the time needed for restoration of competitive sporting activity, as Italian guidelines recommend a period of at least 12 months of suspension [4].

However, a correct approach enables multi-parameter assessment of each subject, diagnosis, type of cardiovascular event, extent of heart disease and success of revascularization. For example, it may be suggested that in the case of diagnosis of stable effort angina with percutaneous revascularization, competitive sport is not suitable for at least 4 weeks after revascularization, which should be longer in the case of unstable angina with percutaneous revascularization [14].

25.5 Conclusions

In patients with heart disease treated with percutaneous revascularization it is recommended to carry out secondary prevention by promoting a change in lifestyle and strict adherence to drug treatment. In this context, programmed physical activity or training are the keys to building a programme of cardiovascular rehabilitation, restoration of daily work life and an improvement in prognosis. Regular physical activity can be the stimulus for patients to face and react positively to their disease, and switching to – but above all maintaining – a healthy lifestyle can lead positively to self-trust, a healthy status, re-entry into society, work, and re-establishment of a normal social life and relations. Beginning a routine physical exercise programme may also normalize major cardiovascular risk factors that were present before the acute event, thus increasing long-term survival. This should definitely be the objective for all our patients and each of us.

References

1. Pelliccia A, Fagard R, Bjørnstad HH et al (2005) Recommendations for competitive sports participation in athletes with cardiovascular disease. Eur Heart J 26:1422-1445
2. Piepoli MF, Corrà U, Benzer W et al (2010) Secondary prevention through cardiac rehabilitation: physical activity counselling and exercise training. Eur Heart J 31:1967-1974
3. Jolliffe JA, Rees K, Taylor RS et al (2001) Exercise-based rehabilitation for coronary heart disease. Cochrane Database Syst Rev 1:CD001800
4. Penco M, Villella A, Griffo R (2010) Cardiopatia ischemica. Med Sport 63:81-85
5. Belardinelli R, Paolini I, Cianci G et al (2001) Exercise training intervention after coronary angioplasty: the ETICA trial. J Am Coll Cardiol 37:1891-1900
6. Faina M, Veicsteinas A, Biffi A et al (2010) Classificazione in relazione all'impegno cardiovascolare. Med Sport 63:9-13
7. Van de Werf F, Bax J, Betriu A et al (2008)Management of acute myocardial infarction in patients presenting with STsegment elevation. The Task Force on the Management of Acute Myocardial Infarction of the European Society of Cardiology. Eur Heart J 29:2909-2945
8. Bassand JP, Hamm CW, Ardissino D et al (2007) Guidelines for the diagnosis and treatment of non-ST-segment elevation acute coronary syndromes. Task Force for Diagnosis and Treatment of Non-ST-Segment Elevation Acute Coronary Syndromes of European Society of Cardiology. Eur Heart J 28:1598-1660.
9. Antman EM, Hand M, Armstrong PW et al (2008) Writing Group to Review New Evidence and Update the ACC/AHA 2004 Guidelines for the management of patients with st-elevation myocardial infarction. J Am Coll Cardiol 51:210-247
10. Anderson JL, Adams CD, Antman E et al (2007) ACC/AHA 2007 Guidelines for the management of patients with unstable angina/non-ST-elevation myocardial infarction: a report of the American College of Cardiology/American Heart Association Task Force on Practice Guidelines developed in collaboration with the American College of Emergency Physicians, American College of Physicians, Society for Academic Emergency Medicine, Society for Cardiovascular Angiography and Interventions, and Society of Thoracic Surgeons. J Am Coll Cardiol 50:1-157
11. Smith SC Jr, Allen J, Blair SN et al (2006) AHA/ACC

guidelines for secondary prevention for patients with coronary and other atherosclerotic vascular disease: 2006 update. J Am Coll Cardiol 47:2130-2139
12. Thompson PD, Buchner D, Pina IL et al (2003) Exercise and physical activity in the prevention and treatment of atherosclerotic cardiovascular disease: a statement from the Council on Clinical Cardiology and the Council on Nutrition, Physical Activity, and Metabolism. Circulation 107:3109-3116.
13. Arena R, Myers J, Williams MA et al (2007) American Heart Association Committee on Exercise, Rehabilitation, Prevention of the Council on Clinical Cardiology, American Heart Association Council on Cardiovascular Nursing. Assessment of functional capacity in clinical and research settings: a scientific statement from the American Heart Association Committee on Exercise, Rehabilitation, and Prevention of the Council on Clinical Cardiology and the Council on Cardiovascular Nursing. Circulation 116:329-343
14. 36th Bethesda Conference (2005) Eligibility recommendations for competitive athletes with cardiovascular abnormalities. J Am Coll Cardiol 19:45

26 Sports Practice in Congenital Heart Diseases

Pier Paolo Bassareo

26.1 Introduction

Congenital heart diseases represent a complex reality on a continuous upwards trend; their incidence is estimated at between 6 and 8 per 1,000 live births [1,2] and new diagnostic methods and modern surgical techniques, in particular, have resulted in an increasingly higher survival rate to adulthood in approximately 80-85% of patients. In this scenario children, teenagers and adults affected by *corrected* (surgically or through interventional techniques) congenital heart diseases to naturally ask to be allowed to undertake sporting activities, both at a recreational and competitive level. Figure 26.1 shows the incidence of congenital heart diseases in live births.

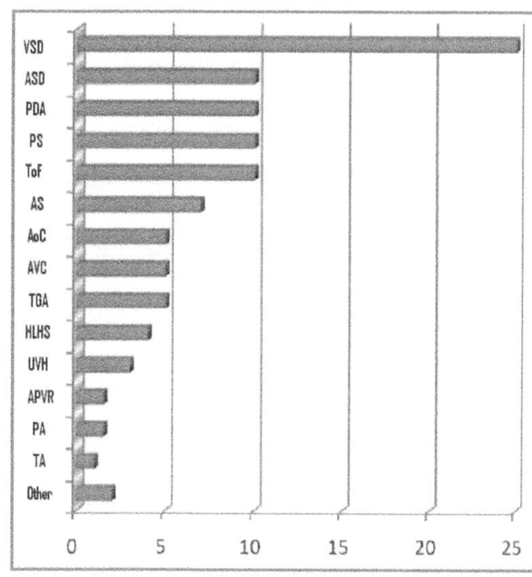

Fig. 27.1 Incidence (%) of congenital heart diseases in live births. *VSD* ventricular septal defect; *ASD* atrial septal defect; *PDA* patent ductus arteriosus; *PS* pulmonary stenosis; *ToF* Tetralogy of Fallot; *AS* aortic stenosis; *AoC* aortic coarctation; *AVC* atrio-ventricular canal; *TGA* transposition of the great arteries; *HLHS* hypoplastic left heart syndrome; *UVH* univentricular heart; *APVR* anomalous pulmonary venous return; *PA* pulmonary atresia; *TA* truncus arteriosus; *Other* Other congenital heart defects

Simplifying for the sake of practicality, congenital heart diseases can be classified as either *simple* or *complex*. *Simple heart defects*, which comprise the majority of diseases addressed by sports physicians, may be further divided into two groups:

1. those characterized by *pulmonary hyperflow* due to left-to-right shunt (such as defects of the interatrial and interventricular septa);
2. those characterized by left and right *ventricular outlet* (such as pulmonary and aortic stenosis).

Complex heart diseases, on the other hand, are represented by less easily identifiable defects frequently accompanied by *cyanosis* due to the presence of a right-to-left shunt with mixing of oxygenated and deoxygenated blood. *Anomalies of the origin and course of coronary arteries,* both congenital and acquired (Kawasaki disease), may also be detected.

Moreover, it should be taken into account that the majority of heart defects, both simple and complex, have an underlying hereditary genetic basis and are often part of syndromic panels; associations with the malformation of other organs and systems should therefore be taken into consid-

P.P. Bassareo (✉)
Department of Cardiovascular and Neurological Sciences
University of Cagliari, Cagliari, Italy

M. Fioranelli and G. Frajese (eds.), *Sports Cardiology*,
DOI: 10.1007/978-88-470-2775-6_26, © Springer-Verlag Italia 2012

eration when assessing the suitability of a patient for recreational and competitive sporting activities (such as, for example, Marfan's syndrome).

26.2 General Criteria for the Identification of Functional Classes in Congenital Heart Patients

In light of the complexity of the diseases in question, the variety of interventions and their possible outcomes, it is essential to emphasize the need for close collaboration between the sports physician and pediatric cardiologist who routinely follow the patient. Indeed, the cardiologist has access, during routine visits, to a considerable part of the medical history and instrumental examinations required for the identification of the functional state of a patient. However, especially for complex heart diseases, these indications will need to be evaluated on a case by case basis, and general criteria for risk stratification may be put forward.

Table 26.1 Eligibility/not eligibility for participation in competitive sports in patients suffering from congenital heart disease

Eligible	Not eligible
1. *Surgical procedure* Fully corrected (anatomically)	Uncorrected or palliative corrected Significant lesions not operated Univentricular hearts Mustard, Senning or Rastelli corrected TGV Arterio-pulmonary shunts
2. *Medical history* Satisfactory NYHA class I	Abnormal Symptoms of severe palpitations/syncope Exercise-induced symptoms (dyspnea, angina, palpitations, syncope) NYHA class II or higher
3. *Physical examination* Satisfactory	Abnormal Hypertension Hepatomegaly, raized venous pressure
4. *ECG/Holter* Satisfactory	Abnormal Ischemia (coronary anomaly, TGV-switch) QRS-duration (Fallot) Significant hypertrophy Significant arrhythmia
5. *Morphology/hemodynamic* Satisfactory	Abnormal Significant rest-lesion Mean transvalvular gradient of aorta >20mmHg Peak transvalvular gradient of the pulmonary artery of > 50mmHg Significant hypertrophy Significant myocardial dysfunction Pulmonary hypertension
6. *Maximal ergospirometry* Satisfactory	Abnormal Values within normal range Chest pain or syncope Significant arrhythmia Ischemia at the ECG

NYHA New York Heart Association; *TGV* transposition of the great vessels; *ECG* electrocardiogram.
Table modified from [3].

In view of the legal implications and high quality of the documents, two European reports will be referred to throughout the present chapter: the *Recommendations for competitive sports participation in athletes with cardiovascular disease* [3], and the *Recommendations for participation in competitive and leisure sports in patients with congenital heart disease: a consensus document* [4], both published by the European Society of Cardiology.

The diagnostic process for a patient should include a complete anamnesis, an accurate objective examination to assess NYHA functional class, and a series of instrumental examinations. Based on these premises, in the patients attending competitive sports, the level of pre-participation screening should be extensive and up to date (Table 26.1) [4]. The latter enhances an objective identification of subjects suitable for sporting activities, potentially at a competitive level, and subjects for whom the practice of sport is not advisable.

26.2.1 Classification of Sporting Activities

Various sporting activities are characterized by different degrees of cardiovascular involvement; the prescription of physical activity, particularly to congenital heart patients, cannot ignore the physiology and pathophysiology of the different types of physical exercise and sport and the cardiovascular effects, acute and chronic, they may trigger.

As far as sporting activities are concerned, reference will made to the *Classification of sports with regards to their type (i.e. dynamic and static) and intensity (i.e. low, moderate, and high)* in the *Recommendations for competitive sports participation in athletes with cardiovascular disease* (Table 26.2) [3]. This classification is intended to provide a schematic indication of the cardiovascular involvement associated with different sports, with an additional warning for those associated with an increased risk of bodily collision and enhanced risk of syncope.

Table 26.2 Classification of sports

	Low dynamic	Moderate dynamic	High dynamic
1 *Low static*	Bowling Cricket Golf Shooting Baseball[1]/softball[1]	Fencing Table tennis Tennis (doubles) Volleyball Squash[1]	Badminton Race walking Running (marathon) Cross-country skiing (classic)
2 *Moderate static*	Auto racing[1,2] Diving[1,2] Equestrian[1,2] Motorcycling[1,2] Gymnastics[1] Karate/Judo[1] Sailing Archery	Field events (jumping) Figure skating[1] Lacrosse[1] Running (sprinting)	Basketball[1] Biathlon Ice hockey[1] Field hockey[1] Rugby[1] Soccer[1] Cross-country skiing (skating) Running (mid/long) Swimming Tennis (single) Team handball[1]
3 *High static*	Bobsledding[1,2] Field events (throwing) Luge[1,2] Rock climbing Waterskiing[1,2] Weight lifting[1,2] Windsurfing[1,2]	Body building[1] Downhill skiing[1,2] Wrestling[1] Snow boarding[1,2]	Boxing[1] Canoeing, Kayaking Cycling[1,2] Decathlon Rowing Speed skating Triathlon[1,2]

[1] Danger of bodily collision; [2] Increased risk if syncope occurs.
Table modified from [3].

It should be noted that, regardless of the cardiovascular involvement of the sport in question, the above stated Recommendations [3,4] identify a group of congenital heart diseases that due to their seriousness and complexity are incompatible with competitive sporting activities. The latter are:

- transposition of the great arteries corrected according to Mustard/Senning techniques;
- congenitally corrected transposition of the great arteries;
- Ebstein anomaly;
- Eisenmenger's syndrome;
- heart diseases with univentricular circulation.

26.3 Simple Congenital Heart Diseases with Pulmonary Hyperflow

26.3.1 Atrial Septum Defects

Atrial septum defects (ASD) account for about 5-10% of all congenital heart diseases [5]. They may be classified in four types (Fig. 26.2):

- *ostium secundum* (1) (50-70% of all ASDs), characterized by a defect of the septal wall around the foramen ovale;
- *ostium primum* (2) (30%), present in defects of endocardial cushions (atrioventricular canal) and located in the lower part of the interatrial septum;
- *venous sinus* (3) (10%), located at the back, frequently around the superior vena cava and rarely around the inferior vena cava;
- *coronary sinus* (1%), characterized by the absence of the roof of the coronary sinus, which therefore communicates openly with the left atrium.

ASDs may be found both as isolated defects and in association with other malformations. *Objectively* a fixed splitting of the second sound, a protomesosystolic ejective murmur on the pulmonary focus and potentially a diastolic rolling hum on the tricuspid focus due to relative stenosis can be observed. An ECG will detect right axial deviation, signs of right ventricular hypertrophy or right bundle branch block (RBBB). A *chest X-ray* will highlight signs of pulmonary hyperflow.

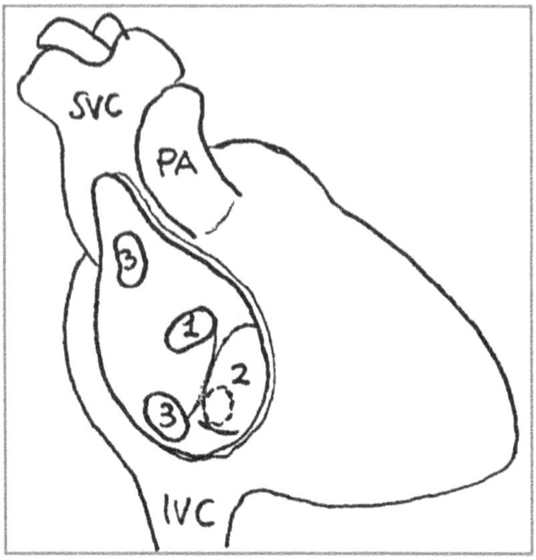

Fig. 26.2 Types of ASD: *1* ostium secundum; *2* ostium primum; *3* venous sinus. *IVC* inferior vena cava; *PA* pulmonary artery; *SVC* superior vena cava

An *echocardiogram* will make it possible to form a diagnosis, evaluate the location, dimension and hemodynamic significance of the defect (significant when Qp/Qs > 1.5) and highlight secondary or associated alterations. A *transesophageal echocardiogram* may be used as a further diagnostic assessment tool preliminary to closure of the defect. Around 80% of small ostium secundum ASDs close spontaneously within the first 4-5 years of life. The majority of patients remain asymptomatic until adulthood. Symptoms such as increased fatigue, a higher predisposition to respiratory infections and growth delays may appear over time. Large uncorrected defects rarely result in cardiac decompenzation in pediatric age; right ventricular insufficiency associated to pulmonary hypertension is more likely to arise in patients over 20-30 years of age. Atrial arrhythmias may also occur and a rare complication is represented by paradoxal embolism.

26.3.1.1 Treatment

As previously mentioned, the majority of patients feature an asymptomatic course not requiring medical treatment. The treatment of atrial arrhythmias does not differ from standard procedures. Closure of the defect may be performed using ei-

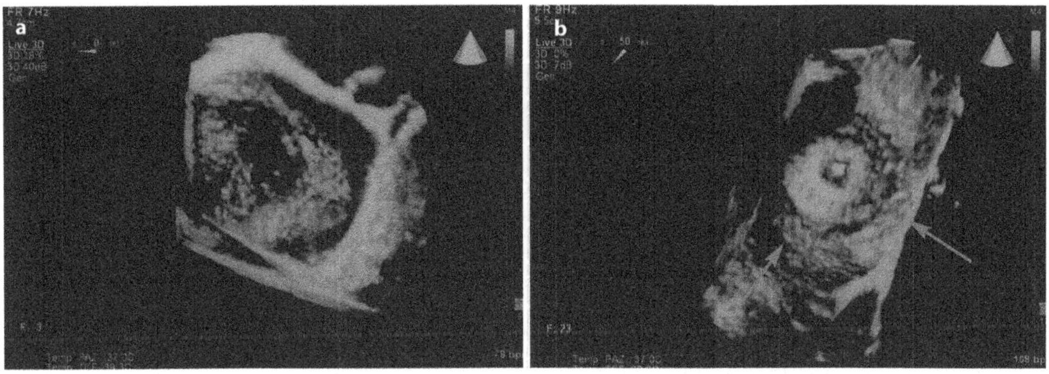

Fig. 26.3 a The 3D transesophageal echocardiogram shows a frontal vision of the ostium secundum interatrial septal defect. b The same defect after percutaneous closure with device (*red arrows*)

ther percutaneous (Fig. 26.3) or surgical techniques, using pericardium or teflon patches, or direct suture, depending on the location and size of the defect. Closure is advisable in the presence of significant (Qp/Qs > 1.5) left-to-right shunt and/or in the presence of right atrial and ventricular enlargement, with or without symptoms. It is still unclear when exactly the closure should be performed: undoubtedly, if no cardiac decompenzation arises, it is advisable to wait at least until 4-5 years of age in order to allow the possibility of spontaneous closure. Patients operated at a later age (after 20-25 years of age) may be subject to an enlargement of the right sections with reduced functional ability after the procedure.

26.3.1.2 Indications for Sports Practice

1. Subjects affected by *non-hemodynamically significant* forms of ASD (i.e. less than 6 mm) can perform all types of sporting activities, except underwater activities with breathing apparatus due to the risk of paradoxical embolism.
2. Subjects with ASD *corrected either surgically or percutaneously* should be revaluated 6 months after the procedure with a follow-up visit (NYHA functional class), chest X-ray, ECG, echocardiogram, cardiac stress test. Suitability for sporting activities will not be recognized in the presence of:
   - persistent and significant enlargement and/or malfunction of the right ventricle;
   - residual pulmonary hypertension;
   - paroxysmal, persistent or permanent supraventricular tachycardia, or symptomatic sinoatrial dysfunction;
   - minimum residual shunt (exclusively for underwater activities with breathing apparatus).

   These patients have to be revaluated yearly.

26.3.2 Ventricular Septum Defects

Ventricular septum defects (VSD) represent the most common cardiac malformation (15-25% of live births) [6]. The interventricular septum consists of a small fibrous (membranous) portion and a large muscular portion that, in turn, can be divided into inlet, outlet and a trabeculated area (muscular in the strict sense of the word). Based on the anatomical location of the defect, the latter can be distinguished as (Fig. 26.4):

- *perimembranous* VSD (70%), located around the membranous septum (Fig. 26.5);
- *muscular* VSD (5-20%), which can be isolated or multiple up to an extreme form known as *Swiss cheese*;
- VSD *of the inlet septum* (5-8%), located near the septal edge of the tricuspid valve;
- VSD *of the outlet septum* (5-7%), located around the infundibular septum (outlet portion); the latter may lead to prolapse of an aortic cusp with subsequent valvular insufficiency.

Small VSDs are generally asymptomatic, whereas moderate and large ones may cause growth delays, reduced effort tolerance, a predisposition to respiratory infections and cardiac de-

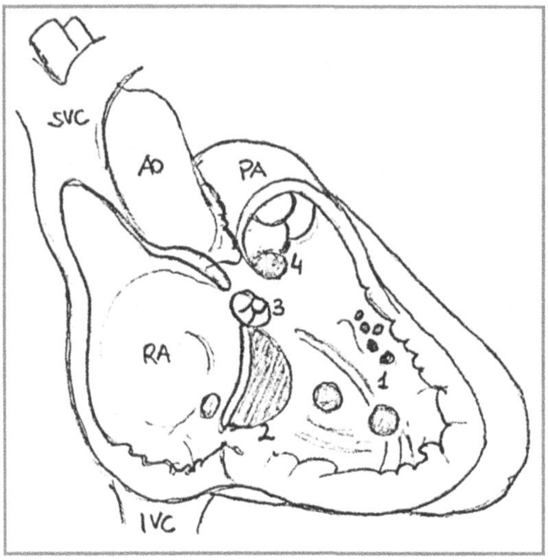

Fig. 26.4 Types of VSD: *1* muscular; *2* inlet septum; *3* perimembranous; *4* outlet septum. *Ao* aorta; *IVC* inferior vena cava; *PA* pulmonary artery; *RA* right atrium; *SVC* superior vena cava

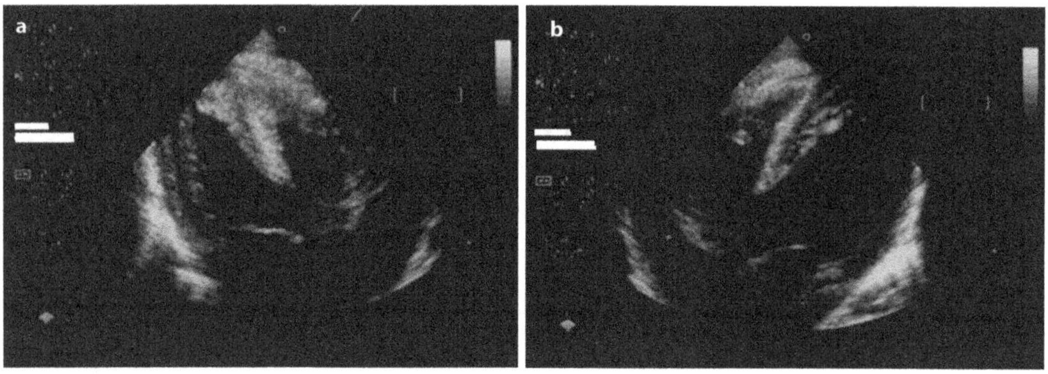

Fig. 26.5 Large perimembranous interventricular defect: a parasternal long axis projection; b apical four-chamber projection

compenzation; if not properly treated, evolution towards pulmonary hypertension or Eisenmenger's syndrome is likely to occur.

Objectively a systolic flutter and holosystolic murmur in the lower-middle sternal region, a second single sound (pulmonary hypertension) and occasionally a decrescendo diastolic murmur caused by aortic insufficiency may be detected. In the eventuality of Eisenmenger's syndrome, cyanosis may be present.

The *ECG* may be normal when dealing with small defects; moderate to large defects will present signs of left ventricular or biventricular hypertrophy. A *chest X-ray* will display an enlargement of the left chambers, growth of the pulmonary vascular tissue and dilation of the main pulmonary arteries. An *echocardiogram* can be diagnostic and assist in the identification of the location, number, size and hemodynamic significance (significant if Qp/Qs >2) of the defects. Small perimembranous and muscular defects may close spontaneously within the first 2-3 years of life and do not tend to grow over time. Defects of the *inlet* and *outlet* septa, on the other hand, generally do not experience spontaneous closure.

26.3.2.1 Treatment

Medical treatment is limited to patients manifesting cardiac decompenzation or pulmonary hypertension. Correction of the defect is preferably performed surgically, through synthetic patches, but in selected cases percutaneous techniques with non-surgical devices may also be used; corrective procedures are advisable if Qp/Qs is > 2 and evi-

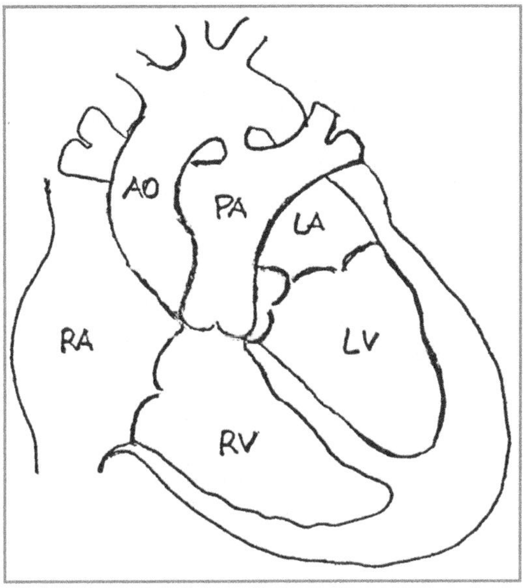

Fig. 26.6 Patency of the arterial duct. *Ao* aorta; *LA* left atrium; *LV* left ventricle; *PA* pulmonary artery; *RA* right atrium; *RV* right ventricle

dence is found of left ventricular overload, in the case of infective endocarditis or endocarditis with Qp/Qs > 1.5 associated with left cardiac decompenzation or pulmonary pressure less than two-thirds of systemic pressure.

26.3.2.2 Indications for Sports Practice

1. Subjects affected by *non-hemodynamically significant* forms of VSD (restrictive defect with left-to-right gradient > 64 mmHg) can perform all types of sporting activities.
2. Subjects with *hemodynamically significant* VSD *corrected surgically or with a device* should be revaluated 6 months after corrective procedure through physical evaluation (NYHA functional class), chest X-ray, ECG, echocardiogram, and cardiac stress test; suitability for sporting activities will not be recognized in the presence of:
   - residual hemodynamically significant VSD;
   - pulmonary hypertension;
   - altered dimensions and functionality of the left ventricle assessed through echocardiogram (particularly for VSD corrected with large patches and/or subjected to ventriculostomy);
   - presence of significant brady- and/or tachycardia at rest and under stress.
3. Subjects with forms of VSD presenting no residual defects may have access to all competitive sporting activities.
   These patients have to be revaluated yearly.

26.3.3 Patency of the Arterial Duct

Patency of the arterial or Botallo's duct (PDA) (5-10% of heart diseases) involves the absence of closure of the arterial connection between the descending aorta and the left pulmonary artery, of fundamental importance during foetal life, which usually experiences spontaneous closure after birth (Fig. 26.6) [7]. *Patients are generally asymptomatic when small ducts are present.* Large ducts determine a considerable left-to-right shunt and can cause frequent infections of the respiratory system, stress dyspnea and hemodynamic compromise resulting in cardiac decompenzation.

Objectively a systolic flutter on the top left parasternal line, an accentuation of the pulmonary component of the second heart sound (pulmonary hypertension) and the characteristic continuous murmur (systo-diastolic) with maximum intensity in the top left parasternal region or left subclavian area may be detected.

The *ECG* may be normal or present signs of left atrial enlargement or left ventricular hypertrophy with overload. A *chest X-ray* will highlight cardiomegaly with enlargement of the left sections and ascending aorta, growth of the pulmonary vascular tissue and possible signs of pulmonary hypertension. An *echocardiogram* is the preferred methodology to assess the presence, size and extent of the shunt or the presence of left atrial and ventricular enlargement.

26.3.3.1 Treatment

Medical therapy (diuretic and digital) is introduced in the eventuality of cardiac decompenzation. Prophylaxis against infective endocarditis/endoarteritis is advisable for all patients, irrespective of duct dimensions. Closure, surgical or percutaneous, is recommended in patients presenting left atrial and/or ventricular dilation or pulmonary hy-

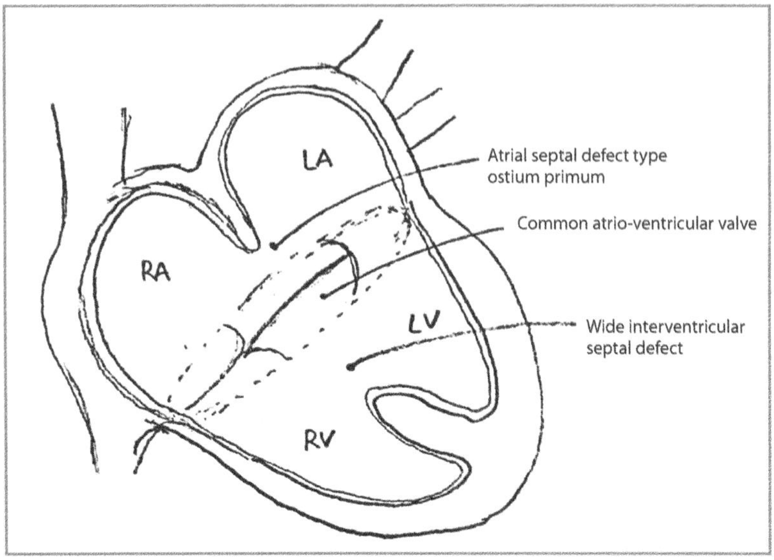

Fig. 26.7 Complete atrioventricular canal (*AV*). *ASD* defect of the interatrial septum, *VSD* defect of the interventricular septum, *LA* left atrium, *LV* left ventricle, *RA* right atrium, *RV* right ventricle

pertension, in case of significant left-to-right shunt or preexisting endoarteritis.

26.3.3.2 Indications for Sports Practice

1. Patients with *small non-hemodynamically significant ducts* may take part in all competitive sporting activities.
2. Percutaneous or surgical closure is advisable in patients with *hemodynamically significant duct* with subsequent reassessment after 6 months through physical examination (NYHA functional class), chest X-ray, ECG, echocardiogram and cardiac stress test; in the eventuality of the absence of pulmonary hypertension and presence of a normal functional ability, patients may be allowed to undertake all sporting activities. These patients need no regular follow up.

26.3.4 Complete Atrioventricular Canal

The atrioventricular canal (AVC) (2% of all congenital heart diseases) is determined by the failed development of the structures deriving from the endocardial cushions (the lower part of the interatrial septum, the rear part of the interventricular septum and the atrioventricular valves) [8].

It may present itself in three different forms (Rastelli's classification):

- *complete* AVC: characterized by the association of ostium primum ASD, non-restrictive VSD of the inlet septum and common atrioventricular valve with *cleft* of the left edge. A number of subclassifications may apply based on the presence and location of the chordae tendinae (Fig. 26.7).
- *partial* AVC: characterized by the presence of ostium primum ASD and *cleft* mitral valve; VSD is not usually present and the mitral and tricuspid valvular rings are separated and placed on the same level;
- *intermediate* AVC: intermediate form consisting in one or more restrictive VSD and two valvular rings.

The AVC, particularly the complete variant, is characterized by a significant left-to-right shunt and pulmonary hyperflow, which, if not corrected at an early stage, may result in pulmonary hypertension, cardiac decompenzation and death within the first 2-3 years of life. It registers a predisposition to relapsing respiratory infections and is extremely common in Down's syndrome patients.

Objectively tachycardia, tachypnoea and signs of cardiac decompenzation, accentuation of the first heart tone and a holosystolic murmur on the lower left parasternal line may be observed. An *ECG* will show a superior QRS axis, first-degree atrioventricular block and right bundle branch block (RBBB). A *chest X-ray* will highlight cardiomegaly, an increase in pulmonary vascularization and signs of pulmonary hypertension. An echocardiogram can be diagnostic and enable the distinction between complete forms and partial and intermediate ones, further to acquiring all anatomic data fundamental for surgical corrective procedures.

26.3.4.1 Treatment

Medical treatment is merely a support tool with a view to surgical correction, which must be performed as soon as possible in complete AVC patients. The preferred procedure is currently a definitive surgical correction (closure of VSD and ASD with a patch and cleft closure with reconstruction of two separate atrioventricular valves).

26.3.4.2 Indications for Sports Practice

AVC patients should be reassessed through physical examination (NYHA functional class), chest X-ray, ECG, echocardiogram, and cardiac stress test as well. In case of:

- absent or mild atrio-ventricular insufficiency;
- no significant subaortic stenosis;
- no significant arrhythmias;
- normal maximal gas exchange measurement;
- normal left ventricular function.

AVC patients may perform all sports, subject to yearly revaluation. Every second year a complete reassessment is needed.

In case of moderate mitral valve regurgitation, the patients may have access only to low to moderate dynamic and static sports.

26.4 Simple Congenital Heart Diseases with Ventricular Outlet Obstruction

26.4.1 Pulmonary Stenosis

Isolated pulmonary stenosis (PS) accounts for around 10% of congenital heart diseases but may be found in association with other defects such as the Tetralogy of Fallot [9]. Stenosis most frequently affects valves; it can also be found around the infundibulum or pulmonary branches (supravalvular, often associated to genetic syndromes (Fig. 26.8). Light valvular stenoses are often asymptomatic; more significant cases may display effort dyspnea and tendency to fatigue.

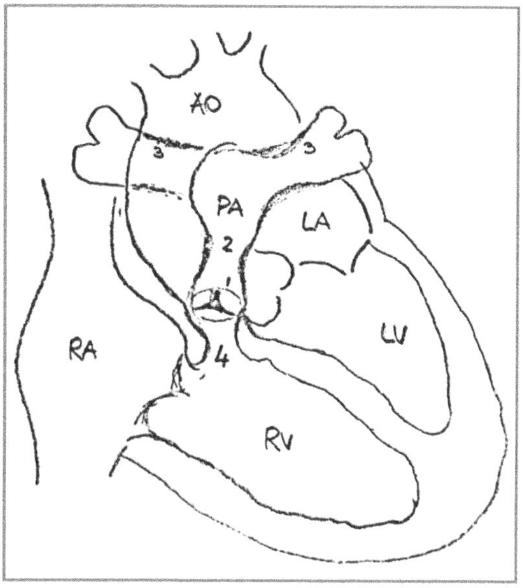

Fig. 26.8 Pulmonary stenosis: *1* valvular, *2* supravalvular, *3* of the distal branches, *4* infundibular. *Ao* aorta, *LA* left atrium, *LV* left ventricle, *PA* pulmonary artery, *RA* right atrium, *RV* right ventricle

Objectively the following may be observed: impulse in right parasternal region, palpatory flutter in top left parasternal region, opening snap of the pulmonary artery and the characteristic ejective systolic murmur on the pulmonary focus, which increases in intensity as the level of the stenosis increases. The ECG in light forms will be normal; in the remaining cases it will show right axis deviation, RBBB and signs of left ventricular hypertrophy. A *chest X-ray* will show post-stenotic dilation of the pulmonary trunk and main branches and cardiomegaly in the presence of cardiac decompenzation. An *echocardiogram* can be diagnostic and make it possible to assess the level of the stenosis and its seriousness based on gradients: stenosis with a peak gradient < 30 mmHg will be considered non significant; moderate between 30 and 50 mmHg and severe if > 50 mmHg. Quality of life in light valvular stenosis patients is almost normal, although the level of the stenosis may worsen over time.

Severe neonatal stenosis left untreated may lead to death. Sudden death may occur during significant efforts in severe stenosis patients.

26.4.1.1 Treatment

Treatment can be surgical (surgical valvotomy) or percutaneous (balloon angioplasty). Percutaneous treatment is the preferred choice for newborns affected by critical stenosis, symptomatic adults with peak gradient > 50 mmHg or average gradient > 30 mmHg and asymptomatic adults with peak gradient > 60 mmHg or average gradient > 40 mmHg. Surgical procedure is the adopted treatment in case of severe stenosis and hypoplastic valvular ring, severe pulmonary insufficiency or sub- or supravalvular stenosis.

26.4.1.2 Indications for Sports Practice

1. In *non-hemodynamically significant* forms no restriction of competitive sporting activities is required;
2. in *moderate forms* patients may be deemed fit for all competitive sporting activities from low to moderate dynamic and static sports;
3. in *severe forms* patients are not allowed to perform any type of sporting activities and should undergo percutaneous or surgical correction;
4. in *corrected (post interventional/post surgical) forms*, subjects should be revaluated 6 months after corrective procedure through physical evaluation (NYHA functional class), chest X-ray, ECG, echocardiogram, and cardiac stress test. They may be deemed fit for low and moderate dynamic and low static sport providing the following criteria are met:
   - residual peak transvalvular gradient between 30 and 50 mmHg;
   - normal functionality of right ventricle;
   - normal ECG or only mild right ventricular hypertrophy.

   These patients need a yearly follow up.

26.4.2 Aortic Stenosis

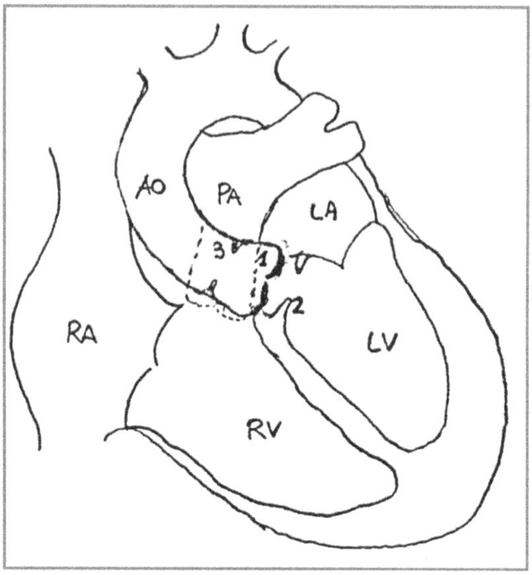

Fig. 26.9 Aortic stenosis: *1* valvular, *2* subvalvular, *3* supravalvular. *Ao*, aorta; *LA*, left atrium; *LV*, left ventricle; *PA*, pulmonary artery; *RA*, right atrium; *RV*, right ventricle

Aortic stenosis (AS) accounts for 7-10% of congenital heart defects [10]. In the majority of cases (70%) obstruction (Fig. 26.9) takes place in the valves and is linked to a malformation or absence of one or more valvular cusps; the most widespread cause of aortic stenosis is a *bicuspid aortic valve*. The obstruction may less frequently be found at a subvalvular level (25%), caused by a membrane, fibrous ring or muscular tunnel; stenosis may more rarely be supravalvular (5%), located just above the valvular level. Aortic stenosis may be associated to other malformations, such as hypoplasia of the ascending aorta and aortic arch, and aortic coarctation. Newborns with critical stenosis show early signs of hypoperfusion and respiratory distress with pulmonary edema and should undergo surgical correction as soon as possible. Patients with light and moderate stenosis are often asymptomatic or present effort intolerance. However all symptoms of aortic stenosis may be observed: dyspnea, effort angina, palpitations and syncope.

Objectively the following may be detected: systolic flutter in jugular pulse, protosystolic click, paradoxical splitting of the second heart sound or complete absence of its aortic component; rough ejective systolic murmur, with irradiation towards neck vessels, sometimes followed by a decrescendo diastolic murmur in case of steno-insufficiency; arterial pressure may be higher in the right arm due to the preferential direction of the stenosis jet towards the anonymous artery in supravalvular stenosis. In severe forms peripheral arterial pulses are small and delayed. The *ECG* can be normal or show signs of left ventricular hypertrophy with or without alterations of repolarization. A *chest X-ray* will highlight normal heart dimensions and post-stenotic dilation of the ascending aorta with prominence of the aortic button. An *echocardiogram* can be diagnostic and allow to assess valve morphology, identify possible sub- or supravalvular diaphragms or membranes and evaluate seriousness of the stenosis. A *dobutamine stress echo* may be useful in stenosis with low gradient and reduced contracting function. A *cardiac stress test* will make it possible to evaluate effort tolerance, the presence of arrhythmia during effort and pressure response. A *cardiac catheterization* will enable an assessment of the characteristic of the stenosis and the concomitant presence of coronary diseases. Symptomatic aortic stenosis has a negative prognosis. Patients with severe aortic stenosis, even if asymptomatic, may incur in sudden cardiac death. Light and moderate valvular stenoses tend to worsen over time. Subaortic stenosis may also display a progressive valvular insufficiency due to the morphofunctional deterioration that the stenosis jet determines on valvular edges.

26.4.2.1 Treatment

The preferred treatment for subvalvular and supravalvular stenosis is surgical procedure. When dealing with valvular stenosis treatment may be percutaneous (balloon valvuloplasty) or surgical. Surgical treatments may differ depending on the patient and range from surgical commissurotomy to valvuloplasty, use of a pulmonary autograft (Ross procedure, which consists in the replacement of the aortic valve with the patient's own pulmonary valve by performing a reimplantation of the coronary arteries and inserting an aortic or pulmonary homograft in pulmonary position), Bentall procedure (positioning of a valvulated tube) when an aneurysmatic dilation of the aorta is associated to the stenosis, simple valvular replacement with mechanical or biological prosthesis.

26.4.2.2 Indications for Sports Practice

1. *Patients with mild aortic stenosis (mean transvalvular gradient less than 21 mmHg)* may be allowed to perform all sports – with exception of high static and high dynamic sports - providing the following criteria are met:
   - absence of significant arrhythmia, syncope, dizziness, or angina pectoris.

   These patients need to be evaluated yearly.
2. *Patients with moderate aortic stenosis (mean transvalvular* gradient between 21 and 49 mmHg) may take part in low dynamic and static sport), with an evaluation every 6 months.

   No competitive sport is allowed in case of the above stated symptoms or left ventricular dysfunction at rest or under stress.

   Exercise testing to look for limiting symptoms seems valuable in predicting the need for surgical intervention in asymptomatic patients and should be performed regularly because of the progressive nature of this lesion.
3. Patients with severe aortic stenosis may not take part in competitive sports.

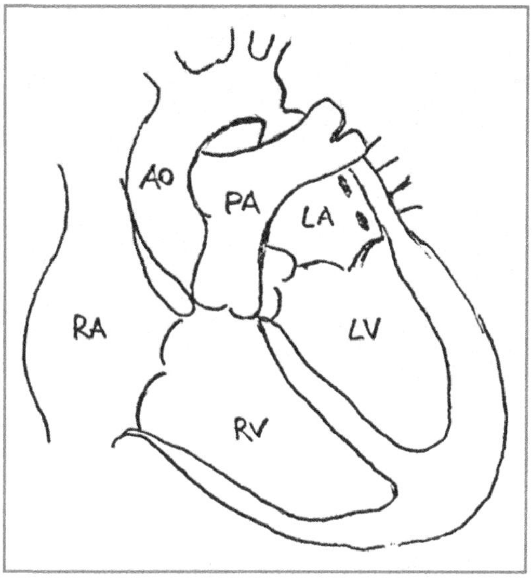

Fig. 26.10 Aortic coarctation. *Ao* aorta, *LA* left atrium, *LV* left ventricle, *PA* pulmonary artery, *RA* right atrium, *RV* right ventricle

26.4.3 Aortic Coarctation

Coarctation of the aorta (CoA) (5-10% of congenital heart diseases) is characterized by a narrowing of the aortic lumen distally to the subclavian aorta, usually in the immediate vicinity of the site of insertion of the arterial duct (Fig. 26.10) [11]. It is

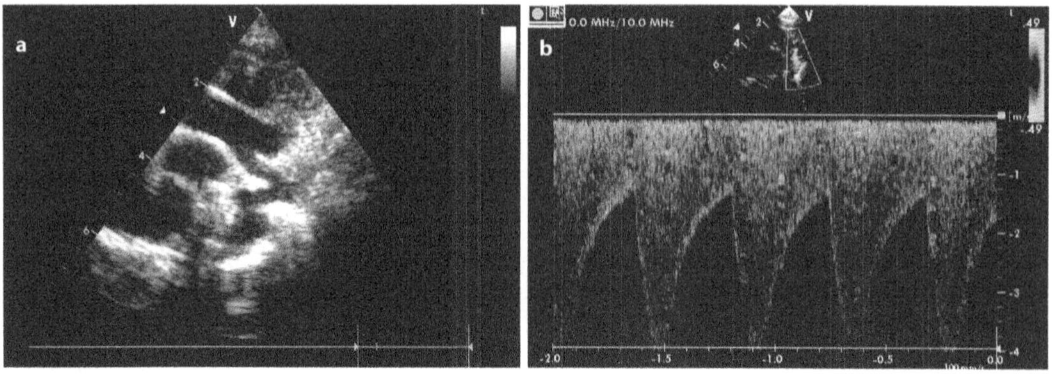

Fig. 26.11 a Severe aortic coarctation with diffuse narrowing of the descending aorta, whose course appears irregular and tortuous (suprasternal projection, in red). a Doppler profile. The elevated systolic gradient (maximum speed higher than 4 m/s) is followed by a "diastolic tail" representing the gradient in question extending for the entire length of the diastole

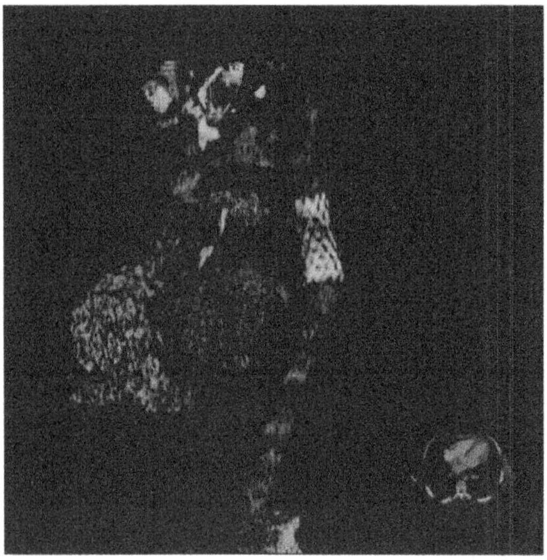

Fig. 26.12 The MRI (sagittal projection) shows the late formation of an aneurysm where the coarcted segment of the aorta had been enlarged by means of a percutaneous angioplasty followed by a stent implantation

often associated to other heart diseases, particularly bicuspid aorta, aortic hypoplasia, DIV etc. Depending on the seriousness of the narrowing and its association with other defects, CoA may be symptomatic or asymptomatic. In more severe cases (Fig. 26.11) symptoms appear during the first week of life and consist in lack of appetite and growth, dyspnea or hemodynamic compromise leading to shock; these patients should undergo surgery as soon as possible. In cases characterized by an isolated defect and a good collateral circulation patients may remain asymptomatic until adulthood, displaying generic symptoms such as weakness or pain to lower limbs after physical exercise; in these cases a diagnosis is performed only occasionally. This approach will only consider the isolated form of the defect.

Objectively the majority of patients present a normal development, although an underdevelopment of the lower body may be observed; lower extremities arterial pulses may be absent or significantly hyposphygmic and delayed compared to radial pulses; systolic arterial hypertension may occur in upper limbs with a considerable differential pressure with lower extremities; a systolic flutter in jugular pulse and an ejective systolic murmur with irradiation towards the back may be detected. An *ECG* will commonly show left axial deviation and left ventricular hypertrophy. A *chest X-ray* will reveal a normal cardiac shadow, dilation of the ascending aorta, *figure 3 sign* (incision of the aorta) and incision of the lower margin of the ribs, linked to the development of collateral circulations. An *echocardiogram* can be diagnostic and enable an evaluation of the size of the coarctation. An *MRI* and *CT Angiogram* will allow to accurately evaluate the anatomy, and presence and size of collateral circulations (Fig. 26.12). Non-operated patients have an average life expectancy of around 35 years, with a 75% mortality in the over 46-year olds. Arterial hypertension, an accelerated coronary disease, stroke, aortic dissection and cardiac decompenzation are common problems to the above-mentioned population. The most frequent causes of death are cardiac decompenzation, aortic rupture/dissection, endocarditis, cerebral hemorrhage and myocardial infarction.

26.4.3.1 Treatment

Treatment of CoA may be percutaneous (balloon angioplasty in isthmic region) or surgical (resection of the coarcted segment through termino-terminal anastomosis, subclavian flap, patch or graft aortoplasty), and it is advisable in the eventuality of peak-to-peak gradient ≥ 20 mmHg or < 20 mmHg, with imaging displaying significant coarctation and collateral circulation. The choice between a percutaneous and a surgical procedure is complex and should be made collegially by expert interventionist cardiologists, pediatric surgeons and cardiologists. The percutaneous procedure is advisable in case of relapsing coarctation with peak-to-peak gradient of at least 20 mmHg.

26.4.3.2 Indications for Sports Practice

Patients suffering from CoA (native or repaired) need to be evaluated through physical evaluation (NYHA functional class), chest X-ray, ECG, echocardiogram, cardiac stress test, and cardiac magnetic resonance imaging.

In absence of systemic hypertension, ischemia on exercise ECG, left ventricular overload, and with both a peak pressure gradient between the upper and lower limbs less than 21 mmHg, and a peak systolic blood pressure during exercise less than 231 mmHg, patients may be allowed to practice all sporting activities from low and moderate dynamic and static sport. A strictly yearly evaluation with a complete reassessment every second year will have to be carried out for these subjects. In evaluating blood pressure in children at rest or during exercise test, it is necessary to take child's age and height in account, using pediatric standard tables.

Those with conduit, interposed graft or on anticoagulant drugs should avoid sports with the risk of bodily collision.

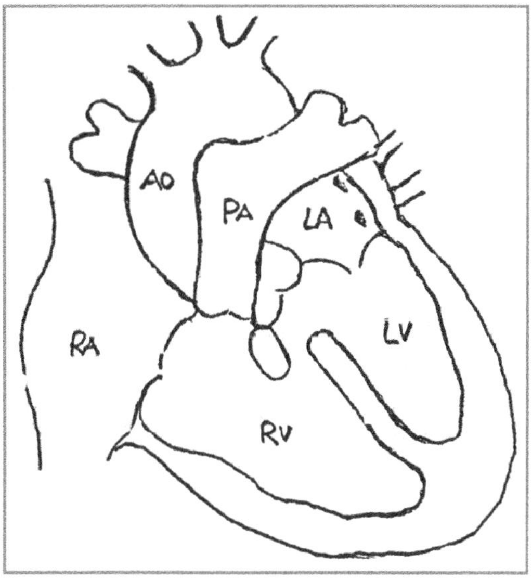

Fig. 26.13 Tetralogy of Fallot. *Ao* aorta, *LA* left atrium, *LV* left ventricle, *PA* pulmonary artery, *RA* right atrium, *RV* right ventricle

26.5 Complex Congenital Heart Diseases

26.5.1 Tetralogy of Fallot

The Tetralogy of Fallot is a heart disease characterized by four main components: subpulmonary infundibular stenosis, defect of the subaortic interventricular septum due to misalignment, aorta overriding the septum and right ventricular hypertrophy (Fig. 26.13) [12]. Corrective surgical procedures are nowadays performed during the first year of life with significantly more positive results than those obtained in the past, when palliative interventions were carried out before reaching a complete correction. The current survival rate to adulthood with satisfactory functional abilities almost reaches 90%; special attention must be paid during the follow-up of these patients: residual pulmonary insufficiency, right ventricular dysfunction and ventricular arrhythmia represent significant prognostic factors in these patients. In view of the results of early complete correction, a more open attitude towards the possibility of practising sports is now adopted, even if in extremely selected cases and after a careful personalized evaluation carried out by highly trained experts. Patients with successfully repaired Tetralogy of Fallot, after having performed physical evaluation (NYHA functional class), chest X-ray, ECG, 24-hours Holter ECG, echocardiogram, and cardiac magnetic resonance imaging may be *allowed to perform sporting activities from low and moderate static and dynamic group* providing the following criteria are met:

- normal or mild right ventricular outflow tract obstruction;
- no more than mild pulmonary insufficiency;
- normal or slightly impaired biventricular function;
- absence of ventricular or atrial arrhythmias.

In case of moderate residual lesion with right ventricular pressure less than 50% of systemic pressure, or residual VSD, or moderate pulmonary regurgitation, but normal biventricular function, only *low static and dynamic sports* are allowed. A yearly follow up is needed, with a complete reassessment every second year. Patients with conduit should avoid sport with risk of bodily collision.

26.5.2 Transposition of the Great Arteries

The transposition of the great arteries (TGA) is a pathology characterized by ventriculoarterial discordance: the aorta, placed on the right side and at the front, originates from the right ventricle, whereas the pulmonary artery originates from the left ventricle (Fig. 26.14) [13]. Two thirds of cases are represented by *simple* forms, which are not associated to other defects. In the past surgical treatment was represented by a *physiological but non anatomical* correction of the defect (Mustard and Senning procedures, characterized by the repositioning of venous returns through an interatrial *baffle*). The preferred surgical intervention is currently the arterial switch (Jatene procedure), in which the two vessels are repositioned correctly and the coronary arteries reimplanted; such an intervention performs *both a physiological and anatomical* correction of the defect and is carried out during the first few days of life, obtaining significantly better results both in terms of mortality rate and late morbidity.

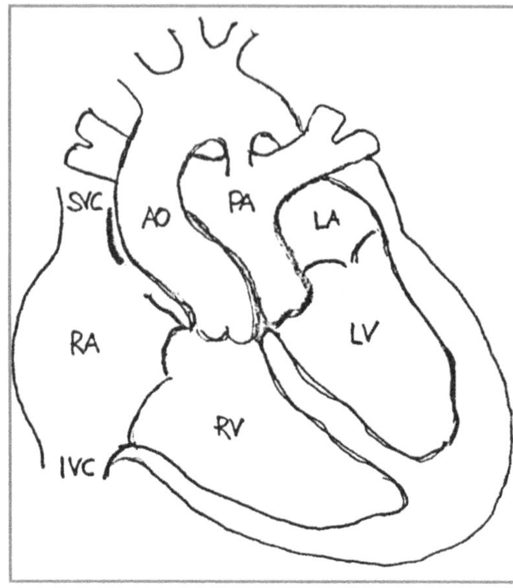

Fig. 26.14 Transposition of the great arteries. *Ao* aorta; *IVC* inferior vena cava, *LA* left atrium, *LV* left ventricle, *PA* pulmonary artery, *RA* right atrium, *RV* right ventricle, *SVC* superior vena cava

Patients corrected through Mustard and Senning procedures may not be allowed to perform any type of competitive sports. However recreational low to moderate dynamic and low static activities are encouraged in carefully selected patients.

In patients corrected with arterial switch the suitability for sporting activities should be assessed through physical examination (NYHA functional class), ECG, echocardiogram, chest X-ray, exercise stress test. In patients with positive outcomes (i.e. without or only mild neo-aortic insufficiency, no significant pulmonary stenosis, no sighs of ischemia or arrhythmia on exercise ECG), all sports are allowed, with exception of high static and high dynamic sports. A yearly follow up is recommended.

26.5.3 Congenitally Corrected Transposition of the Great Arteries

The congenitally corrected transposition of the great arteries (ccTGA) is a complex congenital heart defect characterized by a double atrioventricular and ventriculoarterial discordance: the left atrium is connected to a systemic morphologically right ventricle from which originates the aorta and the right atrium is connected to a morphologically left ventricle from which originates the pulmonary artery [14]. The expression *congenitally corrected* refers to the hematic flow that follows a physiological course even if through anatomically transposed structures. Only 1% of cases present themselves as isolated defects, meaning that in almost all cases one or more associated defects may be observed. Regardless of the latter aspect, two elements that negatively influence the prognosis of these patients may be detected: (1) the presence of a systemic morphologically right ventricle and atrioventricular valve (the right ventricle and the tricuspid valve, often dysplatic, are not *designed* to handle systemic pressure over long periods of time); (2) the location of the atrioventricular node, which very often influences the evolution towards complete atrioventricular block. Although an isolated defect would not require surgical intervention, the constant association to other defects often calls for a surgical correction that varies from patient to patient. *These patients may not be allowed to perform any competitive sporting activities.*

Patients may be allowed to take part in *recreational low to moderate dynamic and low static activities*, only following a personalized evaluation performed by highly trained experts.

26.5.4 Ebstein's Anomaly

Ebstein's anomaly is a rare heart defect (< 1%) characterized by a wide spectrum of anomalies of the tricuspid valve and right ventricle. Its main feature is a downwards displacement of the tricuspid valve with subsequent formation of two cardiac chambers, the first one, supravalvular, being formed by the right atrium and part of the *atrialized* right ventricle, the second one consisting in the remaining portion of the subvalvular right ventricle; the tricuspid valve and its subvalvular apparatus are often affected by dysplasia [15]. It is frequently associated to a number of heart defects (ASD etc.) and arrhythmia due to the presence of accessory beams.

Subjects affected by this *disease may not take part in competitive sport*. Patients may be allowed to take part in *recreational low to moderate dynamic and low static activities*.

26.5.5 Complex Congenital Heart Diseases Corrected with Univentricular Physiology (Fontan Procedure)

The present chapter refers to a group of particularly complex and rather heterogeneous heart defects (tricuspid or mitral valve atresia, double inlet left ventricle, univentricular heart, hypoplastic left or right ventricle and heterotaxy syndromes) that share the impossibility to be subjected to biventricular correction. Their correction through Fontan procedure consists in the repositioning of the systemic venous return towards the pulmonary artery, therefore eliminating any communication between the two circulations. Several changes were carried out to the procedure throughout the years in order to adapt it to the patients' specific conditions [16].

It seems evident that these patients *cannot be allowed to perform any type of competitive sporting activities.*

As far as *recreational instructional activities* are concerned, it is worth bearing in mind that these patients can realistically reach no more than a *good functional ability*, defined by the following characteristics: asymptomatic patient, class NYHA II, absence of residues or enlargement of the right atrium varying from moderate (*classic* Fontan) to absent (total cavopulmonary anastomosis), ejection fraction of the systemic ventricle 40-50%, absent or light atrioventricular valvular insufficiency, effort tolerance and/or physical efficiency 70-80% of normal standards (VO2 max > 25 ml/kg/min), absent or moderate systemic desaturation (85-90%), absence of arrhythmia or supraventricular extrasystole, episodes of supraventricular tachycardia controlled by medical therapy and/or radio frequency ablation procedure, possible normofunctional pacemaker. *These patients may be allowed to take part in recreational activities from low to moderate and low static group.*

26.5.6 Eisenmenger's Syndrome

Eisenmenger's syndrome represents the common final stage of all heart defects with left-to-right shunt, which, if not corrected, may result in irreversible pulmonary hypertension: a simple example is represented by an extensive uncorrected VSD; over time pulmonary hypertension through a left-to-right shunt leads to the development of pulmonary hypertension; when pulmonary pressure becomes suprasystemic the shunt inverts to a right-to-left shunt leading to chronic cyanosis [17]. The above conditions are associated with a series of (pulmonary, cerebral, hematological, arrhythmic, metabolic, infective) complications and life expectancy is significantly reduced. Surgery is not recommended and medical treatment may only be palliative. *These patients cannot be allowed to perform any types of competitive sporting activities.*

As far as *recreational instructional facilities* are concerned, it should be underlined that these patients cannot realistically achieve more than a *good functional ability,* defined by the following characteristics: *good life expectancy over a decade,* more favourable prognosis if < 25 years; slight symptomatic patient, class NYHA II, stable moderate cyanosis (oxygen saturation ≥ 80%); basic heart condition: prevalently simple defects (interventricular defect and, more rarely, ASD, defect of the arterial duct, aortopulmonary window) that may occasionally be complex (pulmonary atresia and interventricular defect etc.); preserved ventricular function; effort tolerance and/or physical efficiency 70-80% of reference standards (VO_2 max 20-25 ml/kg/min); limited arterial desaturation (approximately 70%); absence of arrhythmia and complications or sequences; good control of lab tests: hemoglobin ≤ 18 g%; hematocrit 55-65%; mean corpuscular volume and serum iron within limits (compensated erythrocytosis); normal creatinemia and hyperuceremia. *These patients may be allowed to take part in recreational instructional activities from low dynamic group.*

References

1. Sadowski SL (2009) Congenital cardiac disease in the newborn infant: past, present, and future. Crit Care Nurs Clin North Am 21:37-48
2. Hoffman JIE, Kaplan S (2002) The incidence of congenital heart disease. J Am Coll Cardiol 239:1890-1900
3. Hirth A, Reybrouck T, Bjarnason-Wehrens B et al (2006) Recommendations for participation in competitive and leisure sports in patients with congenital heart disease: a consensus document. Eur J Cardiovasc Prev Rehabil 13:293-299
4. Pelliccia A, Fagard R, Bjørnstad HH, et al (2005) Recommendations for competitive sports participation in atlete with cardiovascular disease. A Consensus document from the Study Group of Sports Cardiology of the Working Group of Cardiac Rehabilitation and Exercise Physiology and the Working Group of Myocardial and Pericardial diseases of the European Society of Cardiology. Eur Heart J 26:1422-1445
5. Porter CJ, Edwards WD (2008) Atrial septal defects. In "Moss & Adams'. Heart disease in infants, children and adolescents (7th ed.)". Allen HD, Driscoll DJ, Shaddy RE, Feltes TF eds. Lippincott Williams & Wilkins, Philadelphia, pp 632-645
6. McDaniel NL, Gutgesell HP (2008) Ventricular septal defects. In "Moss & Adams'. Heart disease in infants, children and adolescents (7th ed.)". Allen HD, Driscoll DJ, Shaddy RE, Feltes TF eds. Lippincott Williams & Wilkins, Philadelphia, pp 667-682
7. Moore P, Brook MM, Hejmann MA (2008) In "Moss & Adams'. Heart disease in infants, children and adolescents (7th ed.)". Allen HD, Driscoll DJ, Shaddy RE, Feltes TF eds. Lippincott Williams & Wilkins, Philadelphia, pp 683-701
8. Cetta F, Minich LL, Edwards WD, et al (2008) Atrioventricular septal defects. In "Moss & Adams'. Heart disease in infants, children and adolescents (7th ed.)". Allen HD, Driscoll DJ, Shaddy RE, Feltes TF eds. Lippincott Williams & Wilkins, Philadelphia, pp 646-666
9. Prieto LR, Latson LA (2008) Pulmonary stenosis. In "Moss & Adams'. Heart disease in infants, children and adolescents (7th ed.)". Allen HD, Driscoll DJ, Shaddy RE, Feltes TF eds. Lippincott Williams & Wilkins, Philadelphia, pp 835-858
10. Schneider DJ, Moore JW (2008) Aortic stenosis. In "Moss & Adams'. Heart disease in infants, children and adolescents (7th ed.)". Allen HD, Driscoll DJ, Shaddy RE, Feltes TF eds. Lippincott Williams & Wilkins, Philadelphia, pp 968- 986
11. Beekman III RH (2008) Coarctation of the aorta. In "Moss & Adams'. Heart disease in infants, children and adolescents (7th ed.)". Allen HD, Driscoll DJ, Shaddy

RE, Feltes TF eds. Lippincott Williams & Wilkins, Philadelphia, pp 987-1004
12. Siwik ES, Erenberg FG, Zahka KG (2008) Tetralogy of Fallot. In "Moss & Adams'. Heart disease in infants, children and adolescents (7th ed.)". Allen HD, Driscoll DJ, Shaddy RE, Feltes TF eds. Lippincott Williams & Wilkins, Philadelphia, pp 888-910
13. Wernovsky G. Transposition of the great arteries (2008) In "Moss & Adams'. Heart disease in infants, children and adolescents (7th ed.)". Allen HD, Driscoll DJ, Shaddy RE, Feltes TF eds. Lippincott Williams & Wilkins, Philadelphia, pp 1038-1086
14. Dyck JD, Atallah J (2008) Congenitally corrected transposition of the great arteries. In "Moss & Adams'. Heart disease in infants, children and adolescents (7th ed.)". Allen HD, Driscoll DJ, Shaddy RE, Feltes TF eds. Lippincott Williams & Wilkins, Philadelphia, pp 1087-1099
15. Epstein ML (2008) Tricuspid atresia, stenosis, and regurgitation. In "Moss & Adams'. Heart disease in infants, children and adolescents (7th ed.)". Allen HD, Driscoll DJ, Shaddy RE, Feltes TF eds. Lippincott Williams & Wilkins, Philadelphia, pp 817-834
16. Hagler DJ, Edwards WD (2008) Univentricular atrioventricular connection. In "Moss & Adams'. Heart disease in infants, children and adolescents (7th ed.)". Allen HD, Driscoll DJ, Shaddy RE, Feltes TF eds. Lippincott Williams & Wilkins, Philadelphia, pp1128-1148
17. Rabinovitch M (2008) Pathophysiology of pulmonary hypertension. In "Moss & Adams'. Heart disease in infants, children and adolescents (7th ed.)". Allen HD, Driscoll DJ, Shaddy RE, Feltes TF eds. Lippincott Williams & Wilkins, Philadelphia, pp1322-1354

27 Sports Practice in Individuals with Cardiac Pacemakers and Implantable Cardioverter-Defibrillators

Filippo Lamberti

27.1 Introduction

The population of patients undergoing implantation of anti-bradycardia systems (pacemaker) or anti-tachycardia systems (implantable defibrillators) is constantly growing. This fact is partially due to the favourable impact of such therapies on cardiovascular mortality, and, in part, to the widening of the indications to implant. The definition of new cardiomyopathies such as Brugada syndrome, long QTs syndromes, short QT syndrome, polymorphic catecholaminergic ventricular tachycardia, etc., has led to the involvement of a relative younger portion of the population as candidates for device implantation, mainly with implantable cardioverter defibrillators (ICD). Moreover, this portion of young patients includes an increasing number of athletes, the majority of whom receive an ICD only on clinically indicated grounds. This event has a great impact in their life, as the presence of an ICD should disqualify athletes from most competitive sports.

Sport participation in patients with implanted devices (pacemakers and/or ICD) is a medical and ethical challenge for the treating physician. Clinicians are more often asked for recommendations regarding what activities are allowed in such patients, particularly in those with ICD. This expectation seems to be evident in young, asymptomatic patients in whom ICD has been prophylactically implanted, but older patients also enquire about this. Clinicians have to address the patient's expectations in sport participation, recognising that there are few data available and that some recommendations seem to be a matter of common sense.

The 36th Bethesda Conference authors themselves recognized that there were significant differences in opinion and little direct evidence to support their recommendations [1]. In any case, limited as it was to competitive athletes, the Conference stated that patients with ICD can participate only in class IA activities such as bowling or golf. Moreover, the desire of the athlete to continue with athletic competitions should not be the primary indication for the use of an ICD. Although these statements are based on a consensus among experts, many courts have recognized guidelines established by national medical associations as evidence of good medical practice.

In any case, it is not clear whether these guidelines should apply to recreational sport activity. In this area, physicians are asked to solve the dilemma between the patient's wishes and his/her heart disease.

27.2 Sport Activity and Heart Disease: General Considerations

The adequacy of a sport activity in a patient with heart disease should be evaluated based on:

- the type of cardiovascular response to the demands of the specific sport activity;
- the specific cardiovascular diagnosis and its pathophysiological consequences;
- the level of sports participation.

Exercise may broadly be divided into two

F. Lamberti (✉)
Electrophysiology Department
"San Eugenio" Hospital, Rome, Italy

M. Fioranelli and G. Frajese (eds.), *Sports Cardiology*,
DOI: 10.1007/978-88-470-2775-6_27,

types: dynamic (isotonic) and static (isometric) [2]. The former involves changes in muscle length and joint movements with rhythmic muscular contractions that develop relatively small intramuscular forces, and the latter requires little or no change in muscular length or joint movement with the development of large intramuscular forces. Obviously no sport is only dynamic or static, but the two components combine differently in various sporting activities. For example, distance running has low static and high dynamic demands; on the other hand, water skiing has low dynamic and high static demands, while rowing has high static and dynamic demands.

The cardiovascular response to static or dynamic exercise differs. Dynamic exercise performed with a large muscle mass causes a marked increase in oxygen consumption. There is a substantial increase in cardiac output, heart rate, stroke volume and systolic blood pressure; a moderate increase in mean arterial pressure; and a decrease in diastolic blood pressure. Also, there is a marked decrease in total peripheral resistance. Static exercise, in contrast, causes a small increase in oxygen consumption, cardiac output and heart rate, and no change in stroke volume. Moreover, there is a marked increase in systolic, diastolic and mean arterial pressure and no appreciable change in total peripheral resistance. Thus, dynamic exercise primarily causes a volume load on the left ventricle, whereas static exercise causes a pressure load. In conclusion, both dynamic and static exercise increases factors that are important in determining myocardial oxygen demand.

As mentioned above, there are heart diseases that intrinsically limit the level of sports participation. The residual ejection fraction and NYHA function class determine this limit. When the limit is also evident to the patient, it is easier to find a reasonable level of exercise for him/her. In a different setting, where that limitation is absent or not evident, what is reasonable to the physician may to be the same as what is reasonable to the patient. Moreover, in patients with ionic cannel dysfunction (channelopathies), where a structural damage of the cardiac pump function is found, ICD appears to be, in patients' view, the only conditioning factor, much more than the disease itself.

A clear definition of the level of sports participation may be difficult and ambiguous. In fact, as the definition of a *competitive athlete* seems clear, it is not the same for non-competitive, recreational athletes. The authors of the 36th Bethesda Conference define a competitive athlete *as one who participates in an organized team or individual sport that requires regular competition against others as a central component, places a high premium on excellence and achievement, and requires some form of systematic (and usually intense) training*. The authors point out that competitive sports are regarded as a distinct lifestyle and *an important component of competitive sports activity concerns whether athletes are able to properly judge when it is prudent to terminate physical exertion*. They state that all other forms of sports participation should be viewed as recreational sport activity, even if there are subjects who engage in sports activity for recreation, but who are very competitive, for example, the twice-a-week tennis player, the employee who plays on his/her company's softball team, or the runner who jogs several times per week and occasionally races to improve his/her time. In such cases the difference between competitive and recreational athletes may simply be semantics.

27.3 Sports Activity and Patients with ICD

The postulated risks of sport activity in patient with ICDs are:

1. increased frequency of arrhythmic episodes;
2. potential failure of anti-tachycardia therapy in the treatment of ventricular arrhythmias;
3. potential injury or death resulting from a loss of consciousness or device therapy (shock);
4. potential damage to the implanted system (device and/or electrodes).

27.4 Sports Activity and Incidence of Ventricular Arrhythmias

The role of sports activity in the onset of arrhythmic events should be considered in patients with any cardiomyopathy, particularly those treated with ICDs.

Some evidence suggests that sports activity *per se* increases the risk of SCD. In the Physician's Health Study, exercise substantially increased the risk of SDC [3]. In a series of young subjects who died suddenly, the relative risk of SCD among athletes was 2.5 higher compared to non-athletes; the majority of episodes occurred during exercise.

It seems quite likely that sports will increase the rate of arrhythmic events in patients with cardiomyopathy and the risk of shock in patients with ICD.

In about half of patients with HCM, ventricular arrhythmias and SCD episodes are associated with exercise. Exertion usually provokes ventricular arrhythmias in ARVD. In a review of idiopathic ventricular fibrillation, 15% of patients had the arrhythmic event while exercising.

In long QT syndrome, exercise, particularly swimming, has been associated with SCD and syncope. In CAD patients, vigorous exercise is associated with a significant risk of SCD and acute myocardial infarction, but the lasting benefit of exercise in lowering such risks is well known. In patients with congenital abnormalities of the coronary arteries, nearly all deaths are related to exercise.

Less evident is the role of exercise in increasing the risk of arrhythmic events in patients with Brugada syndrome. In such patients the arrhythmic events are much more commonly related to relative bradycardia, as it occurs, for example, while sleeping. Moreover, it is known that typical ECG abnormalities for the syndrome may disappear during exercise, however a potential role of hyperthermia related to exercise has been mentioned as a potential cause of arrhythmias in such patients.

Although there is no direct evidence, it is likely to hypothesise that, in patients with the above mentioned diseases treated with an ICD, exercise may provoke arrhythmias that require device activation, potentially in a repetitive manner.

This potential event has to be weighed with the fact that many of these patients are young subjects who are frequently asymptomatic, prophylactically given an ICD implantation, and who wish to continue their previous bountiful life, including sporting activity. While shocks decrease quality of life, so abstention from sport may do too.

27.5 Sports Activity and the Efficacy of Anti-tachycardia Therapy

Another point to consider is whether an ICD can effectively terminate ventricular arrhythmia during exercise. There are a few and inconclusive examples in literature of this argument.

In experimental studies, patients were treated with epinephrine at doses mimicking exercise during ICD implantation, finding that defibrillation thresholds were minimally increased and the first shock efficacy was reduced while performing defibrillation threshold testing.

Moreover, it has been reported that the defibrillation threshold is higher and the first shock efficacy is lower in the morning when the levels of catecholamine are highest.

On the other hand, animal studies demonstrated a beneficial effect of epinephrine in lowering the defibrillation threshold and favouring cardioversion. In fact, studies with multisite action potential recordings have demonstrated that epinephrine increased spatial synchronization and reduced the dispersion of refractoriness during ventricular arrhythmias.

Potentially, exercise may increase the risk of shock failure.

However, direct evidence is inconclusive.

The failure of shock in the treatment ventricular arrhythmias has been reported in two patients, one of whom died of intractable ventricular tachycardia during a treadmill test.

On the contrary, in a group of patients with HCM treated with ICD implantation, effective shocks were documented during exercise: eight during competitive and twelve during non-competitive sports. In another series of 36 shocks delivered during vigorous exertion, none of them were ineffective.

To date the largest series is a survey by Lampert et al., who retrospectively surveyed members of the Heart Rhythm Society regarding their experiences with ICD patients, focusing on those participating in any form of sport, whether competitive or non-competitive [4].

Although 40% of respondents reported caring for patients with ICD receiving shocks during exercise, only four episodes of shock failure were actually documented. In any case, none of these ineffective shocks was associated with death.

In conclusion, to date it is not possible to determine if the risk of shock failure is higher during exercise than other situations. From the data of Lampert's survey, this risk does not appear to be high.

27.6 Sports Activity and Patient Injury

The risk of injury in patients with ICD due to loss of consciousness induced by ventricular arrhythmia or a fall induced by shock seems to be more concrete.

This risk is clearly related to the type of exercise performed. It seems quite evident that arrhythmic syncope or a fall due to involuntary muscle contraction induced by shock may have more dangerous consequences while performing extreme sports (i.e. hang gliding, diving, rock climbing, etc.) than brisk walking. However, a fall for the same reasons may not be less dangerous when cycling or running.

In any case these are commonsense suggestions, as there are no data to assess a relative safe sport in such patient populations.

In the survey by Lampert, although shock delivery during exercise was relatively common, responding physicians reported very few cases of injury related to syncope or ICD shock. Only 1% of physicians reported cases of injury. There were six cases of minor injury (bruising, laceration, soft tissue damage) and three case of major injury. The latter consisted of head injuries in two patients (while running and on treadmill, respectively) and one neck injury while hunting. Two deaths were reported, one of which occurred on a treadmill.

27.7 Sports Activity and System Damage (Device and Electrodes)

Damage of the implanted device and/or of the electrodes may actually be a more consistent event.

System damage can occur or be a consequence of repetitive muscle contractions or direct trauma in contact sports, or collision with a contusive object (ball, disc, etc.).

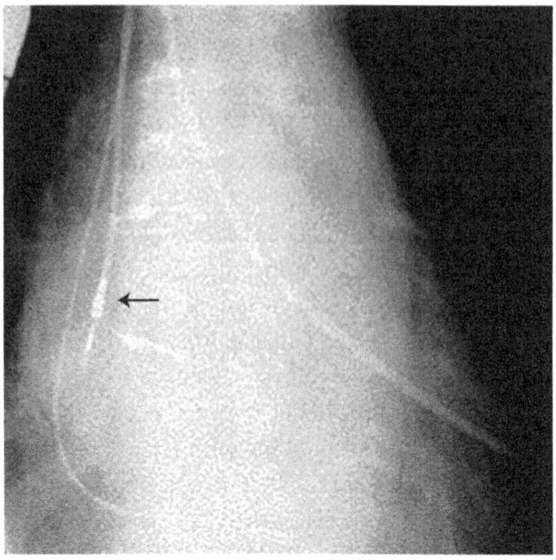

Fig. 27.1 Chest X-ray (AP projection) in a patient with a dual-chamber ICD: A macroscopic dislodgment of the atrial lead (*arrow*) is evident

Table 27.1 Common signs of lead dislodgment

Pacing: transient or fixed loss of capture
Sensing: transient or fixed loss of sensing
Electric therapy not delivered
Inappropriate therapy delivery

Many sports require vigorous and often repetitive pectoral muscle contractions, which lead to significant traction on the electrodes. Long lasting traction may provoke electrode dislodgment and subsequently system failure. This failure often requires surgical system revision. Electrode dislodgment causes system malfunction through a loss of sensing or pacing or both in the heart chamber where the electrode(s) is/are positioned. Gross electrode dislodgment can easily be detected on chest X-rays (Fig. 27.1). More often we deal with micro-electrode dislodgment, identifiable only by telemetric system checks (Table 27.1). Moreover, ventricular electrode dislodgment, on which defibrillation coils are inserted, may impair cardioversion therapy (anti-tachycardia pacing or shock) in cases of ventricular arrhythmias. In such conditions, surgical revision of the implanted system is mandatory. Much more frequently, repetitive muscle contractions cause electrode fractures or crushing or an insulation breach (Fig. 27.2). These

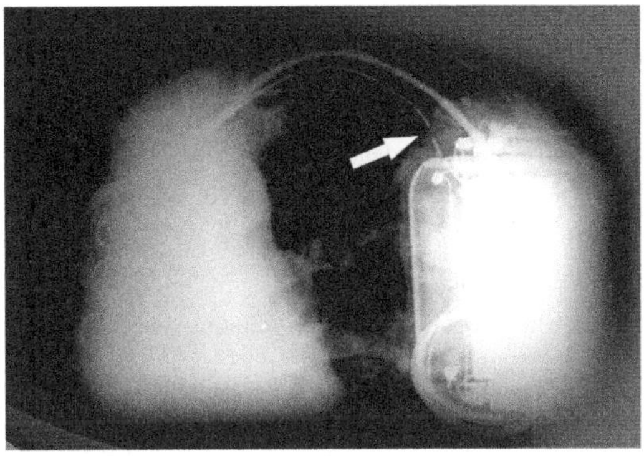

Fig. 27.2 Chest X-ray (AP projection) in a patient with ICD: The fracture of a conductor (*white arrow*) is clearly evident

forms of damage may occur at any electrode level. In any case, they tend to concentrate where there is a high point of stress or a high pressure point. The following are the points of higher pressure upon the lead: suture sleeve and tricuspid valve, but more frequently at the 1st rib – at the clavicle level where there is a consistent area of mechanical stress (Fig. 27.3). Electrode fracture may be recognized on an X-ray, but more frequently it is highlighted on telemetric system checks showing no intermittent or erratic sensing, intermittent loss of capture or abnormally high or low impedance. Electrode fracture or crushing may result in the delivery of inappropriate antiarrhythmic therapy for the device, i.e. shock, due to the input of noise in the circuit which is incorrectly interpreted as ventricular arrhythmias (Fig. 27.4). Sports more frequently associated with such complications are: weight lifting, rowing, golf, tennis, etc.

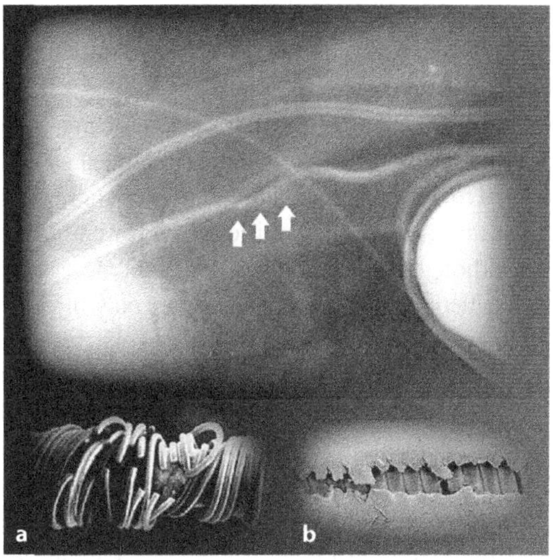

Fig. 27.3 Upper panel: X-ray documentation of an electrode crush (*white arrows*) at 1st rib and clavicle level (subclavian crush). Lower panel: magnification of a break point with the involvement of electric spirals (a) or insulation only (b)

If such complications are more common in patients with ICD who exercise than in those who do not, it is not clear. In Lampert's survey, 28 electrode fractures and dislodgments were reported, sixteen occurring in patients who exercise with weight lifting, five with golf, two with tennis, and one each with swimming, water skiing and hunting.

In the same report system damage by direct

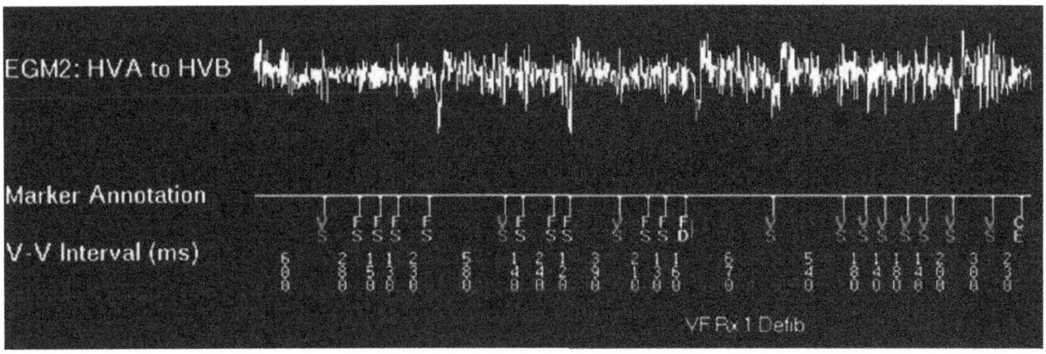

Fig. 27.4 Electrocardiogram analysis of a recorded episode: failure in sensing in a patient with ICD and right ventricle electrode fracture: note the presence of artefacts on ventricular signal (EGM2) due to noise entrance in the circuit. The very short intervals (V-V interval) between recorded electrocardiograms are incorrectly diagnosed as ventricular fibrillation by the device (FS on Marker Annotation) with inappropriate shock delivery (*CE*)

trauma occurred when practicing football, basketball, hockey, skiing, cycling, golf, baseball and softball.

Available data suggest that there is no safe sport for any patient with ICD. Clinical judgment is warranted for each patient, taking into account his/her heart disease and the specific sport desired [5].

Although the 36th Bethesda Conference states that patients with ICD can participate only in Class IA sport activity such as bowling or golf, the reality seems to be significantly different. In Lampert's survey only 10% of responding physicians adhered to this statement. In fact 71% of them reported caring for patients with ICD who participate in sport, including vigorous exercise, and about 40% stated that they were aware of at least one patient engaged in competitive athletics. Only 45% of the interviewed physicians clearly prohibited any sport at competitive level. Basketball, running and skiing are the most reported sporting activities. Criteria on which a large number of the responding physicians based their evaluation of sports participation restrictions were: the EF and the underlying heart disease, without taking in account the device itself.

In conclusion, few data are available to establish safety in sports participation for patients with ICD. Although there are theoretical reasons to restrict patients with ICD from participating in sports, in reality a wide part of this population takes part in sport at any level, with a relatively low rate of adverse events. In any case, cardiologists have to be aware that the population of patients with ICD is strongly heterogeneous and by this their judgment cannot be generic and standardized [6]. ICDs should not be viewed as universally protective devices that allow unlimited athletic participation. Any physician should have a fully informed discussion about the risks and benefits of a particular sporting activity with the patient and his/her family. An analysis of the environment in which the activity takes place may be useful, with a suggestion of more protective conditions in which the staff or colleagues are fully aware of the patient's status. In patients who will to perform sport at competitive recreational level, a treadmill test may be useful to test the susceptibility of ventricular arrhythmias to exercise and to evaluate device capability in distinguishing ventricular arrhythmias from sinus tachycardia, in order to avoid inappropriate shocks. Moreover, physicians should teach patients to monitor heart rate and stop at a target rate; the implantation of dual chamber ICDs with improved arrhythmia discrimination algorithms should be preferred. Finally, a more frequent and complete telemetric device check-up is advisable to recognize malfunction or system damage (Table 27.2).

Table 27.2 ICD telemetric control checklist

Battery voltage status
Circuit status
Pacing/sensing/impedance tests
Efficacy of electric therapies delivered
EGM analysis of recorded arrhythmic episodes
EGM amplitude stability
Correlation between patient's symptoms and recorded episodes

27.8 Sports Activity and Patients with Pacemakers

Patients with pacemakers have less limitation in sports participation than patients with ICD. In the absence of a structural heart disease, patients with pacemakers carry a risk of ventricular arrhythmia similar to that of the general population. The true limit to sports participation is the potential damage of the implanted system related to exercise. The 36th Bethesda Conference also recognized that athletes treated with pacemakers should not engage in competitive sports with a danger of bodily collision because such trauma may damage the pacemaker system. As for ICD, system damage may involve the device and/or the electrodes. Many considerations about this that are mentioned above (patients with ICD) are also valid for pacemakers. The consequences of device malfunction depend on the heart chamber involved (atrium or ventricle), the presence or not of spontaneous electrical activity (i.e. junctional, ventricular escape rhythm), the duration of loss of electrical stimulation (transient or prolonged). Severe consequences of device malfunction are syncope or death due to asystole. Patient injury may occur due to a fall secondary to syncope. It is stated that limiting more extreme sporting activities is less evident, i.e. diving is allowed within the limits of the device's pressure resistance.

27.9 Conclusion

There are few data regarding the adequacy and safety during sports of patients with implanted devices, particularly those with ICD. Although decisions regarding how we choose to view risk in our lives are rarely entirely rational, by quantifying the risks of sports for individuals with ICDs, we will give patients the information necessary to make an informed decision [7]. Recognising that there are few data available and that some recommendations seem to be a matter of common sense, clinical judgment is warranted for each patient. Correct and complete information, shared choices and professional experience should be the cornerstones of our action.

References

1. Maron BJ, Zipes DP, et al (2005) 36th Bethesda Conference eligibility recommendations for competitive athletes with cardiovascular abnormalities. J Am Coll Cardiol 45:1312- 1375
2. Mitchell JH; Haskell W, Snell P et al: Task Force 8: Classification of Sports (2005). JACC Vol. 45, No. 8,1364–7
3. Albert CM, Mittleman MA, Chae CU, et al (2000) Triggering of sudden death from cardiac causes by vigorous exertion. N Engl J Med 343:1355–1361
4. Lampert R, Cannom D and Olshansky B (2006) Safety of sports participation in patients with implantable cardioverter defibrillators: a survey of Hearth Rhythm Society members. J Cardiovasc Eletrophysiol 17:11-15
5. Fogel RI (2006) Athletes and ICDs: what to do when the clinical community disagrees with the "experts". J Cardiovasc Eletrophysiol 17:16-17
6. Lampert R, Cannom D (2008) Sport participation for athletes with implantable cardioverter –defibrillators should be an individualized risk-benefit decision. Heart Rhythm 5:861-863
7. Ropeik D, Gray G (200) Risk: A Practical Guide for Deciding What's Really Safe and What's Really Dangerous in the World Around You. Boston: Houghton Mifflin

Other Clinical Indications: Sports Practice in Individuals with Patent Foramen Ovale and in Patients Undergoing Non-Coronary Interventional Procedures

28

Ilaria Dato, Rocco Vergallo, Antonella Tommasino and Italo Porto

28.1 Sports Practice in Patients with Patent Foramen Ovale

28.1.1 Anatomical and Pathophysiological Notes

Patent foramen ovale (PFO) is an anatomical variant characterized by the incomplete fusion of septum I to septum II, which causes a communication between the right and left atria close to the fossa ovale (Fig. 28.1), sometimes associated to other abnormalities of the interatrial septum, such as atrial septal aneurysm (ASA) or microfenestrations of the interatrial fibrous septum.

In intrauterine life, PFO allows the oxygenated blood from the placenta to flow from the umbilical veins to the aorta, bypassing non-functional foetal lungs. After birth, the increase in right atrial pressure causes a functional closure of foramen ovale and, in most individuals, an anatomical closure of the PFO too within the first year of life, by fusion of the two membranes. However, in about 25% of people this fusion is not complete [1]. This defect can lead to a transient right-to-left shunt during all the conditions in which right atrial pressure exceeds left atrial pressure (e.g., during the Valsalva manoeuvre). As a consequence, pulmonary filters could fail and the direct passage of venous blood into the arterial circulation could cause the *paradoxical embolism* phenomenon.

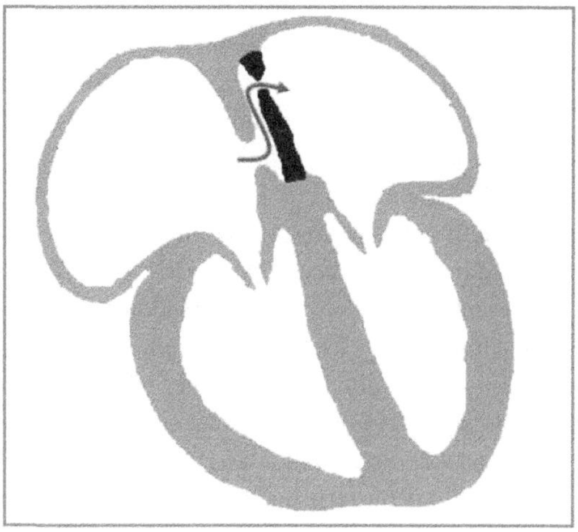

Fig. 29.1 Schematic representation of the heart, which shows the incomplete fusion of septum I to septum II, with a communication between the right and left atria close to the fossa ovale

The presence of PFO has been associated with the following pathological conditions:

- cryptogenic stroke [2];
- migraine [3];
- decompression sickness in scuba divers [4];
- obstructive sleep apnea [5];
- platypnea-orthodeoxia [6];
- multi-infarct dementia [7];
- cerebral embolism following orthopedic knee surgery [8].

Among these conditions, the first three play the most important role and will be described below.

I. Porto (✉)
Cardiovascular and Neurological Department
San Donato Hospital
Arezzo, Italy

M. Fioranelli and G. Frajese (eds.), *Sports Cardiology*,
DOI: 10.1007/978-88-470-2775-6_28, © Springer-Verlag Italia 2012

28.1.2 PFO and Cryptogenic Stroke

The cause-effect relationship between PFO and cryptogenic stroke, in particular when it is associated with ASA, is derived from several observations [9]. Firstly, the incidence of PFO in patients with cryptogenic stroke (more than 50%) was significantly higher than in the general population [10]. Interestingly, Mas et al. observed a significantly higher incidence of recurrent cerebrovascular events in patients with the association of PFO and ASA, despite antiplatelet therapy [11]. Percutaneous closure of the PFO by dedicated devices was superior to medical therapy alone in reducing recurrent cerebrovascular ischemic events [12]. Systematic reviews of non-randomized studies reported a lower annual recurrence rate of these events in patients undergoing percutaneous closure of the PFO (0-5%) than in those receiving medical therapy alone (4-12 %) [13]. Moreover, this benefit seems to be superior in young individuals and in the presence of ASA [14].

Currently, the only completed randomized study is the CLOSURE I trial, recently published in the New England Journal of Medicine, in which 910 patients with cryptogenic stroke or transient ischemic attacks were randomized to receive medical therapy (325 mg aspirin and/or warfarin daily with a target INR of 2 to 3) or PFO percutaneous closure using the STARFlex device (NMT Medical, Boston, MA) along with antiplatelet therapy (75 mg clopidogrel daily for 6 months and 325 mg aspirin daily for 2 years). After 2-years of follow-up, PFO percutaneous closure was not superior to medical therapy in the *intention-to-treat* analysis. The cumulative incidence of the primary end point, composite of stroke or transient ischemic attack, was 5.5% in the closure group compared to 6.8% in the medical therapy group (adjusted hazard ratio, 0.78; 95% confidence interval, 0.45 to 1.35; P=0.37). Other studies with different designs and tested devices (PC trial, CLOSE, RESPECT, REDUCE) are in progress, with many enrolment problems due mainly to young patients' preference to be treated by percutaneous methods, and due to the need for enrolling a large population in order to observe statistically significant results, considering the low annual incidence of cerebral ischemic events.

28.1.3 PFO and Migraine

Migraine is a relatively frequent pathological condition, which affects about 12% of people [15]. PFO prevalence in individuals affected by migraine with or without aura is considerably high (about 50%). The pathophysiological mechanism seems to be the passage of microemboli and vasoactive substances through the PFO [16].

Several case studies have demonstrated a resolution or marked improvement of migraine in a large number of patients (up to 80%) treated by percutaneous closure of the PFO. However, this observation has not been confirmed by the randomized, double-blind MIST trial, published in Circulation in 2008, in which 147 patients with PFO and migraine were enrolled and randomized to percutaneous PFO closure with the STARFlex device (NMT Medical, Boston, MA) or to medical therapy plus a sham procedure (skin incision in the groin) [17]. At the 3-month follow-up visit, no significant difference was found for primary endpoints (migraine headache ceszation, 3/73 vs. 3/74, p=0.51) or secondary endpoints (change in the severity, frequency and characteristics of migraine) between the two groups.

There are other randomized studies in progress (PRIMA, PREMIUM, ESCAPE, MIST II), which promise to clarify the cause-effect relationship between PFO and migraine.

28.1.4 PFO and Decompression Sickness (DCS)

PFO seems to play a role in the pathogenesis of the DCS during scuba activities. Indeed, during scuba diving with the use of compressed air-supplied regulators, because of the increased pressure due to the dive, air components (in particular, oxygen and nitrogen) dissolve in the bloodstream and soak into the tissues. In the decompression phase, during the ascent, dissolved nitrogen gradually returns to the gaseous state and is released through the lungs. The amount of dissolved nitrogen is strictly related to the depth and duration of the dive and to the ascent speed. Generally, close respect for the so called *decompression tables* allows nitrogen to move back from the tissues to the blood by forming small blebs of gas that are released through the pulmonary capillaries into the expired air. However, in presence of a PFO, the contact between venous and arterial blood allows these blebs to enter the systemic circulation and embolise to peripheral tissues (paradoxical embolism), causing decompression sickness (DCS). Several studies [18-20] reported an increased incidence of PFO (up to 62%) in DCS with neurological involvement. Neurological symptoms of DCS occurring within 30 minutes after the ascent in scuba divers who carefully respect safety norms are generally associated with the paradoxical embolism phenomenon. These symptoms have to be distinguished from those in individuals who do not perform a scuba diving within the safety curve, which are generally associated with considerable production of blebs in the tissues, but not to paradoxical embolism.

However, it is important to consider that about 25% of people are affected by PFO, which can cause a right-to-left shunt, but a considerably lower rate of scuba divers develop DCS. In particular, the Divers Alert Network (DAN) Europe estimated that the risk of DCS for a scuba diver is 1/42000 for dives deeper than 30 meters, and 1/7000 for dives deeper than 30 meters. Therefore, most scuba divers will never experience DCS. However, DAN recommends strict adherence to the safety rules of scuba diving in individuals with diagnosed PFO in order to avoid action that would further the passage of blebs in the systemic circulation.

28.1.5 Diagnosis

Following the clinical suspicion of PFO it is appropriate for patients to undergo instrumental diagnostic procedures in order to confirm the defect and define its severity.

Transthoracic echocardiography is the simplest diagnostic method, but it is able to identify only very large defects. More accurate information can be derived from the use of contrast echocardiography, which allows detection of the passage of the contrast medium injected into a peripheral vein from the right atrium to the left atrium, during the Valsalva manoeuvre. The *gold standard* for the diagnosis of PFO, however, is contrast transesophageal echocardiography, which enables both confirmation of the defect and a clear description of its anatomical details and functional relevance, by counting the number of blebs passing through the defect during the Valsalva manoeuvre (Fig. 28.2). Finally, further information can be obtained by transcranial Doppler, which is able to detect a paradoxical shunt during the Valsalva manoeuvre by counting the *hits* generated in the middle cerebral artery after intravenous injection of the contrast medium. It is a simple diagnostic method with considerable screening utility, but it should only be performed along with transesophageal echocardiography due to its inability to provide information about either PFO anatomical features or other possible associated anomalies.

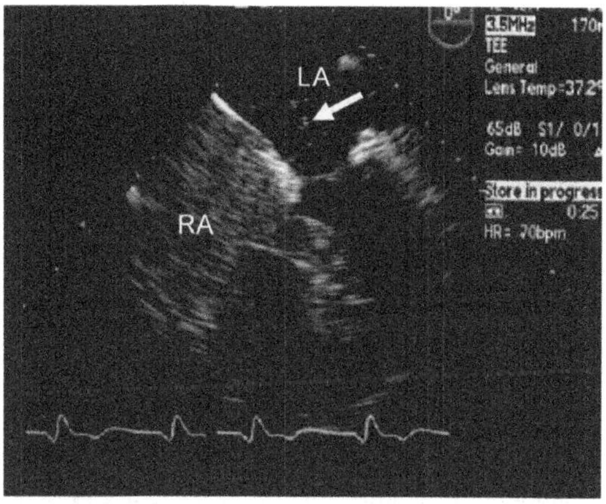

Fig. 28.2 Contrast transesophageal echocardiography. Evidence of the passage of blebs from the right atrium to the left one (*arrow*) in a patient with PFO. *LA* left atrium, *RA* right atrium

In the case of a patient with PFO and a cerebral ischemic event, however, it may not be easy to find objective confirmation of the cause-effect relationship between the two conditions: in fact, this relationship is *confirmed* only by the detection of thrombotic materials within the defect; it is *presumptive* if there are thrombotic events in the venous circulation of patients with PFO and no otherwise explanation of the cerebral ischemic events; finally, the relationship remains *uncertain* if no signs of venous thrombosis can be observed. Moreover, it is important to perform systematic screening for prothrombotic states, which could explain the predisposition to venous thrombosis.

28.1.6 Prophylactic Medical Treatment of Paradoxical Embolism in Patients with PFO

In patients with PFO or ASA without previous cerebral ischemic events, prophylactic medical treatment of paradoxical embolism is not indicated. On the other hand, prophylactic medical treatment is recommended for patients with PFO who have already experienced a transient ischemic attack (TIA), or stroke, without the evidence of other causes of ischemia (*cryptogenic* events). Treatment for these patients is generally with oral anticoagulants or antiplatelet agents. There is no agreement, however, on which treatment is most effective or on the ideal duration of medical therapy after a cerebral ischemic event.

28.1.7 Percutaneous Closure of PFO

The first percutaneous closure of an interatrial defect was performed by King in 1974, using a double umbrella of Dacron [21]. Since then, an increasing interest in this approach has led to a very large number of percutaneous treatments and to the development of several types of dedicated devices. Among the closure systems, there are the Sideris buttoned device, the Sideris self-centering device (Custom Medical Devices, Amarillo, TX), the Angel Wings device (Microvena Corporation, White Bear Lake, MN) and the Cardioseal device (NMT Medical, Boston, Massachusetts). Technical difficulties with implantation, uncontrolled release and the inability of retrieval due to the form and structure are some of the main disadvantages of these devices. The Amplatzer PFO Occluder (AGA Medical, Plymouth, Minn.) overcomes most of these drawbacks due to its controlled release system and the ease of implantation and retrieval after dislodgement. Therefore, it is one of the most used devices despite its cumbersome structure and its Nitinol composition, an alloy with a high nickel content. In the last years, new devices with a lower amount of this metal (Helex, W.L. Gore & Assoc., Flagstaff, Arizona, USA) or improved bioabsorbability (Biostar, NMT Medical, Boston, Massachusetts) have been developed in order to be used in patients with nickel allergy. Regardless of the employed device, the rate of success in terms of residual shunt is of almost 100% [22]. The most frequent complications are arrhythmias, mainly supraventricular, and bleeding from the puncture site. In addition, thrombus development at the site of the device can occur with an incidence ranging from 1 to 7% depending on the different studies and used devices, as assessed by transesophageal echocardiography some weeks after implantation [23].

The American Guidelines for the Prevention of Stroke in Patients With Stroke or Transient Ischemic Attack (2010) [24] recommend antiplatelet therapy in patients with PFO and a previous cerebral ischemic event (class IIa, level of evidence B), if there are no other pathological conditions requiring oral anticoagulant therapy (class IIb, level of evidence B). Percutaneous closure of PFO can be considered in patients who have recurrent cerebral ischemic events despite optimal medical therapy (class IIb, level of evidence C).

28.1.8 Sports Practice in Patients with PFO

In Italy, the practice of scuba sports with the use of compressed air-supplied regulators in individuals with PFO is forbidden by the COCIS (Comitato Organizzativo Cardiologico per l'Idoneità allo Sport), whilst all the other sports and scuba activities in apnoea patients are allowed. In the absence of an evident interatrial shunt, the presence of ASA alone does not modify the criteria for sports practice [25-26]. In patients undergoing percutaneous closure of the PFO, a cardiology follow-up at 6 months along with a standard ECG, 24-hour Holter monitoring and transthoracic echocardiography is necessary to obtain a fitness certification for sports practice. Moreover, contrast transesophageal echocardiography and/or contrast transcranial Doppler are required to exclude spontaneous or post-Valsalva manoeuvre residual shunt, which is a contraindication for scuba diving practice [27]. Finally, since the risk of late complications in patients undergoing percutaneous closure of the PFO is not well known, long-term echocardiography follow-up is recommended in order to detect any mitral and/or aortic valve dysfunction, pulmonary and systemic venous obstruction, or atrial wall *erosion* [28].

28.2 Sports Practice in Patients Undergoing non-Coronary Interventional Procedures

28.2.1 Left atrial appendage closure

The left atrial appendage is the site of thrombus origin in over 90% of patients with non-valvular atrial fibrillation. In the last years, new devices and techniques for percutaneous closure of the left atrial appendage have been developed, in order to reduce the incidence of cerebral thromboembolism and to avoid oral anticoagulant therapy.

The main study that tested this particular technique is the PROTECT AF (Watchman Left Atrial Appendage System for Embolic Protection in Patients with Atrial Fibrillation) [29]. This study evaluated the efficacy and safety of the percutaneous closure of the left atrial appendage compared with warfarin therapy in patients with non-valvular atrial fibrillation. Enrolled patients were randomized in a non-inferiority trial, at a ratio of 2:1 for percutaneous closure of the left atrial appendage with the Watchman device or with warfarin treatment (target INR was between 2 and 3). The primary efficacy endpoint (stroke, cardiovascular or unexplained death and systemic embolism) was similar in the two groups of patients, one treated with the device and one treated with warfarin. In particular, cardiovascular or unexplained death and hemorrhagic stroke were less frequent in the group treated with the device than in the one with warfarin therapy, while the incidence of any type of stroke and overall mortality were not different in the two groups. Regarding the primary safety endpoint, percutaneous closure was associated with more procedural complications (severe pericardial effusion requiring surgical drainage, 4.8%, periprocedural stroke mainly for gas embolism, 1.1%, embolization of the device, 0.6%). Both in the device group (in which patients were also treated with warfarin for a limited period, followed by the combination of aspirin plus clopidogrel, and then with aspirin alone in the long term) and in the warfarin group, major bleeding events (3.5% vs. 4.1%) and hemorrhagic strokes (0.2% vs. 2.5%) occurred. In conclusion, PROTECT AF showed that percutaneous closure of the left atrial appendage was a therapeutic option in patients with non-valvular atrial fibrillation, even if a non-negligible risk of periprocedural complications was present. However, further studies are clearly needed to assess the effectiveness and safety of this technique.

28.2.1.1 Sports Practice in Patients Undergoing Left Atrial Appendage Closure

COCIS does not provide indications about sports activity in patients undergoing percutaneous closure of the left atrial appendage. The assessment of suitability for competitive sports should be performed on a case-by-case basis. Probably the same criteria used for arrhythmias can be applied, taking into consideration, however, the presence of a device in the left atrium (echocardiographic assessment of correct positioning).

28.2.2 Percutaneous Angioplasty of Peripheral Arterial District

28.2.2.1 Carotid Artery Disease

The most common cause of carotid stenosis is represented by atherosclerosis. Generally, atherosclerotic plaques are located at the level of the carotid bifurcation or at the origin of the internal and external carotid arteries. Stenoses of the carotid bifurcation and of the internal carotid artery are, in hemodynamic terms, the most important, since they are strongly associated with transient ischemic attacks (TIA), or strokes. This association is well documented.

Diagnosis

On physical examination, a vascular murmur in the neck region, a sign of carotid stenosis, can generally be found. In the instrumental diagnosis of carotid stenosis the most useful exam is echo-color-Doppler, as it allows to identify the lesion and to assess its severity and characteristics. Angio-CT and angio-MR provide useful diagnostic completion, allowing the study of the aortic arch, in view of a possible revascularization procedure.

Treatment

The most common indications for revascularization of carotid vascular disease are: stenosis >60% in asymptomatic lesions and >50% in symptomatic lesions (recent TIA / stroke) [30]. Treatment options are carotid endoarterectomy (CEA) and carotid percutaneous stenting (CAS). During the last years, several authors have focused their attention on the comparison between CEA and CAS, in order to identify the treatment of choice for carotid stenosis. Currently, the medium-term results of two large studies, which compare CEA and CAS in patients with symptomatic carotid stenosis, have been made available. In the EVA-3S study (Endoarterectomy Versus Angioplasty in Patients with Symptomatic Severe Carotid Stenosis) [31], the risk of ipsilateral stroke after 4 years of follow-up was similar and very low for both procedures (1.26% for CEA and 1.37% for CAS), while CEA demonstrated a significantly decreased risk of periprocedural stroke and death compared to CAS (3.9% vs. 9.6%). The SPACE study (Stent-Protected Angioplasty versus Carotid Endoarterectomy) [32], which enrolled 1214 patients, showed similar data. There were no significant differences between the two treatments at the follow-up visit after 2 years: mortality was 6.3% for CAS and 5.0% for CEA, while ipsilateral stroke occurred in 2.2% of patients with CAS and in 1.5% of patients with CEA.

Recently, the results of the CREST study (Carotid Revascularization Endoarterectomy vs. Stenting Trial) [33] have been published. This study, which included over 2,500 patients for a mean follow-up period of 2.5 years, is the largest randomized trial in this area, and its primary end-point was the incidence of stroke, myocardial infarction, death from any cause during the periprocedural period and death from any ipsilateral stroke during the follow-up period. The CREST study detected similar results regarding the primary end-point among the patients treated with stenting and those treated with endoarterectomy (7.2% and 6.8%, respectively; HR 1,11; IC 95%, 0,81-1,51; $p = 0,51$), and no differences about sex or symptomatology of the stenosis. At 4 years, the incidence of stroke or death was higher in patients treated with stenting than in those treated with endoarterectomy (HR 1.50, $p = 0.03$), while the rate of myocardial infarction was higher in patients treated with endoarterectomy (1.1 vs. 2.3%, $p = 0.03$). In clinical practice, therefore, the proper selection of patients for surgery or for endovascular treatment remains controversial.

28.2.2.2 Lower Extremity Artery Disease

Lower extremity artery disease (LEAD) can be defined as the atherosclerotic involvement of an arterial trait that can range from the terminal portion of the aorta to the distal arteries of the foot. This disease predominantly affects male patients and usually occurs after 40-50 years of age.

The most common clinical manifestation is the intermittent claudication, a cramping pain caused by muscular ischemia while walking, which usually decreases until it disappears with rest. There is a strong relationship between the location of the pain and the site of the atherosclerotic disease: the involvement of the aortoiliac axis usually corresponds to a pelvic pain extending to the buttock and thigh, while superficial femoral artery disease is associated to a calf pain. If the disease affects the leg arteries, the pain is mostly located to the foot, often matched to trophic lesions, an index of critical ischemia.

There are several classifications of LEAD and currently the most widely used is that of Leriche-Fontaine:

- stage I: asymptomatic/silent arteriopathy;
- stage II: intermittent claudication;
  - IIa: pain-free walking distance >200 m;
  - IIb: pain-free walking distance <200 m;
- stage III: ischemia at rest;
- stage IV: trophic lesions possibly leading to gangrene.

Diagnosis

The patient's medical history and physical examination are usually enough to guide the diagnosis of LEAD, and they could already identify the site and severity of arterial lesions or the presence of aneurysms. The medical history should not be focus on an assessment of vascular involvement, but should detect risk factors for atherosclerosis (smoking, dyslipidemia, hypertension, diabetes) and other related diseases (heart or cerebrovascular disease, respiratory and kidney failure, anemia, polycythemia, hypercoagulability states, etc.).

The physical examination starts with the analysis of the cutaneous and muscular trophism, and with the evaluation of the presence of edema, trophic lesions or scars of previous ulcers. Then it involves palpation of the abdominal aorta and of arterial pulses of the lower limbs (femoral, popliteal, anterior and posterior tibial, foot). Tibial pulses require a particular attention: in a small number of healthy subjects they may not be palpable, while sometimes they could be detectable even in case of intermittent claudication caused by isolated lesions of the aorto-iliac or femoral axis. Finally, the presence of murmurs during auscultation can provide useful additional information.

Echo-color-Doppler is first-choice for patients with multiple-level vascular disease, since it shows the site and degree of the arterial lesion causing the symptoms, and the possible association with aneurysms. Tomographic methods, such as angio-CT and angio-MRI, allow morphological (association with aneurysmal disease, presence of dissection) and qualitative (calcifications) evaluation of the vessels, and both of them are able to create three-dimensional reconstructions of large segments of the vascular system. However they still have to be considered second-level examinations. The availability of new multi-slice equipment has significantly increased the sensitivity and specificity of angio-CT. Angiography is an invasive examination, and it is limited by non-negligible morbidity (0.1%) and mortality (0.16%) rates, although the incidence of complications has been reduced after the employment of non-ionic contrast media and improved introducer sheaths. This examination is currently no longer indicated in the initial diagnostic phase, but only when revascularization is planned.

Treatment

LEAD is essentially treated with endovascular (percutaneous transluminal angioplasty) and/or surgical (bypass or endoarterectomy) revascularization. The choice depends on many factors, starting from the lesion site.

With regard to aorto-iliac axis disease, the recommendations of the TransAtlantic inter-Society Consensus (TASC), published in 2000 and subsequently amended in 2007 [34], indicate a preference for traditional bypass surgery in cases of:

- multiple unilateral stenoses involving the common iliac artery, external iliac artery or common femoral artery (usually >10 cm);
- unilateral occlusion involving both the common iliac artery and external iliac artery;
- bilateral occlusion of the external iliac artery;
- spread/diffuse disease involving the aorta and both common iliac arteries;
- iliac stenoses associated with abdominal aortic aneurysm or with lesions requiring aorto-iliac surgery.

Percutaneous transluminal angioplasty (PTA) with or without stent placement is advized, on the other hand, in cases of:

- single stenosis < 3 cm of the common or external iliac artery (uni- or bilateral);
- single stenosis with a length of between 3 and 10 cm, not extending to the common femoral artery;
- total stenosis or two stenoses < 5 cm of the common or external iliac artery, not extending to the common femoral artery;
- unilateral obstruction of the common iliac artery;
- bilateral stenoses of the common and/or of external iliac artery with a length of between 5 and 10 cm, not extending to the common femoral artery;
- unilateral occlusion of the external iliac artery, not extending to the common femoral artery;
- unilateral occlusion of the external iliac artery, extending to common femoral artery;
- bilateral obstruction of the common iliac artery.

Continuous improvements in the equipment and in endovascular techniques have occurred in recent years, leading to excellent intraprocedural and medium/long-term results, and causing a gradual increase in indications for percutaneous angioplasty.

With regard to the *femoropopliteal axis*, the best revascularization technique is still under discussion. Although endovascular techniques are gaining popularity, they are still burdened by high re-stenosis rates, and therefore by a greater need for reintervention compared to traditional surgery.

According to the recommendations by TASC [34], femoropopliteal PTA is indicated in cases of single stenoses or occlusions < 3 cm, not involving the origin of the superficial femoral artery or the distal popliteal artery. Surgery is instead to be preferred in cases of complete occlusion of the common femoral artery, extending occlusion of the superficial femoral artery and complete occlusion of the popliteal artery.

A consensus is lacking on the most appropriate revascularization treatment in cases of:

- stenosis or occlusion with a length of between 3 and 10 cm, not involving the distal popliteal artery;
- calcified stenoses < 3 cm;
- multiple and obstructive stenoses in series (< 3 cm each);
- single lesions or multiple lesions not extending to the tibial arteries;
- single stenosis or occlusion > 10 cm;
- multiple stenoses or occlusions with a length of between 3 and 5 cm, with or without calcifications.

In these unclear situations, the benefit/risk ratio of one revascularization technique compared to another has to be assessed on a case-by-case basis.

With regard to diseases of the *arteries below-the-knee* (anterior and posterior tibial arteries, tibioperoneal trunk, peroneal artery), revascularization is generally reserved for patients with critical ischemia, with the aim to restore the flow in at least one of the leg vessels, in order to facilitate the healing of the trophic lesions and prevent limb loss. Beyond revascularization, pharmacological therapy also plays an important role; it is based on anti-platelet agents, statins and prostanoids, and is particularly indicated in cases of refractory ischemia. [35]

28.2.2.3 Aortic Diseases

Abdominal aortic aneurysm (AAA) is the most common disease affecting the aorta. The therapeutic choice is usually still surgical, consisting of the insertion of a Dacron prosthesis sutured to the edges of the aneurysmal area. However, surgery is burdened by a discrete perioperative mortality (3% in elective interventions), and by a variable incidence of infections, hernia, vascular accidents, renal and respiratory failure. Recent introduction of endoprosthesis (stent-graft) has totally changed the treatment of this disease. The indications for endoprosthesis implantation, which were initially limited to surgical patients with high perioperative risk for respiratory failure, liver cirrhosis, severe heart diseases, Parkinson's disease and hostile abdomen because of previous surgeries, have been extended due to encouraging follow-up results. At the present time, the placement of aortic endoprosthesis may be therefore considered a valid alternative to traditional surgery [36].

28.2.2.4 Sports Practice in Patients Undergoing Angioplasty of the Peripheral Arteries and Aortic Endoprosthesis

No clear indications exist about sports activity in patients with peripheral vascular disease. These patients are often compromized and have multiple comorbidities (renal failure, heart diseases), therefore the possibility of practicing sports appears to be quite limited. In hemodynamically stable and asymptomatic patients, with verified documentation of good functioning of the stent or of the positioned endoprosthesis, suitability for sports activity of the A group (low physical demands) may be granted. The issue of the suitability is secondary to a cardiology examination, with baseline and exercise ECG, echocardiogram, echo-color-Doppler study of the vascular district of interest and eventually angio-CT/MR. The patient has to be strictly followed with periodical clinical and instrumental exams, in order to assess the risk and extent of atherosclerotic disease. In any case, suitability cannot be granted until at least 12-18 months after any acute event or any revascularization procedure. In most patients, playful and healthy physical activity as part of a psychophysical rehabilitation is allowed.

References

1. Hagen PT, Scholz DG, Edwards WD (1984) Incidence and size of patent foramen ovale during the first 10 decades of life: an autopsy study of 965 normal hearts. Mayo Clin Proc 59:17-20
2. Lamy C, Giannesini C, Zuber M, et al (2002) Clinical and imaging findings in cryptogenic stroke patients with and without patent foramen ovale: the PFO-ASA Study. Atrial Septal Aneurysm. Stroke 33:706-11
3. Del Sette M, Angeli S, Leandri M, et al (1998) Migraine with aura and right-to-left shunt on transcranial Doppler: a case-control study. Cerebrovasc Dis 8:327-30
4. Wilmshurst, P (1997) Patent foramen ovale and decompression illness. SPUMS J 27:82-3
5. Agnoletti G, Iserin L, Lafont A, et al (2005) Obstructive sleep apnoea and patent foramen ovale: successful treatment of symptoms by percutaneous foramen ovale closure. J Interv Cardiol 18:393-5
6. Kerut EK, Norfleet WT, Plotnick GD, et al (2001) Patent foramen ovale: a review of associated conditions and the impact of physiological size. J Am Coll Cardiol 38:613-23
7. Angeli S, Carrera P, Del Sette M, et al (2001) Very high prevalence of right-to-left shunt on transcranial Doppler in an Italian family with cerebral autosomal dominant angiopathy with subcortical infarcts and leukoencephalopathy. Eur Neurol 46:198-201
8. Sulek CA, Davies LK, Enneking FK, et al (1999) Cerebral microembolism diagnosed by transcranial Doppler during total knee arthroplasty: correlation with transesophageal echocardiography. Anesthesiology 91:672-6
9. Homma S, Sacco RL, Di Tullio MR, et al (2002) Effect of medical treatment in stroke patients with patent foramen ovale: patent foramen ovale in Cryptogenic Stroke Study. Circulation 105:2625-31
10. Lechat P, Mas JL, Lascault G, et al (1988) Prevalence of patent foramen ovale in patients with stroke. N Engl J Med 318:1148-52
11. Bogousslavsky J, Garazi S, Jeanrenaud X, et al. Stroke recurrence in patients with patent foramen ovale: the Lausanne Study. Lausanne Stroke with Paradoxal Embolism Study Group. Neurology 1996; 46: 1301-5.
12. Windecker S, Wahl A, Nedeltchev K, et al (2004) Comparison of medical treatment with percutaneous closure of patent foramen ovale in patients with cryptogenic stroke. J Am Coll Cardiol 44:750-8
13. Khairy P, O'Donnell CP, Landzberg MJ (2003) Transcatheter closure versus medical therapy of patent foramen ovale and presumed paradoxical thromboemboli: a systematic review. Ann Intern Med 139:753-60
14. Wohrle, J (2006) Closure of patent foramen ovale after cryptogenic stroke. Lancet 368:350-2
15. Azarbal B, Tobis J, Suh W, et al (2005) Association of interatrial shunts and migraine headaches: impact of transcatheter closure. J Am Coll Cardiol 45:489-92
16. Wilmshurst, P, Nightingale S (2001) Relationship between migraine and cardiac and pulmonary right-to-left shunts. Clin Sci (Lond) 100:215-20
17. Dowson A, Mullen MJ, Peatfield R, et al (2008) Migraine Intervention With STARFlex Technology (MIST) trial: a prospective, multicenter, double-blind, sham-controlled trial to evaluate the effectiveness of patent foramen ovale closure with STARFlex septal repair implant to resolve refractory migraine headache. Circulation 117:1397-1404
18. Germonpre P (2005) Patent foramen ovale and diving. Cardiol Clin 23:97-104
19. Honek T, Veselka J, Tomek A, et al (2007) Paradoxical embolization and patent foramen ovale in scuba divers: screening possibilities. Vnitr Lek 53:143-6
20. Harrison D, Lloyd-Smith R, Khazei A, et al (2005) Controversies in the medical clearance of recreational scuba divers: updates on asthma, diabetes mellitus, coronary artery disease, and patent foramen ovale. Curr Sports Med Rep 4:275-8
21. King TD, Thompson SL, Steiner C, et al (1976) Secundum atrial septal defect. Nonoperative closure during cardiac catheterization. JAMA 235:2506-9
22. Wahl, A, Meier B. Patent foramen ovale and ventricular septal defect closure. Heart 2009; 95: 70-82
23. Wahl A, Krumsdorf U, Meier B, et al (2005) Transcatheter treatment of atrial septal aneurysm associated with patent foramen ovale for prevention of recurrent paradoxical embolism in high-risk patients. J Am Coll Cardiol 45:377-80
24. Furie KL, Kasner SE, Adams RJ, et al (2011) Guidelines for the prevention of stroke in patients with stroke or transient ischemic attack: a guideline for healthcare professionals from the american heart association/american stroke association. Stroke 42:227-76
25. Picchio FM, Colonna PL, Daliento L, et al (2001) Criteria for work capacity evaluation, adequacy for specific jobs, attitudes towards physical activity and sports, and insurance eligibility in subjects with congenital cardiopathy. Ital Heart J Suppl 2:46-77
26. Graham TP Jr, Driscoll DJ, Gersony WM, et al (2005) Task Force 2: congenital heart disease. J Am Coll Cardiol 45:1326-33
27. Helber U, Baumann R, Seboldt H, et al (1997) Atrial septal defect in adults: cardiopulmonary exercise capacity before and 4 months and 10 years after defect closure. J Am Coll Cardiol 29:1345-50
28. Warnes CA, Williams RG, Bashore TM, et al (2008) ACC/AHA 2008 Guidelines for the Management of Adults with Congenital Heart Disease: a report of the American College of Cardiology/American Heart Association Task Force on Practice Guidelines. Circulation 118:e714-833
29. Reddy VY, Holmes D, Doshi SK, et al. Safety of percutaneous left atrial appendage closure: results from the Watchman Left Atrial Appendage System for Embolic Protection in Patients with AF (PROTECT AF) clinical trial and the Continued Access Registry. Circulation 2011; 123: 417-24
30. Tendera M, Aboyans V, Bartelink ML, et al (2011)

ESC Guidelines on the diagnosis and treatment of peripheral artery diseases: document covering atherosclerotic disease of extracranial carotid and vertebral, mesenteric, renal, upper and lower extremity arteries: the Task Force on the Diagnosis and Treatment of Peripheral Artery Diseases of the European Society of Cardiology (ESC). Eur Heart J 32:2851-906
31. Mas JL, Trinquart L, Leys D, et al (2008) Endarterectomy Versus Angioplasty in Patients with Symptomatic Severe Carotid Stenosis (EVA-3S) trial: results up to 4 years from a randomized, multicentre trial. Lancet Neurol 7:885-92
32. Eckstein HH, Ringleb P, Allenberg JR, et al (2008) Results of the Stent-Protected Angioplasty versus Carotid Endarterectomy (SPACE) study to treat symptomatic stenoses at 2 years: a multinational, prospective, randomized trial. Lancet Neurol 7:893-902
33. Brott TG, Hobson RW 2nd, Howard G, et al (2010) Stenting versus endarterectomy for treatment of carotid-artery stenosis. N Engl J Med 363:11-23
34. Norgren L, Hiatt WR, Dormandy JA, et al (2007) Inter-Society Consensus for the Management of Peripheral Arterial Disease (TASC II). Eur J Vasc Endovasc Surg. 33 Suppl 1:S1-75
35 Arain SA and White CJ (2008) Endovascular therapy for critical limb ischemia. Vascular Medicine 13:267-79
36 Prinssen ME, Verhoeven LG, Jaap B et al (2004) A Randomized Trial Comparing Conventional and Endovascular Repair of Abdominal Aortic Aneurysms. N Engl J Med 35:1607-18

Cardiac Rehabilitation

29

Mara Piccoli and Giovanna Giubilato

29.1 Introduction

The approach to cardiovascular disease must currently be focused on the prevention of acute illness and the control of disease progression, because an increasing incidence of this disease is observed, especially in its chronic form. Each year, an estimated 785,000 Americans will suffer from a new acute coronary syndrome, and 470,000 will have a recurrent attack, with an increase in health expenditure (23.5% of pharmaceutical expenditure for cardiovascular disease). In 1993 the World Health Organization defined cardiac rehabilitation as "the sum of activities required to favourably influence the underlying cause of the disease, as well as to ensure patients the best possible physical, mental and social conditions so that they may, by their own efforts, preserve or resume, when lost, as normal a place as possible in the life of the community".

Cardiac rehabilitation, as a multidisciplinary form of intervention in patients with heart disease, has two purposes:

1) to facilitate the return to normal life through physical assessment (prognostic stratification – low risk, medium, high – and therapeutic setting), physical activity counselling, personalized physical training, and psychosocial and vocational counselling;
2) to prevent disease progression, through the implementation of an active lifestyle, assessment of aggressive cardiac risk factors and tailored secondary prevention programmes.

M. Piccoli (✉)
Cardiology Unit
Policlinico "Luigi di Liegro", Rome, Italy

29.2 Historical Notes

- *Bed rest:* Until the 1950s [1], bed rest was widespread in cardiology practice and, in accordance with general medicine findings, the affected organ had to be rested in order to recover adequately. Prolonged bed rest was basic treatment for victims of cardiac events. Therefore, patients suffering from a heart attack remained in bed for 4-6 weeks after the event, and in some cases stair climbing was prohibited for up to one year, and cardiac patients were defined as a chronic invalids for the rest of their lives. This social representation is deeply rooted in the collective imagination, and after a heart attack patients tended to become invalids and non-productive members of society.
- *Armchair treatment:* In bedridden patients, clinical observation showed the negative effects of prolonged rest. It emphasized the deterioration of physical and psychological conditions, with a high incidence of constipation, thrombophlebitis, osteoporosis, pneumonia, atelectasis, depression and psychological stress among patients and their caregivers. Some doctors therefore suggested transferring patients from their bed to an armchair as soon as possible, arguing that a sitting position with the feet on the ground decreased venous return and cardiac work. However, this development in the treatment of heart disease barely influenced the social representation of cardiac patients,

M. Fioranelli and G. Frajese (eds.), *Sports Cardiology*,
DOI: 10.1007/978-88-470-2775-6_29,

who continued to be considered as weak and incapable of carrying out physical exertion. This altered representation is largely responsible for a socio-cultural process that enhanced disability in these patients.

- *Early mobilization:* During the 1970s, early mobilization transformed cardiology practice. This finding emanated from new knowledge in the field of cardiac physiology: physicians recognized that the heart was a muscle, intimately connected to all the body's muscles and to pulmonary function. It was sensitivity to deconditioning, but also the more generalized deconditioning of the body's muscles, that compromized patients' rehabilitation.

The resistance, however, to enable patients with myocardial infarction to carry out activities that require some physical effort could be explained by this social representation of the heart as fragile and vulnerable. At the beginning of the 1980s, the exercise test became part of the routine physical examination of patients with myocardial infarction for risk stratification, and this made it safer for physicians to advise gradual resumption of daily activity and work.

However, the view of cardiac patients as weak is hard to eliminate, and this explains why early rehabilitation programmes have been developed only in few selected centres.

29.3 Size of the Problem: What and Who

An effective strategy for the secondary prevention of cardiovascular risk factors is not implemented in 50% of American patients suffering from cardio-cerebrovascular events [2]. Only 14-35% of patients suffering from acute ischemic events and 31% of those undergoing coronary bypass grafting surgery (especially since rehabilitation centres treat medical and post-surgical sequelae) attend rehabilitation centres. Many factors limited referral and enrollment [3]: patient oriented (minority, old age, low educational and socio-economic status, limited social support), medical (comorbidities, musculoskeletal pathology), and healthcare system (lack of referral, program availability, limited facilitation of enrollment). In Italy, the situation [4] is not any better (Fig. 29.1)

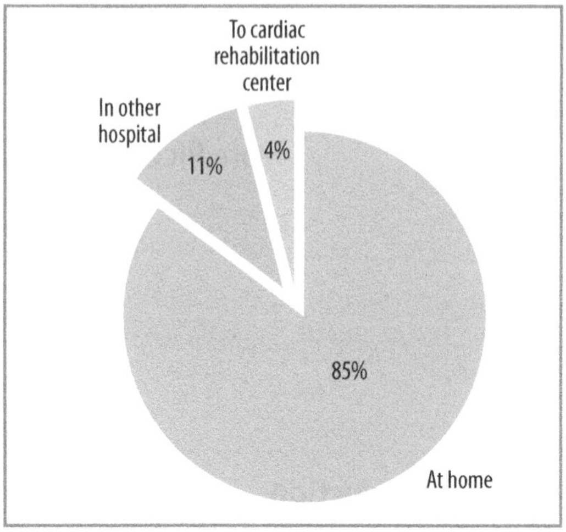

Fig. 29.1 Approach to cardiac rehabilitation after myocardial infarction in Italy. BLITZ study [3]

Rehabilitation programmes for patients with cardiovascular disease can be performed in hospitals, day hospitals, outpatient clinics and at home. For planning the best choice of rehabilitation, it is therefore necessary to consider a number of variables, such as population aging, the highest number of interventional procedures, and not least any administrative and organizational problems concerning the national healthcare system [5-6]. But more specifically, in addition to a physical evaluation of the patient, other variables must be considered, such as the place of residence, patient autonomy and ability to attend rehabilitation centres, mobility and other logistical factors, which are specific to patients and for rehabilitation centres.

In Italy (ISYDE data registry [7]) there has been an increase in hospital rehabilitation in recent years compared to rehabilitation in outpatient settings, primarily because it is the most common form of response to cardiac patients and those undergoing complex cardiac surgery, including the elderly and those with comorbidities (Fig. 29.2).

In fact, in cardiology and cardiac surgery departments, hospital stays are decreasing and the aim is to manage acute diseases and interventional solutions (with a high probability of early discharge and readmission). It is performed with lit-

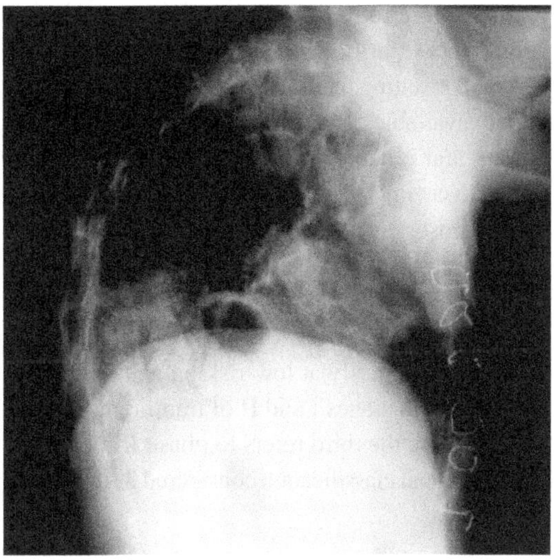

Fig. 29.2 Radiological evaluation of a patient undergoing cardiac surgery. The team must possess multidisciplinary competence to treat this high-risk population and to allow patients an appropriate return home

tle attention to prognostic stratification and *counselling* for the resumption of daily activities, and frequently there is an inadequate setting for secondary prevention. This behaviour leads to an increase in readmissions, with a consequent rise in health-care costs (Fig. 29.3).

What is needed when cardiac patients are discharged from hospital [8-9]?

- a quick and safe return to active life;
- intensive management of complications and comorbidities;
- prognostic stratification, optimization of the therapeutic setting and long-term follow-up;
- an effective secondary prevention programme.

29.4 Patients Referrals for Cardiac Rehabilitation

As demonstrated by Philip A. Ades, all hospitalized patients with diagnosed coronary heart disease should be systematically evaluated by a specialist in preventive cardiology and cardiac rehabilitation [10].

Currently, eligible candidates for cardiac rehabilitation programmes are:

1) post-acute phase:

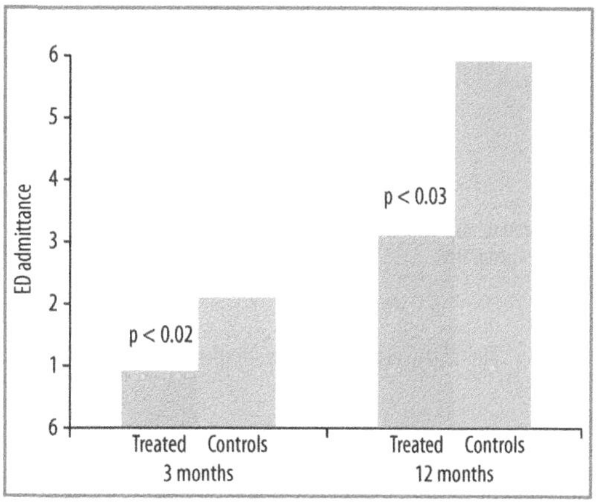

Fig. 29.3 Reduction in hospital readmissions in patients > 65 yrs after myocardial infarction undergoing to cardiac rehabilitation [8]

- ischemic heart disease.
  - acute myocardial infarction;
  - coronary angioplasty;
  - coronary bypass grafting surgery.
- outcomes of cardiac surgery:
  - valve surgery;
  - heart transplant.
- heart failure including monitoring (optimising therapy and recovery).
- patients with rate-responsive pacemakers or implantable defibrillators.

2) chronic phase:

- stable ischemic heart disease;
- valvular disease for therapeutic evaluation and timing of surgery;
- chronic heart failure;
- peripheral vascular disease.

29.5 Pathophysiological Mechanisms and Programmes

It has been noted that physical training, part of the overall rehabilitation programme, slows the progression of atherosclerosis. This occurs due to several mechanisms. An increase in flow-mediated *sheer stress* on the artery walls during exercise causes an improvement in endothelial function associated with increased synthesis, release, and duration of action of nitric oxide. Levels of C-reactive

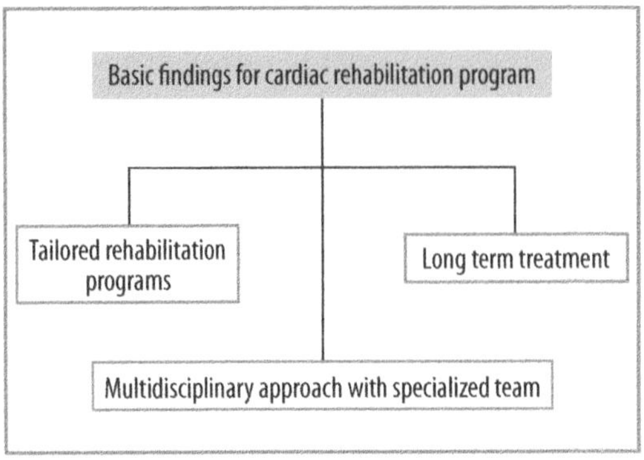

Fig. 29.4 Cardiac rehabilitation program must be structured, with multidisciplinary management to the improve quality of care for patients with heart disease

protein, a marker for inflammation, are reduced with exercise. A benefit is also seen for the lipid profile (decreased triglycerides and increased HDL), blood glucose profile (improvement in insulin resistance and glucose homeostasis) and blood pressure. Endurance exercise can reduce oxygen consumption and lower the heart rate during exercise, with a consequent rise in the ischemic threshold. Peak oxygen consumption is an independent predictor of long-term survival in both the normal population and cardiac patients. There is also favourable modulation in terms of the sympatho-vagal balance resulting from an increase in RR variability and baroreceptor sensitivity. Improved recovery of heart rate was also observed after exercise training in the first minute after exercise; this indirect indicator of vagal tone is a powerful predictor of mortality in patients with coronary artery disease.

In addition to physical exercise, rehabilitation programmes provide intensive monitoring of cardiovascular risk factors through nutrition counselling, for obesity, dyslipidemia, diabetes mellitus and hypertension management. Moreover, adherence to and compliance with prescribed drug therapy for secondary prevention improved.

Recommendations to return to work and psychological support are elements for the management post-acute event depression (heart attack and/or cardiac surgery), anxiety and social isolation, in addition to the benefits to the quality of life.

Currently, cardiac rehabilitation is divided basing on clinical patient complexity. Intensive rehabilitation is referred to patients with acute and subacute disease at high or medium risk, mainly in hospital or setting that must have a physician immediately available and accessible for medical consultations and emergencies. Intermediate rehabilitation aim at intermediate risk patients in low and middle post-acute stage of the disease, to play both structures as residential and outpatient. Extensive rehabilitation or maintenance, which represents the long-term maintenance of the rehabilitation program, aim primarily at low-risk patients. First two correspond to stages I and II of traditional classification, while the third refers to phase III.

Traditional classification considered 3 stages [11].

29.5.1 Rehabilitative Phase I

Acute phase. Duration: 3-4 days; Coronary Intensive Care Unit): this includes a physical assessment of the patient and evaluation of the rehabilitation setting. Patient mobilization should be initiated as early as possible to prevent complications related to immobilization syndrome: breathing exercises are recommended with mobilization, initially passive exercises, followed by active exercises, always under monitoring.

29.5.2 Rehabilitative Phase II

Convalescence phase. Duration: 2-8 weeks; in specialist rehabilitation centres, in day-hospitals or outpatient facilities.

This phase is reserved for stable patients with no associated cardiac or pathological situations that my lead to absolute or relative contraindications against physical activity. It includes:

1. clinical care to prevent complications;
2. exercise test;
3. risk stratification;
4. choice of exercise programme (with monitoring related to the risk category);
5. health education for aggressive modification of risk factors.

In this phase physical activity is very important and is administered for its training effect and should therefore exhibit specific characteristics: tailored frequency, intensity and duration.

Many elements can be evaluated in order to adapt training programmes for patients:
1. clinical history;
2. peri-and post-operative complications;
3. physical examination;
4. modifiable risk factors (smoking, sedentary lifestyle, nutrition, stress);
5. presence or absence of cognitive diseases;
6. respiratory function;
7. echocardiogram, chest X-ray, exercise/cardiopulmonary test results;
8. age, sex, risk level, comorbidities and physical activity compliance.

In patients with ischemic heart disease, training reduces the heart rate and blood pressure with an increase in the ischemic threshold. This event is particularly desirable because ischemic events tend to occur with increasingly higher workloads. Finally, it is effective for secondary prevention in that it reduces atherosclerosis progression.

Each exercise training session should begin with a warm-up (exercise designed to raise heart rate and body temperature), training exercise (breathing exercises, stretching, aerobics and body free isotonic exercises), and end with a cool-down (mild exercise designed to slowly decrease heart rate and body temperature).

Isotonic exercise requires less myocardial effort infarction and, therefore, a reduced demand for oxygen, compared to isometric.

Warm-up is preparation for exercise of the cardiovascular and muscular systems. The objective is:
1. to mobilize the major joints;
2. to minimize the possibility of stretching diseases;
3. to increase O_2 transport to the muscle groups by vasodilatation;
4. to increase coronary blood flow by reducing the risk of ischemia.

Training is very important and must always be conducted aerobically to enable oxidative metabolism and minimise lactate accumulation.

Cooling down aims to restore the initial value of the heart rate, blood pressure and respiratory rate, and is also needed to treat muscle fatigue, remove heat, metabolize lactic acid, and to prevent the occurrence of cardiovascular disorders such as hypotension, due to vasodilation-induced arrhythmias and decreased venous return to the heart.

Physical activity will be continuous (endurance training) and of alternating intensity (interval training). A progressive increase in training parameters depends on a number of variables, to adjust exercise progression easier is heart rate (HR).

HR training can be determined indirectly using the theoretical maximum heart rate [(220 - age) or nomograms adjusted for age and sex], or directly by means of a maximum symptom-limited exercise test (HR max effort]). For example:

Theoretical max HR = 220-60 = 160 bpm years
60% HR max = 96 bpm
80% HR max = 128 bpm
Training heart rate range = 96-128 bpm
max HR = 155 bpm effort
60% HR max = 93 bpm
80% HR max = 124 bpm
Training heart rate range = 93-124 bpm.

The Karyonen Method can be used to calculate the heart rate reserve (HRR). Whereas the base frequency of the subject is zero, it is possible to calculate the percentage intensity of training using the difference between the maximum heart rate at rest and upon effort. For example:

Resting HR = 70 bpm
Max HR = 150 bpm effort
60% RFC = 0.6 x (150-70) = 48 bpm
80% RFC = 0.8 x (150-70) = 64 bpm
Training heart rate range = 118-134 bpm.

Phase II concludes with an examination of the results of rehabilitation procedures using:
- functional assessment (measured in ml O_2/kg/min or mets or watts) with exercise testing. It is measured as patient physical ability by three elements:
  - maximum aerobic capacity;
  - endurance;
  - individual perception of effort (Borg scale).
- psychological evaluation to quantify the degree of adaptation to the disease and to analyse factors that influence compliance with rehabilitation treatment and reintegration work.
- work evaluation to compare the approximate energy expenditure required for work (and

leisure), with maximum activity reached during aerobic exercise testing.

On discharge from Phase II information will be provided on:

- home-exercise programs;
- behavioural habits to control cardiovascular risk factors.

In addition, the patient must have been instructed how to control his or her own heart rate and blood pressure.

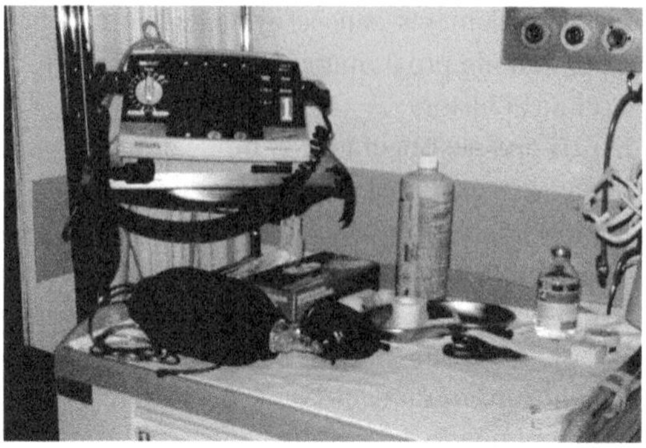

Fig. 29.5 The presence of a complete and efficient kit for emergencies must be an integral part of every cardiac rehabilitation programme

29.5.3 Rehabilitative Phase III

Maintenance phase. duration: life; at home, in outpatient centres or gyms). The secondary prevention programme must be continued. Cardiac patients decide whether to continue with structured programmes (in specialized centres), self-managed programmes (at home) or planned controls (periodical medical tests). This phase coincides with clinical follow-up, which is responsible for checking that the educational health program is not neglected by patients and their families.

29.6 Cardiovascular Risk of Rehabilitation Programmes

The safety of rehabilitation programs supervized by physicians has been documented [12-13]. The occurrence of adverse cardiovascular events during exercise supervized by medical staff in the current rehabilitation programs is approximately 1/50,000 to 1/120,000 patients/hour (2 fatalities reported in the literature for 1.5 million patients/hour of exercise).

This is also due to more extensive procedures for risk stratification in coronary artery disease to identify patients at high risk, who require, in addition to medical supervision, careful cardiac monitoring during exercise training (Fig. 29.5).

The percentage of people who maintain a sufficient physical activity level remains high in the months following structured intervention programmes (80% at 3 months, 60-70% at 6 months), but then falls to 45-55% after one year and continues to drop. Encouragement and support from car-

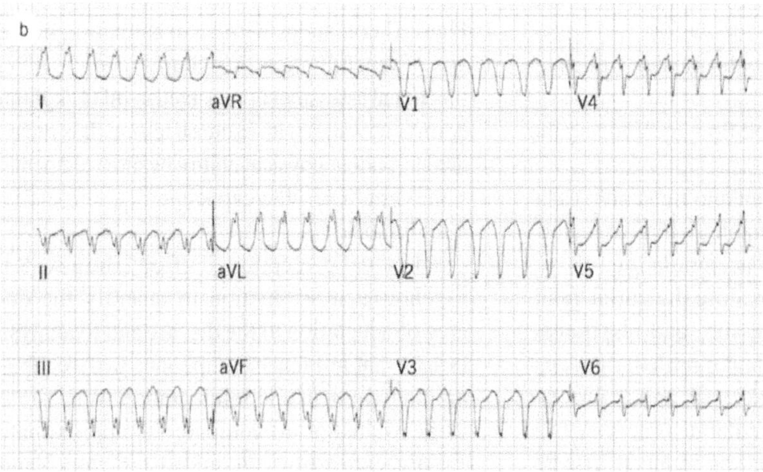

Fig. 29.6 Uncontrolled arrhythmia is absolute contraindication to rehabilitation. It may be considered rehabilitation only after arrhythmia is controlled by drugs and/or electrical therapy

diologists is therefore necessary to reinforce adherence to continued physical activity.

29.7 Contraindications

Physical training is contraindicated in the first week after acute myocardial infarction, unstable angina or during phases of reduced ischemic threshold, and during uncontrolled supraventricular and ventricular arrhythmias (Fig. 29.6) [14-15]. In patients undergoing coronary angioplasty with or without stent placement during the procedure or those with vascular injury, the start of rehabilitation treatment will be delayed until the resolution of vascular damage. All patients with heart failure with symptoms at rest may delay rehabilitation training until the clinical condition allows it. In patients undergoing cardiac surgery, major limitations resulting from comorbidities must be properly treated to optimize the rehabilitation programme: anemia (Hb < 8 g/dl), circumferential pericardial effusion, excessive drainage from the surgical wound, atrial fibrillation, complex sepsis.

29.8 A Particular Aspect of Cardiac Rehabilitation: Heart Failure

In recent years, strong rationale data based on pathophysiology and controlled clinical trial results [16-19] have constantly increased rehabilitation practice in patients with chronic heart failure (CHF).

The basic aims in patients with CHF are:

- clinical stabilization and treatment optimization;
- functional autonomy recovery and physical training through specific tailored interventions;
- health education and motivational counselling;
- behavioural intervention;
- adequate follow-up.

Rationale for the need for physical conditioning in patients with chronic heart failure (CHF) is based on two general concepts. First, these patients are significantly limited and require important medical care. Second, they may also benefit from modest increases in exercise capacity during their daily activities, with a great benefit in their quality of life (Table 29.1). On the other hand, there are many similarities in pathophysiology between heart failure patients and deconditioning patients.

Both conditions are characterized by:

- changes in peripheral hemodynamics (increase in vascular resistance, impaired oxygen use during exercise);
- autonomic system altered control (activation of the neuro-hormonal system of compenzation: renin-angiotensin system, sympathetic system over-activation, vagal system reduction and reduced baroreflex sensitivity);
- reduced functional capacity (reduced exercise tolerance and peak oxygen consumption);
- abnormal muscle mass (reduced mass and composition);
- depressed psychological state (reduced activity and sense of well being).

Traditionally, exercise has been contraindicated in patients with CHF. At the end of the 1980s, the first studies showing the benefit on exercise tolerance, increased peripheral blood flow, and the balance of the sympathetic system by exercise in these patients without side effects, were published. It has been shown to increase oxygen consumption

Table 29.1 Results of the exercise in left ventricular dysfunction and chronic heart failure: clinical evidence by ELVD-CHF Trial [18]

	Training (45 patients)		Control group (44 patients)	
	Baseline	6 months	Baseline	6 months
Clinical score	7.0 ± 2.7	5.3 ± 2.1*	7.2 ± 2.1	7.2 ± 2.1
Symptoms perceived during daily physical activity	13.4 ± 1.8	10.9 ± 1.3*	13.8 ± 1.4	13.4 ± 1.8

Data are expressed mean ± SD. For clinical score and symptoms perceived during daily physical activity, low score is better. Reproduced with permission from [18].
*p < 0.01

at maximum effort, improve hemodynamics and the central autonomic control system by reducing the tone of the sympathetic system and increasing vagal tone. The most recent studies demonstrated an improvement in neuro-hormonal hyperactivity [18-19].

In light of these results, the therapeutic role of physical activity in these patients is evident. In summary, the benefits of training in the CHF are:

- ventilation: the most evident training effect is an increase in oxygen consumption, which is a reproducible sign of improvement in functional capacity. More recent acquisitions show that training creates more efficient ventilation. In fact, this reduces the minute ventilation for each workload. The mechanism is not yet clear. This hypothesis considers the reduction in lactate levels, with an improvement in blood flow in the muscles during exercise, or an improvement in oxygen extraction from the muscle, as well as improved muscle metabolism.
- Autonomic control and neuro-hormonal activation: training improves the autonomic system by reducing sympathetic tone and increasing vagal tone. This modification may explain the reduction in ventricular arrhythmias and levels of angiotensin, aldosterone, vasopressin and atrial natriuretic peptide, which is related to the progression of heart failure.
- Effects on quality of life: negative impacts n functional limitations are well known; patients, by training, become more toned and therefore better at carrying out their daily leisure activities with increasing independence. Physical conditioning improves scores in quality of life tests for dyspnea, fatigue, and general well-being, and makes it easier to carry out daily activities [18].
- Central hemodynamic: Studies show that there is no change in cardiac output at rest and during exercise after treatment for physical therapy (exercise) in patients with left ventricular dysfunction. Physical activity improves diastolic function in dilated and hypertrophic cardiomyopathy.
- Skeletal muscle: The primary role of peripheral alterations in the onset of symptoms of exercise limitation in patients with heart failure is supported by the finding that the training effect is mediated primarily by improving peripheral muscle function:
  - training induces an increase in blood flow to the lower limbs;
  - training induces various structural changes in the peripheral muscle (increase in mitochondria volume and fibre size, increase in capillary density, improved endothelial function);
  - training improves muscle metabolism.

29.9 Conclusions

Cardiac rehabilitation significantly and positively affects the physical health status and quality of life of a patient with heart disease. Quality of life is recent but, with good reason, a basic parameter for optimal recovery of the individual.

To continue with an exercise programme is not simple: it is important to involve and prepare patients and their families, and to ensure the motivation and commitment of all healthcare staff involved. Physical activity must be appropriate, including aerobic exercise, which privileges isotonic exercise and allow sufficient monitoring, to achieve maximum of positive effects.

The construction of a good doctor-patient relationship based on trust and mutual respect is fundamental. There is no single solution adaptable to all patients with different family situations or social, educational and cultural backgrounds. To be effective, a rehabilitation programme must be tailored and adapted to the interests and wishes of the patient, in order to obtain the best results, especially in the long term.

References

1. Certo CM (1985) History of cardiac rehabilitation. Phys Therapy 65(12):1793–1795
2. Brown TM, Herandez AF, Bittner V, Cannon CP, et al (2009) Predictors of cardiac rehabilitation referral in coronary artery disease. JACC 54:515–21
3. Di Chiara A, Chiarella F, Savonitto S, Lucci D, Bolognese L, De Servi S, Greco C, Boccanelli A, Zonzin P, Coccolini S, Maggioni AP; BLIT Investigators (2003) Epidemiology of acute myocardial infarction in the Italian CCU network: the BLITZ study. Eur Heart J 24(18):1616–29

4. Balady GJ, Ades PA, Bittner VA, Franklin BA, Gordon NF, Thomas RJ, Tomaselli GF, Yancy CW (2011) Referral, enrolment and delivery of cardiac rehabilitation/secondary prevention programs at clinical centers and beyond. Circulation 124:2951–2960
5. Audelin MC, Savage PD, Ades PA (2008) Changing clinical profile of patients entering cardiac rehabilitation/secondary prevention programs: 1996 to 2006. J Cardiopulm Rehabil Prev 28(5):299–306
6. Grace SL, Russell KL, Reid RD, Oh P, Anand S, Rush J, Williamson K, Gupta M, Alter DA, Stewart DE (2011) Cardiac Rehabilitation Care Continuity Through Automatic Referral Evaluation (CRCARE) Investigators. Effect of cardiac rehabilitation referral strategies on utilization rates: a prospective, controlled study. Arch Intern Med 14;171(3):235–41
7. Tramarin R, Ambrosetti M, De Feo S, Griffo R, Maslowsky F, Diaco T; Gruppo Italiano di Cardiologia Riabilitativa e Preventiva, Piepoli M, Riccio C (2008) The Italian Survey on cardiac rehabilitation 2008 (ISYDE 2008): study presentation. G Ital Cardiol (Rome) 9(7):497–503
8. Bondestam E, Breikss A, Hartford M (1995) Effects of early rehabilitation on consumption of medical care during the first year after acute myocardial infarction in patients > or = 65 years of age. Am J Cardiol 75(12):767–71
9. Goel K, Lennon RJ, Tilbury RT, Squires RW, Thomas RJ (2011) Impact of Cardiac Rehabilitation on Mortality and Cardiovascular Events After Percutaneous Coronary Intervention in the Community. Circulation 123(21):2344–52
10. Ades PA (2001) Cardiac rehabilitation and secondary prevention of coronary heart disease. N Engl J Med 345(12);892–902
11. Griffo R, Urbinati S, Giannuzzi P, Jesi AP, Sommaruga M, Sagliocca L, Bianco E, Tassoni G, Iannucci M, Sanges D, Baldi C, Rociola R, Carbonelli MG, Familiari MG; Gruppo di Lavoro dell'Agenzia per i Servizi Sanitari Regionali,; Istituto Superiore di Sanità; Piano Nazionale Linee Guida; Gruppo Italiano di Cardiologia Riabilitativa e Preventiva, Cristinziani GR, Amari C, Richichi I, Alessandrini F, Mordenti F, Mauro B, Mozzetta S, Miglioretti M, Buchberger R, Cammarano R, Sampaolo L, Pellegrini L, Rusticali B, Mele A, Ceci V, Chieffo C, Bolognese L, Schweiger C, Michielin P, Baglio G, Nobile A, Scrutinio D, Vigorito C (2008) Italian guidelines on cardiac rehabilitation and secondary prevention of cardiovascular disease: executive summary. G Ital Cardiol (Rome) 9(4):286–97
12. Van Camp SP, Peterson RA (1986) Cardiovascular complications of outpatient cardiac rehabilitation programs. JAMA 256:1160–1163
13. Franklin BA, Bonzheim K, Gordon S, Timmis GC (1998) Safety of medically supervized outpatient cardiac rehabilitation exercise therapy. A 16-year follow-up. Chest 114:902–906
14. Thompson PD (2005)Exercise prescription and proscription for patients with coronary artery disease. Circulation 112:2354–2363
15. Beswick AD, Rees K, Griebsch I, Taylor FC, Burke M, West RR, Victory J, Brown J, Taylor RS, Ebrahim S (2004) Provision, uptake and cost of cardiac rehabilitation programmes: improving services to under-represented groups. Health Technol Assess 8(41):iii–iv,ix–x,1–152
16) Davies EJ, Moxham T, Rees K, Singh S, Coats AJ, Ebrahim S, Lough F, Taylor RS (2010) Exercise based rehabilitation for heart failure. Cochrane Database Syst Rev (4):CD003331
17. Piepoli MF, Davos C, Francis DP, Coats AJ; ExTraMATCH Collaborative (2004) Exercise training meta-analysis of trials in patients with chronic heart failure (ExTraMATCH). BMJ 328(7433):189
18. Giannuzzi P, Temporelli PL, Corrà U, Tavazzi L; ELVD-CHF Study Group (2003) Antiremodeling effect of long-term exercise training in patients with stable chronic heart failure: results of the Exercise in Left Ventricular Dysfunction and Chronic Heart Failure (ELVD-CHF) Trial. Circulation. 108(5):554–9
19. Flynn KE, Piña IL, Whellan DJ, Lin L, Blumenthal JA, Ellis SJ, Fine LJ, Howlett JG, Keteyian SJ, Kitzman DW, Kraus WE, Miller NH, Schulman KA, Spertus JA, O'Connor CM, Weinfurt KP; HF-ACTION Investigators (2009) Effects of exercise training on health status in patients with chronic heart failure: HF-ACTION randomized controlled trial. JAMA 301(14):1451–9

Index

The manufacturer's authorised representative in the EU is Springer Nature Customer Service Centre GmbH, Europaplatz 3, 69115 Heidelberg, Germany. If you have any concerns regarding our products, please contact ProductSafety@springernature.com

Printed and bound by CPI Group (UK) Ltd, Croydon, CR0 4YY
30/09/2026
02225436-0020